# Lapps and Labyrinths

## Saami Prehistory, Colonization and Cultural Resilience

# Lapps and Labyrinths

## Saami Prehistory, Colonization and Cultural Resilience

NOEL D. BROADBENT
WITH CONTRIBUTION BY JAN STORÅ

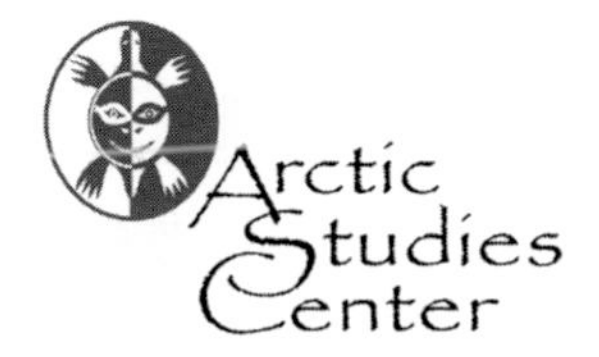


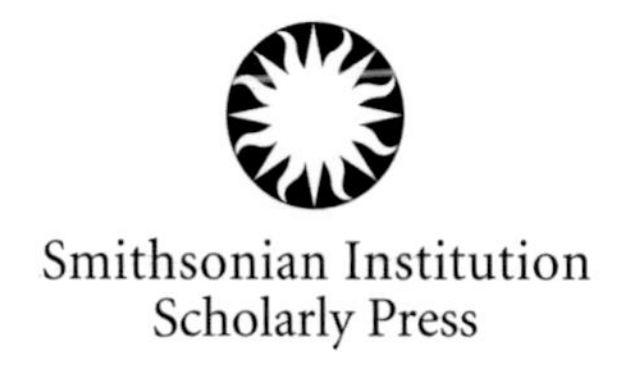

Smithsonian Institution
Scholarly Press

WASHINGTON, D.C.
2014

Published by the ARCTIC STUDIES CENTER
Department of Anthropology
National Museum of Natural History
Smithsonian Institution
P.O. Box 37012, MRC 112
Washington, D.C. 20013-7012
www.mnh.si.edu/arctic

In cooperation with
SMITHSONIAN INSTITUTION SCHOLARLY PRESS
P.O. Box 37012, MRC 957
Washington, D.C. 20013-7012
www.scholarlypress.si.edu



*Cover image:* A painting of a bear burial marked by an antler-sheathed Saami spear. Ossian Elgström, 1930 (Norrbotten Museum). Colors used on cover inspired by the Saami flag.

**Library of Congress Cataloging-in-Publication Data:**
Broadbent, Noel.
Lapps and labyrinths : Saami prehistory, colonization and cultural resilience / Noel D. Broadbent ; with contribution by Jan Storå.
p. cm.
"Published by Arctic Studies Center, National Museum of Natural History Smithsonian Institution . . . in cooperation with Smithsonian Institution Scholarly Press."
Includes bibliographical references and index.
1. Sami (European people)—Sweden—History. 2. Sami (European people)—Sweden—Antiquities. 3. Coastal archaeology—Sweden. 4. Sweden—Antiquities. 5. Antiquities, Prehistoric—Sweden. I. Arctic Studies Center (National Museum of Natural History). II. Title.
DL641.L35B76 2010
948.5'0049455—dc22 2009028011

ISBN 978-0-978846-06-0 (cloth)
ISBN 978-1-935623-64-9 (pbk)
ISBN 978-1-935623-36-6 (ebook)

Printed in the United States of America

⊗ The paper used in this publication meets the minimum requirements of the American National Standard for Permanence of Paper for Printed Library Materials Z39.48–1992.

# Contents

# Director's Note

Scandinavian archaeology has a long and revered history leading back to the foundation of scientific archaeology pioneered by Christian Thomson, a Dane who devised the three-age classification system (Stone, Bronze, Iron Ages) and Oscar Montelius, a Swede who first developed the seriation method of relative dating based on style-change through time. In the 1940s Gutorm Gjessing, a Norwegian, was one of the first to begin promoting social interpretation of archaeological remains, a view later developed by Frederik Barth, a Norwegian, by developing the anthropological theory of social boundaries as expressed in visible signaling of material culture, style and design. In *Lapps and Labyrinths* Noel Broadbent, an American who lived and taught for many years in Sweden, carries this tradition of archaeological innovation into the problematic field of historical ethnicity – in this case the social and territorial history of the Swedish Saami.

I visited many of the sites discussed in this book with Noel in 1984, before their significance had become obvious from his excavations of the past decade. Like Noel, I spent many years conducting "boulder-field" archaeology in a similar subarctic environment, central and northern Labrador. I had found this work exceedingly frustrating because the corrosive nature of subarctic soils and transient nature of the sites resulted in poor artifact preservation and recovery. One was often left with elaborate maps of sites and structures of a people whose culture and identity remained unknown or conjectural. One could easily describe the architectural forms, but determining who they were was frequently elusive. Broadbent's careful excavation techniques and ingenious analytical methods have turned the archaeology of boulder-field sites from a confusing conundrum to a coherent picture that overturns a century of conventional archaeological wisdom about Saami origins, settlement systems and adaptation. For the first time the ubiquitous but inscrutable boulder sites lining the raised beaches and terraces of Sweden's northern Baltic coast sites have been shown to be the remains not of recent Germanic pioneers but of people who must have been ethnic Saami – but Saami living a very different life than known from historical records.

Integrating archaeological finds with an array of anthropological data, place-names, history, religion, geography and ecology, Broadbent has produced a revolutionary new synthesis that indicates a former, long-term Saami occupancy of the North Swedish coast and outlines a model of culture change and acculturation stimulated by the northward advance of Germanic-Swedish farmers and fishermen. Rather then viewing this history as one of ethnic confrontation and geographic and political isolation – processes that have characterized Saami relations with the Swedish state during recent centuries and continue today – Broadbent reconstructs a Late Medieval period characterized by processes of accommodation, cultural exchange and demographic mixing. Only later did institutionalized nation-state policies begin to exclude Saami rights from traditional coastal territories and resources. In time those policies resulted in the re-definition of Saami ethnicity and identity into the reindeer herder of the upper river valleys, interior lakes and mountain zones where most Saami had lived exclusively since the 1700s.

Noel Broadbent's research raises many questions that call for further study. More data are needed from other regions of the Baltic coast; correlations are needed between archaeological remains and Lappish place-names in Sweden south of the study area. Relations between traditional Saami shamanic religion, bear cults and medieval Christian practices need exploring. Coastal and interior archaeological sites need more comparative study. Broadbent's work lays out a new paradigm that powerfully calls into question the established version of Swedish and Saami histories as separate and apart; it sets forth a new conception of social history for the North Baltic, and perhaps even the greater North Nordic region, in which the Saami have to be seen as more important players in the history of their respective modern states than previously accorded through history and ethnology.

For these reasons this work should be of interest not only to archaeologists and culture historians of northern regions but to students of anthropology, history, linguistics, political science and native studies. It is a work in the broadest of anthropological tradition and breaks new ground in the application of archaeological and anthropological methods to issues of modern concern. While dealing with the history of a small Saami population in a restricted area of the northwestern Baltic, the historical situation that transpired following the appearance of newcomers in their lands has been experienced by many indigenous peoples around the world. In this sense Broadbent's *Lapps and Labyrinths* has broad application and demonstrates the value of anthropological studies for balancing the dominance of history in native studies. This work is in the best tradition of Scandinavian archaeology and breaks new ground for science and society.

*William W. Fitzhugh, Director*
*Arctic Studies Center*
*Smithsonian Institution*

# Foreword

Saami bear burials seem to retain their magic, even today. They are eye-openers, being such explicit expressions of Saami identity. They clearly tell that the Saami were here! This insight gave Noel Broadbent a new direction in his research – one that he had not expected. The same befell me in 1970. As the archaeologist in charge at Västerbotten County Museum in Umeå, northern Sweden, I was commissioned to investigate a bone find on an island in Lake Storuman in Lapland. This turned out to be a well-preserved bear burial, not older than 250 years. Up to then I was specialised in the metal techniques of the Scandinavian Viking Age. But just like Noel, I became fascinated by Saami cultural history. A totally new world opened up before me. I still have that fascination, and it surprises me that more Swedish archaeologists have not been affected in the same way. Since then, I have worked with Saami archaeological material and its relationship to Scandinavian culture, initially with material from undisputed Saami areas – that is, the inland regions north of the River Ångermanälven. But in 1982, I realised that a cemetery from the eleventh and twelfth centuries, much further south at Vivallen in northwestern Härjedalen (excavated in 1913), must also be Saami – nobody was more astonished than myself. Two hearths from the ninth and thirteenth centuries typical of Saami huts were found nearby and we excavated a hut foundation as well as other remains from the eleventh century. This led to an interdisciplinary project of early Saami culture and its relationship to the Scandinavian (Germanic/Nordic) culture in the central part of the Scandinavian Peninsula. This project showed that the Saami had been there at least 2,000 years and had extended south of there to about the 60th parallel. The book *Möten i gränsland: samer och germaner i Mellanskandinavien* (Encounters in Border Country: Saami and Germanic Peoples in Central Scandinavia) was published by the Swedish Museum of National Antiquities in 1997.

The history of the Saami in central Scandinavia has also become important regarding one of the most extensive court cases in Sweden, about the rights of the Saami in Härjedalen to let their reindeer graze in winter on private land. The Saami lost their case in 1996 and on appeal in 2002, but this case has recently (2009) been accepted by the European court of justice. For over a century, the dominant standpoint had been that the Saami had only relatively recently immigrated into this area and that they had not reached their southernmost territories until the eighteenth century. A newer view, and the role of the Saami in Swedish prehistory, is possible today. This is in reality a return to views prevalent for most of the nineteenth century, namely that the Saami have a very long history, not only in northern, but also in central Scandinavia. All available source materials lead to the conclusion that Saami cultures emerged out of local hunter-gatherer cultures, just as Noel has argued for coastal Västerbotten. New genetic research tells its own story, showing that there are many connections between today's Saami and the first people to arrive in Scandinavia more than 10,000 years ago.

Swedish archaeology developed out of the seventeenth century goal of demonstrating our national greatness. Unfortunately, there are still attitudes within Swedish archaeology that can be characterized as ethnocentric, nationalistic and chauvinistic. The ethnic pluralism that once existed in Sweden has all too often been overlooked in favour of a one-sided focus on "Swedish" prehistory. As a consequence, people without their own written histories are often left defenceless in the courts. Many Swedish archaeologists still look upon Saami culture as static and inferior – even as non-definable. If the archaeological material does not coincide with historically known Saami culture, they find it hard to imagine that it can be Saami. It will be a long time before the "new" ways of looking at the role of the Saami in the historical process filters through to the government and the general public. The museums – and even more so, the schools – have much to do in this regard. Even in local archaeological exhibits in northern Sweden the Saami are most often presented as an exotic minority of the eighteenth and nineteenth centuries, while the visitor gets the impression that it is the Scandinavian farmer whose culture extends back to the Stone Age – not the other way around.

The research work mentioned above has up till now almost totally concentrated on mountain and forest areas in the inland of Scandinavia. The Bothnian coast(land) in Sweden and its Saami connections were on the whole unknown. The research results by Professor Broadbent and his colleagues are therefore a minor revolution in our knowledge of the Saami past. *Lapps and Labyrinths* presents new interpretations of Saami prehistory in Sweden as well as innovative interdisciplinary methods and theoretical approaches to the study of ethnicity in archaeology. A large number of surveys, excavations and analyses are put into the context of long-term ecological and cultural changes. The study of Lapp place-names has not previously been the object of this kind of project and opens the door to much future archaeological research.

*Lapps and Labyrinths* is easy to read, and the hypotheses and conclusions are well argued in simple to understand language. The excellent illustrations are in no small measure part of the book's impact – they are pedagogical enough to be accessible to the broader public and for use in schools. To conclude, *Lapps and Labyrinths* is an important contribution to Saami and Swedish prehistory, to the history of northern Europe and to indigenous studies everywhere.

*Inger Zachrisson, Ph.D.*
*Associate Professor of Archaeology and Curator emerita*
*Museum of National Antiquities*
*Stockholm*

# Preface

This book is the culmination of an academic journey that started in 1979 when I completed my doctoral dissertation at Uppsala University, followed by a seven-year stint as the Director of the Center for Arctic Cultural Research at Umeå University. My own academic ambitions took a back seat when I moved to Washington, D.C., in 1990, and for six years I managed other people's research at the National Science Foundation (NSF). Three individuals that deserve my appreciation for those amazing years are the late Dr. Peter Wilkniss (Director, Polar Programs), Dr. Jerry Brown (Head, Arctic Section), and Dr. Robert Corell (Director, Geoscience).

In 1996, I was awarded the Chair of Archaeology at Umeå (later merged with Saami Studies) and for seven years commuted between Umeå and Washington, D.C. Many exciting things happened during my tenure, one of which was the Northern Crossroads (*Möten i norr*) Project. This Bank of Sweden–funded project energized the department on multiple fronts and provided full-time salaries for a post-doctoral position and nine doctoral students (including one in Stockholm and one in Lund), but unfortunately, once again, left me with little research time of my own. I chose to finally resign that position late in 2003, a decision that ironically brought my own original research ambitions back to life. With the generous support of NSF starting in 2004, I could move forward at last, and this has resulted in the book you now hold in your hands.

I came to know and work with many Nordic Saami and Saami organizations such as the Nordic Saami Council and the Swedish Saami National Organization (SSR), and through the NSF Office of Polar Programs, I was able to travel widely in Alaska. In the latter instance, I would like to acknowledge Julie Kitka, President of the Alaska Federation of Natives; Dr. Ray Barnhardt and Dr. Oscar Kawagley, University of Alaska, Fairbanks; Caleb Pungowiyi (former president of the Inuit Circumpolar Conference); Amy Craver, Alaska Native Science Commission (now with the National Park Service); and Patricia Cochran, Alaska Native Science Commission (former president of the Inuit Circumpolar Conference). Thanks to these contacts my research started to evolve into a deeper appreciation of the meaning of knowledge to the people of the North. This is where my journey has led me. My scholarly life has literally been divided by worlds apart, both geographically and spiritually, and I have found peace in the wisdom that has now brought me full circle, and to a more meaningful completion of this project than I had originally envisioned. I trust this can serve not only the interests of the archaeological community and the development of the field, but of those who are invested in understanding the past – teachers, policy makers and all who live in the North.

## Pronunciation and Saami Orthography

Swedish has three letters at the end of the alphabet that are unfamiliar to English speakers: "å" is pronounced like *o* in *fore* (long) and like *o* in *yonder* (short); *"ä"* is pronounced like *ai* in *fair* (long) and like *e* in *best* (short); *"ö"* is pronounced like *eu* in the French *deux*, and before an *r* like *u* in *fur*, or like an *e* in *her*. The "ö" in Swedish is written as "ø" in Danish and Norwegian and *å* can be written as *aa* in Danish. In order to avoid confusion regarding Saami spellings, which are often Swedish versions of Saami words in older literature (e.g., Manker 1960), Lule Saami orthography, as summarized in Rydving (1995), has been used. Exceptions to this are quotations or references to North Saami sources, such as *sijdda* (South Saami) versus *siida* (North Saami).

# Acknowledgements

There are many people I would like to thank in Sweden: Professor Bertil Almgren at Uppsala University, who had so welcomed me to the Department of Nordic and Comparative Archaeology, and saw me through the completion of my dissertation; the late Docent Hans Christiansson, who brought me into the Swedish North; Professor Evert Baudou, who encouraged me to join the Department of Archaeology in Umeå and was instrumental in the establishment of the Center for Arctic Cultural Research; Professor Lars Beckman, the late Umeå University Rector; Umeå University Director Dr. Dan Brändström, later Director of the Bank of Sweden Tercentenary Fund; the late Professor Håkan Linderholm, M.D., with whom I helped organize the 7th International Conference on Circumpolar Health – all of whom truly understood the value of international research in Sweden.

Academic colleagues for whom I also feel a special fondness are Professor Åke Hyenstrand, Professor Phebe Fjellström and Professor Mats Malmer. These old friends are gone now, but not forgotten. I wish to also acknowledge Carina Lahti (the heart and soul of the Department of Archaeology in Umeå), Professor Bozena Werbart, Professor Birgit Arrhenius, Docent Anders Carlsson, Docent Patrik Lantto and Margareta Axelson, stalwart friends over the years. Dr. Lana Troy (Professor of Egyptology in Uppsala) has been my de facto editor-at-large, whipping me into grammatical shape and maintaining my intellectual rigor. Film-maker and photographer Boris Ersson (Luleå) has been a great collaborator in recent years. Docent Inger Zachrisson (Swedish National Historical Museum) is an icon of Saami archaeology in Sweden, having stood her ground when most others did not. I am honored by her foreword. Together with Dr. Inga-Maria Mulk (former director of the Ájtte Mountain and Saami Museum, Jokkmokk) and Dr. Ingela Bergman (director of the Silver Museum in Arjeplog), she has laid the groundwork for this project and others like it.

The wonderful years and productive collaboration at the Center for Arctic Cultural Research were made possible by Professor Roger Kvist and Dr. Rabbe Sjöberg. Both made invaluable contributions to this book through their research in the Seal Hunting Cultures Project, and Rabbe rendered my field drawings into fine ink illustrations. Elaine Reiter, while a student at Northern Virginia Community College, transformed many of the figures into Photoshop® masterpieces. My interns: Kim Consroe at George Washington University, Jacquelyn Graham at the University of Minnesota, together with Dr. Katherine Rusk helped produce great reconstructions and maps. Intern Aza Derman, The Bronx, helped with my bibliography using EndNote®. Dr. Pam Stern (formerly of Sterling College) gave early critiques of my manuscript and has made many helpful suggestions; and Cara

Seitchek and especially Ginger Strader (Smithsonian Scholarly Publications Manager) worked on the final edits. Unless otherwise noted, all translations, figures, tables, and photographs and conclusions are by the author, who is solely responsible for their content. The aerial photographs are published with the permission of the Swedish Department of Defense.

Special thanks naturally go to my colleagues Britta Wennstedt Edvinger, and Jan Storå (Osteological Research Laboratory, Stockholm University). Britta and Kjell Edvinger (*Arkeologicentrum i Skandinavien AB*) facilitated new excavations at Grundskatan in 2004 and an international field school at Hornslandsudde in 2005. Britta and I have co-authored a number of articles through this project and her knowledge of Saami prehistory has been invaluable. Her contributions are particularly important in Chapter 8 (Rituals and Religion). Jan has done wonders with the animal bones, bringing many aspects of the investigation to life. He has made a major contribution to this book and all the osteological tables, figures and analyses are his work, none of which have been published before. Eva Hjärthner-Holdar, Director of the Geoarkeologiska Laboratoriet, and her colleagues in Uppsala (Eva Grandin, Emma Grönberg and Daniel Andersson) have advanced our knowledge of northern iron working through their analytical reports. Imogen Poole (Utrecht) and David Black (University of Western Michigan) have revealed the identities of trees hidden in bits of charcoal, Johan Linderholm, soil chemistry, and Karin Viklund, macrofossils (both Umeå University). Thanks also to Ulf Lundström (Skellefteå Museum) for his inspirational manuscript on Saami place-names and eskers in Skellefteå.

There are a number of people to thank here at the Smithsonian, many of whom have read my texts: Dr. Dan Rogers, Dr. Don Ortner, Dr. Bill Honeychurch (now at Yale), Dr. Torben Rick, Dr. Mary Jo Arnoldi, Dr. Bruno Frohlich, Dr. Candace Greene, Dr. Mindy Zeder, Ann Kaupp and Kathleen Adia. Marcia Bakry helped with the illustrations, as did Beatrix Arendt. My sincere gratitude also goes to my colleagues of many years at the Arctic Studies Center: Dr. Bill Fitzhugh, Dr. Stephen Loring and Dr. Igor Krupnik. For the financial support that made this all possible, the National Science Foundation's Arctic Social Sciences Program and its Director Anna Kerttula. These years at the Department of Anthropology and the National Museum of Natural History have been among the most enjoyable and stimulating of my career. Finally last, but hardly least, thanks to my patient wife Elaine and our daughter Rosanna, who was born in Uppsala and has been on Swedish archaeological sites before she could walk, and Greg Lavallee, who has been my in situ information technology expert.

Thank you one and all!

*Noel D. Broadbent*
*Washington D.C.*

# List of Figures

# List of Tables

# Lapps and Labyrinths

Saami Prehistory, Colonization and Cultural Resilience

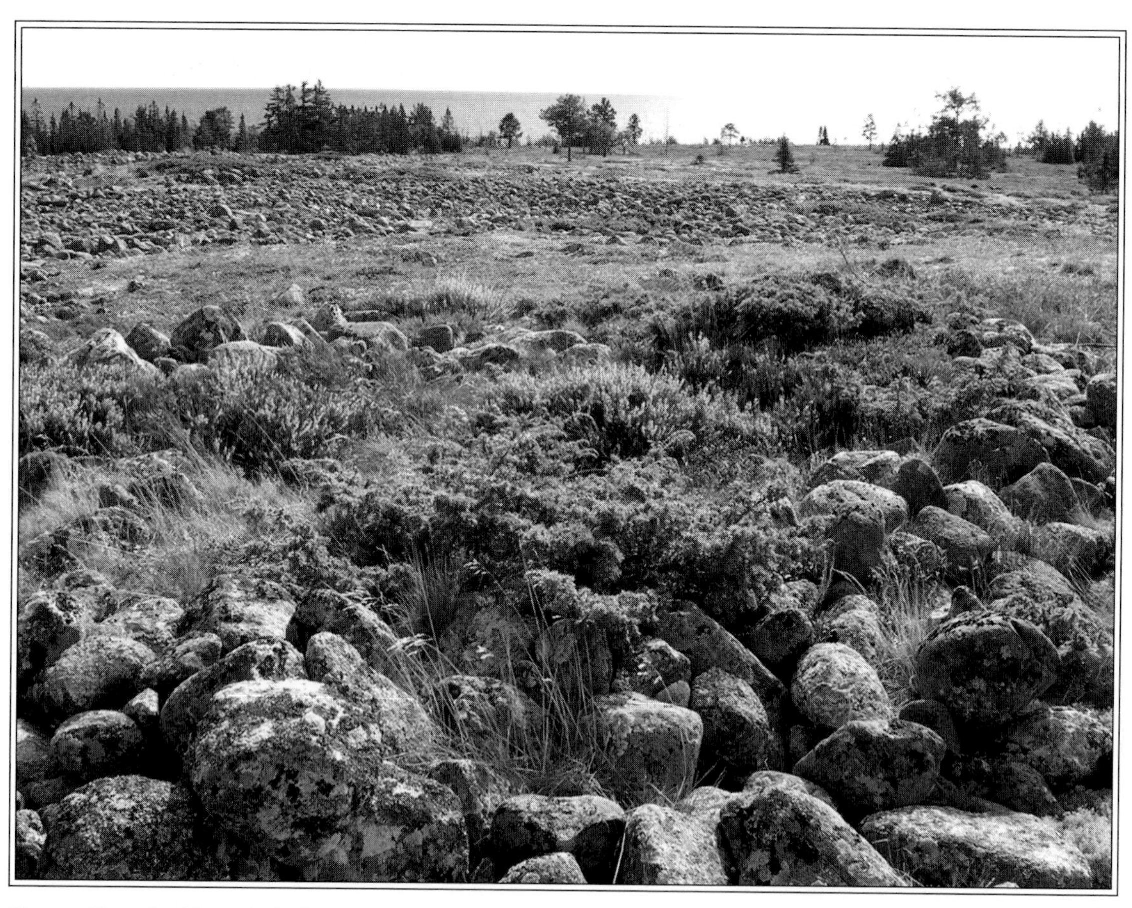

*Figure 1. View of seal hunters' dwelling (Hut B) lying 19 meters above present sea level on Stora Fjäderägg Island, Västerbotten.*

1

# Introduction and Narrative Context

The Viking Age (ca. A.D. 800–1100) is one of the most fascinating periods of European history. This was the juncture between prehistory and written history in northern Europe and for the first time we could know more about these ancient societies than mere artifacts could convey. The Norse Sagas and other accounts tell us not only about Scandinavian exploits, but also about the indigenous reindeer people of the north they called Lapps. These people, whose self-designation is Saami, were experts in northern travel technologies, including skis, sleds and sewn and riveted boats of the types that brought the Swedish Vikings down Russian rivers to Constantinople, and that were still used by coastal fishermen in Norway and sealers on the Gulf of Bothnia in the twentieth century (Schefferus 1673:280–282; Bonns 1988; Eldjarn and Godal 1988; Westerdahl 1995a; Mulk and Bayliss-Smith 2006a:65–79).

Far from being a marginalized backwater, most of the forces of European history and medieval mercantilism played out in this northern region of hunter-gatherers, herders, farmers and traders. Flexible patterns of kinship and social alliances, diverse economic strategies and highly effective travel technologies facilitated remarkable contacts with the outside world; hundreds of Viking Age objects that reflect a vast Eurasian trading network have been found at Saami offer sites in Swedish Lapland (cf. Serning 1956; Zachrisson 1984).

The interplay of different cultural influences, with impulses coming from both the east and the south, is what makes the Nordic region among the most dynamic of the Circumpolar North.[1] These interactions are the key to understanding Saami origins, locked not into antiquated ideas of great migrations, but of indigenous societies that pursued their own historical destinies and adapted over thousands of years to environmental, technological and cultural changes.

The maritime perspective is in equal measure essential for understanding Nordic prehistory and history. Seas almost completely encompass the Scandinavian Peninsula (Norway and Sweden) and extend along most of the length and breadth of Finland. The coasts and larger waterways were the principal means of travel to the north, south and east, and the thousands of lakes, streams and rivers were the arteries that sustained Nordic life. These bodies of water provided abundant sources of fish and marine mammals and the ameliorating effects of the maritime climate made the Nordic region, at the same latitude as Alaska, a part of agrarian Europe.

The Saami are best known today as nomadic herders living in the interior and in northernmost regions of Norway, Sweden, Finland and northwestern Russia – but this was not always the case. This book addresses the issue of Saami ethnogenesis, the origins of Saami cultural identities, through the archaeology of the Swedish Bothnian coast. The title of this book introduces two terms that bring these Saami origins to the forefront. The first of these is "Lapp." The existence of more than 1,100 place-names referring to Lapps in Sweden, of which 87% are on the Bothnian coast, is a reflection of the history of contacts between the Saami and other groups. These places are of great importance for understanding the development of modern Saami identity (refer Chapter 2 regarding the origin of this name).

The second term is "Labyrinth," referring to hundreds of stone circles found around the Gulf of Bothnia. The labyrinths were Christian symbols in this region and are associated with medieval and later historic fishing sites. They were manifestations of Swedish colonization, the power of the church that came with it, and the point at which a balanced relationship started to turn into one of suppression, setting the pattern that changed the course of northern history from the fourteenth century onward. This linguistic and cultural evidence helps to frame the archaeological narrative in both time and space.

The archaeological project focuses on the County of Västerbotten about 800 km north of Stockholm. Comparisons are also made at sites along a 500 km stretch of the Bothnian coast to within 300 km of Stockholm. This north to south transect encompasses areas of likely Saami settlement and extends to areas of Germanic/Scandinavian settlement during the period A.D. 1–1500. This line also intersects the Mid-Nordic region, which spans across the Scandinavian Peninsula from the Norwegian coast in the west to Finland in the east. The northern part of this coastal region has been discussed by other authors (Grundberg 2001, 2006), primarily with regard to Germanic and medieval history, but also as "Saamiland" (cf. Bergvall and Persson 2004; Åhrén 2004:63–89; Erikson 2004:151–186; Westerdahl 2004:111–139). This was a major zone of cultural interaction with both Saami and Germanic settlements (cf. Ramqvist 1983; Liedgren 1992; Gullberg 1994; Zachrisson 1988, 1991, 1992, 1995, et al. 1997a).

Many ideas about the Saami have derived from evolutionary theories that held that societies not only evolved from the primitive to the civilized – nomadic herders were intermediate between hunters and farmers – but that these cultures still exist as living fossils. The Saami were consequently seen as an exotic society, representing a second stage of cultural development. The interactions of northern peoples over thousands of years challenge these evolutionary ideas in a multitude of ways. Resiliency, the ability to adapt to change, has entailed cultural and economic heterogeneity. The harsh environments of the north have necessitated economic diversity, collaboration between groups, and shifts from sedentary to more mobile settlement systems and back again. The same is true regarding technologies, and it is among the northern hunter-gatherers, for example, that we find some of the first metallurgy of the Nordic region (Hjärthner-Holdar 1993). Saami prehistory is a remarkable example of northern resiliency, and resilience theory is central to this archaeological analysis, including discussions of long-term human environmental interactions and social change.

## Vikings, Dwarves and Giants

Worldviews also met and merged as the shamanistic beliefs of the circumpolar world became deeply entrenched in the Nordic psyche, finding form in the religion of the Vikings (Dubois 1999; Price 2002). There are also examples where the meeting of these two peoples resulted in the stuff of folklore. The Nordic fascination with dwarves, trolls and giants may have grown out of early contacts between the Saami and the Norse (Nilsson 1866:153–157; Saressalo 1987). The master ironsmith of Norse mythology, Völundr/Weland, was descended from dwarves and was the son of the Finn

[Saami] King. He made the magic sword, Gram, and the rings, which were portals to other worlds,[2] as popularized in Tolkien's *Lord of the Rings*. Volundr was also a shaman who hunted reindeer, and presumably bears, on skis (Bæksted 1970:228–231).

Giants entered the academic discourse as late as the 1970s in a discussion of the "Stalo" creatures of Saami folklore. The Stalo were interpreted as steel-using Norse giants involved in reindeer hunting in the mountain foothills of Sweden and Norway (Kjellström 1976). Although the Saami and the Norse were almost certainly actively involved with each other in the exploitation of these alpine resources (cf. Sommerseth 2004; Bergstøl 2004), there is little reason to assume that this kind of interaction inevitably involved hostilities and subordination. On the contrary, there is much evidence of interdependencies, not least in hunting, but also in religion.

## What Is the Cultural Identity of the Saami?

Nomadic reindeer herding, the dominant symbol of Saami identity today, is the legal basis for their recognition as a cultural group by Swedish authorities. But what happens to Saami rights when nomadic herding, considered as an economic sector on par with forestry and tourism in Sweden (Broadbent and Lantto 2008), is not part of the equation? Above all, how do our misconceptions about the past influence the policies and decisions of lawmakers, courts and governments?

The more information we have about Saami culture, the more complex the question of "Saaminess" becomes, and there are no simple answers. That there are nine Saami languages across four nations suggest that there could be just as many answers as to where and how Saami identities were formed. Archaeological analysis does not deal with living individuals but rather with physical remains, and there are many opinions regarding the difficulties of connecting archaeological evidence to Saami ethnicity (Kleppe 1977; Reymert 1980; Odner 1983; Werbart 2002; Hansen and Olsen 2004; Wallerström 2006). Although there is much controversy regarding the issue, nearly all agree that the most relevant question is not "who was first," but how did the Saami and the north Scandinavians become who they are today? The criteria of Saami identity in archaeology, notwithstanding genetic and linguistic arguments, most often encompass economies (hunters/herders versus farmers); religious expressions, such as burial practices and grave forms, offer sites and other types of sacred places; material culture (artifacts, dress, etc.); social organization, especially the so-called *sijdda/siida* (a basic settlement unit of Saami society); dwelling types, the *kåta/goahte*; and common territory (Ränk 1948; Reymert 1980; Yates 1989; Zachrisson 1997b:189–220; Hansen and Olsen 2004:18–45). These criteria can be somewhat self-fulfilling, however, as they are partly based on historically known Saami culture in Lapland. They tend to reinforce the idea that this culture was relatively recent, uniform and limited in extent.

Ethnic membership is often based on subjective, non-empirical, arbitrary and emotional principles or issues, sometimes in ways that outsiders cannot understand (Kent 2002:4–5). While ethnicity may rest on a universal predilection of humans to select positively in favor of their own kinsman, it is also variable because of the diverse cultural meanings that people in different historical circumstances have drawn upon in interpreting this predilection (Keyes 1981:6–8). The cultural characteristics marked as emblematic of ethnic identity also depend upon interpretations of mythical ancestors and symbolic beings, including animals. In this respect, consideration of spiritual entities becomes an essential part of analysis, at least from the archaeological perspective, of the physical by-products of ritual behaviors.

## The Testimony of a Bear . . .

My archaeological investigations started out as a straightforward study of seal hunting during the Iron Age in the North Bothnian region of Sweden and Finland (Broadbent 1987a, 1987b, 1989a, 1989b, 1991, 2000). As this region is outside of Lapland, I admittedly initially gave little thought to Saami prehistory. In fact, Saami archaeology in Sweden seemed at the time to be an exotic field connected with interior and alpine regions and with reindeer, not with seals. It took a second research project to fully connect this coastal material to the Saami past (Broadbent 2004b, 2006; Wennstedt Edvinger and Broadbent 2006; Broadbent and Wennstedt Edvinger n.d.).

The turning point in my own thinking grew out of a single archaeological discovery. This find, buried in the corner of a Viking Age dwelling on the North Bothnian coast, consisted of the bones of a brown bear (Broadbent and Storå 2003). These bones were not ordinary food residues as found in cooking hearths, but bones that had been carefully selected, systematically placed and then sealed under a stone cairn on the floor of a dwelling. This deposition of bones seemed incongruous and yet, as I came to realize when they proved contemporary with the hearth, was one of the most revealing finds of the project. This was a ritual bear burial of South Saami type.

Bear ceremonialism was widespread in the Circumpolar Region and is well documented among Finno-Ugrian hunters and herders (Schefferus 1673; Reuterskiöld 1912; Hallowell 1926; Haavio 1952; Paproth 1964; Zachrisson and Iregren 1974; Bäckman and Hultkrantz 1978; Edsman 1994; Mebius 2003). The bear also figured in Germanic Iron Age funerary contexts in middle Sweden, Gotland, Öland, southwest Norway and the Åland Islands, where the dead were sometimes buried lying on or wrapped in bear skins, of which only phalanges remain (Petré 1980). This practice was common over much of Northern Europe and has been associated with the graves of elites (Schönfelder 1994). Post-mortem bear rites and burials, as practiced by the Saami, were an entirely different kind of phenomenon conducted out of respect for the animal, to ask for forgiveness for the killing, for the protection of the body and, ultimately, for rebirth and renewal (Hallowell 1926:154). Saami bear burials connected the human and animal worlds through this cult. They have been dated to as early as A.D. 200 and as recently as the nineteenth century (Myrstad 1996), but these bear rites may be thousands of years older in the Nordic region.

So what were these Saami doing on the Bothnian coast, and what happened to them? This was a culture that disappeared a century before the demise of the Norse settlers on Greenland, and two centuries before Columbus sailed into the New World. This is also a contested landscape, in reality and in peoples' minds. The fate of these Saami is one of the most fascinating questions of the investigation.

## The Power of Historical Narratives

Saami and Scandinavian relations are not just an academic matter, however, and relate to historical narratives and the formation of the Swedish state. The Saami, like most indigenous peoples, have been characterized more by history than by prehistory (Olsen 1994:20–30, 1998). Historical narratives and myths were nearly always created to sanctify unity and establish historical precedence in the nation-building process (Carr 1986; Hodder 1991; Richards 1992; Kramer 1997), and the beginnings of Nordic archaeology were intimately connected with this political process. In the seventeenth century, the father of Swedish antiquarianism, Olof Rudbeck, went so far as to propose that the Nordic Peninsula had been an island, and that Sweden was the mythical Atlantis. A national registry of rune stones, grave mounds and antiquities was initiated as evidence of a glorious Nordic past (Klindt-Jensen 1975; Baudou 2004). Sweden had been embroiled in the Thirty Years' War and their prowess in warfare was believed by German Catholics to be due to Saami sorcery, and indeed, the Saami had been feared since Viking times for their supposed witchcraft. Trials of Saami suspected of sorcery were initiated in the seventeenth century and later (Sköld 1993:64–81). Johannes Schefferus' *Lapponia* (The History of Lapland) published in 1673 and later translated into German and English in 1673–1682, was undertaken as a response to such allegations and to facilitate the Christian mission. Schefferus was not an historian per se, but a professor of rhetoric and, significantly, government at Uppsala University.

Prominent nineteenth-century Swedish prehistorians were otherwise quite open to the legitimacy of the Saami past. Sven Nilsson, who was a professor of Natural History at Lund University, is credited with one of the first scientific studies of prehistory in the country. In his *Skandinaviska Nordens Ur-Invånare* (The Aboriginal Populations of Nordic Scandinavia), Nilsson wrote:

> *After numerous investigations, I came to the conclusion that the people who used the stone tools were a Hyper-boreal (polar) tribe, to which I count the Lapps and that these peoples lived on the coasts of southern Sweden in a manner similar to that of the Greenlanders and other Eskimos in America. These peoples, of which the Lapps are the last survivors, were forced into the mountains of the Scandinavian North, but had in the most ancient times not only lived in the southern parts of this country, but probably in the rest of northern and Western Europe, Denmark, northern Germany, the British Isles and parts of France. (1866:106)*

These ideas were followed up on and given better focus by Oscar Montelius in three papers at the International Congress of Anthropology and Prehistoric Archaeology in Stockholm (Montelius 1876a, 1876b, 1876c). Montelius and Hans Hildebrand in Sweden and Oluf Rygh in Norway coined the terms "Arctic Stone Age" and "Lappish Stone Age" with regard to the slate and quartz cultures of the northern parts of both countries. Montelius charted the north to south distributions of flint, slate and bronze artifacts in order to demonstrate the existence of two cultural regions (1876a:191, 1876c: 511). With reference to von Düben's *Om Lappar och Lappland* (On Lapps and Lapland) from 1873, Montelius rejected the idea that the Lapps were all over southern Sweden and Europe, and instead believed they came in from the far north and around the Gulf of Bothnia during the period they were using bone, quartz and slate tools. With the acquisition of metallurgy they expanded southward to the 61st parallel and reached their maximum territorial extent following the Black Death in 1350. They were subsequently largely assimilated, while others retreated into the mountain regions in the west (Montelius 1876a:195). Montelius's ideas were remarkably perceptive for his day.

Inger Zachrisson (1997a:11–20) has divided the history of ideas about Saami prehistory into four phases. In the period 1820–1860, scholars like Nilsson believed that the Lapps were a Nordic *urbefolking* who once lived all over Scandinavia. The period 1860–1900 was characterized by ideas about "two Stone Age cultures," one in the north and one in the south. The third phase (1900–1970s) had more racial overtones. In 1919, Oscar Montelius shifted from his earlier cultural-historical ideas to seeing the Lapps as a race (Montelius 1919). Another of the early pioneers of Swedish archaeology, Gustaf Hallström, was convinced that the Stone Age cultures of northern Sweden were of Scandinavian origin and that the Lapps had immigrated much later (Hallström 1929).

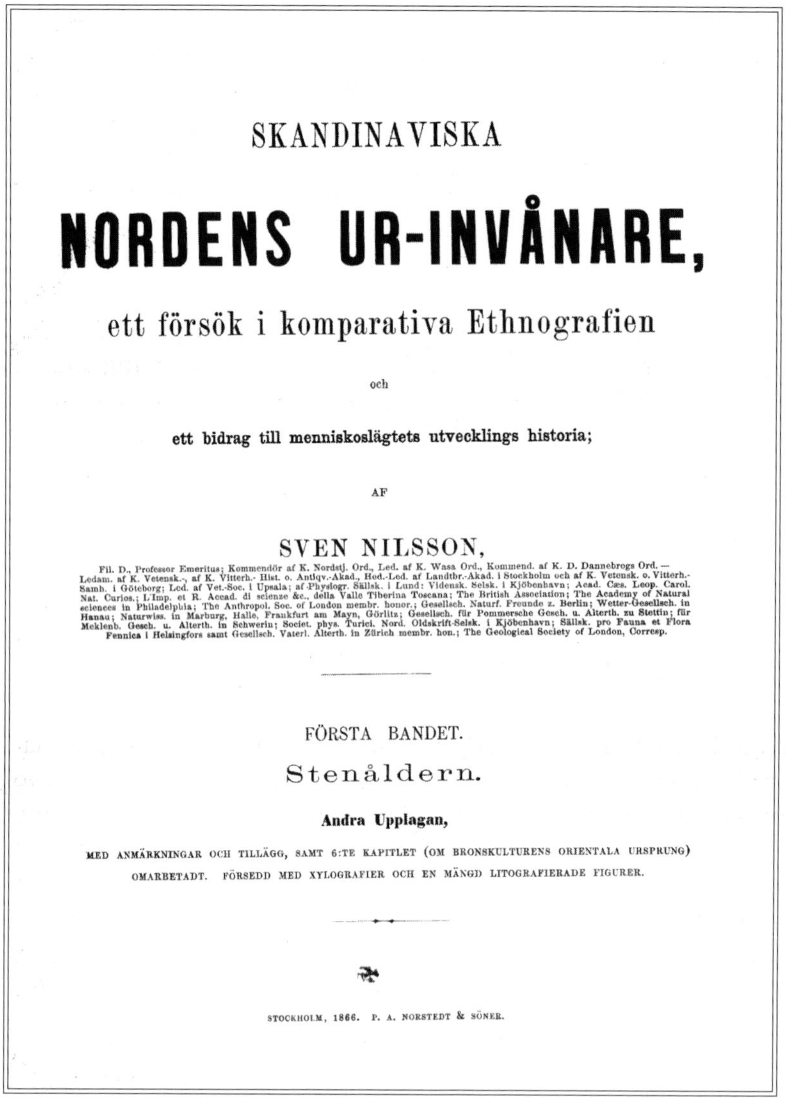

SKANDINAVISKA

# NORDENS UR-INVÅNARE,

ett försök i komparativa Ethnografien

och

**ett bidrag till menniskoslägtets utvecklings historia;**

AF

SVEN NILSSON,

Fil. D., Professor Emeritus; Kommendör af K. Nordstj. Ord., Led. af K. Wasa Ord., Kommend. af K. D. Dannebrogs Ord. — Ledam. af K. Vetensk.-, af K. Vitterh.- Hist. o. Antiqv.-Akad., Hed.-Led. af Landtbr.-Akad. i Stockholm och af K. Vetensk. o. Vitterh.-Samh. i Göteborg; Led. af Vet.-Soc. i Upsala; af Physiogr. Sällsk. i Lund: Vidensk. Selsk. i Kjöbenhavn; Acad. Cæs. Leop. Carol. Nat. Curios.; L'Imp. et R. Accad. di scienze &c., della Valle Tiberina Toscana; The British Association; The Academy of Natural sciences in Philadelphia; The Anthropol. Soc. of London membr. honor.; Gesellsch. Naturf. Freunde z. Berlin; Wetter-Gesellsch. in Hanau; Naturwiss. in Marburg, Halle, Frankfurt am Mayn, Görlitz; Gesellsch. für Pommersche Gesch. u. Alterth. zu Stettin; für Meklenb. Gesch. u. Alterth. in Schwerin; Societ. phys. Turici. Nord. Oldskrift-Selsk. i Kjöbenhavn; Sällsk. pro Fauna et Flora Fennica i Helsingfors samt Gesellsch. Vaterl. Alterth. in Zürich membr. hon.; The Geological Society of London, Corresp.

FÖRSTA BANDET.

Stenåldern.

**Andra Upplagan,**

MED ANMÄRKNINGAR OCH TILLÄGG, SAMT 6:TE KAPITLET (OM BRONSKULTURENS ORIENTALA URSPRUNG) OMARBETADT. FÖRSEDD MED XYLOGRAFIER OCH EN MÄNGD LITOGRAFIERADE FIGURER.

STOCKHOLM, 1866. P. A. NORSTEDT & SÖNER.

*Figure 2. Front plate of Vol. I (The Stone Age) of Sven Nilsson's* The Aboriginal Population of Nordic Scandinavia: An Attempt at Comparative Ethnography and a Contribution to Humankind's Evolutionary History *(second edition, 1866).*

In the 1980s, new ideas started developing in Norway inspired by social anthropology. Knut Odner and Bjørnar Olsen, influenced by the theories of Frederik Barth (1969), began characterizing Saami ethnogenesis as the result of cultural interactions, including collaboration and conflict (Odner 1983; cf. Olsen 1994) – more specifically, local hunters in North Norway and Finland with metal-producing agrarian groups from central and eastern Russia (Jørgensen 1986; Jørgensen and Olsen 1988). Hansen and Olsen (2004:36–42) pushed this process of "cultural consolidation" back to the Early Metal Age/Bronze Age.

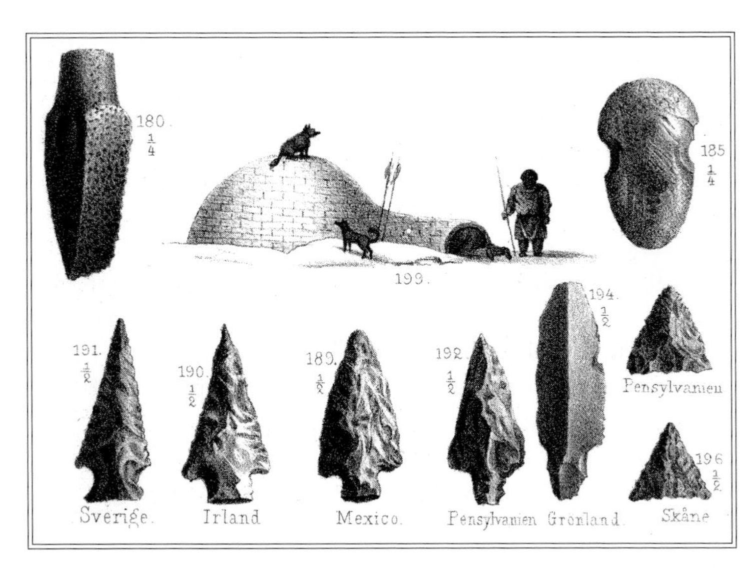


*Figure 3. Plate VIII showing artifacts from Sweden, Ireland, Mexico, Greenland and Pennsylvania together with an Eskimo igloo (Sven Nilsson 1866).*

Against this background, I have been struck by how much Saami and Nordic cultures had in common in northern Sweden, and how much the Saami had contributed to Swedish culture. Many Saami offer rites and ritual practices, for instance, mirror Germanic Iron Age practices, and vice versa. Hunting and land-use patterns are remarkably similar throughout the Stone, Bronze and Iron Ages. The northern hunter-gatherer past is even expressed in historic times by the organization of farmsteads on the Bothnian coast (Roeck-Hansen 2002) and through beliefs about forest spirits (Rathje 2001:162–174). There is abundant evidence of long-term continuity in coastal Västerbotten.

Cultures can change relatively quickly but still retain cognitive structures that transcend race, economy, material culture and even religion (Goody 1977; Banton 1981; Lloyd 1990; D'Andrade 1995). The ways northern societies related to their environments, both natural and human, are therefore central to our understanding of the origins of identities (Berkes and Folke 1998; Berkes 1999; Ingold 2000). Oral histories, stories, myths and sagas are the verbal repositories of these memories. The bear rites and stories about dwarves and Stalo giants are examples of this phenomenon. They are so-called *longue durée* manifestations of cultural identity (cf. Braudel 1949; Thomas 1996; Redman and Kinzig 2003). Long-term continuities have also been described as the "cultural trajectories" of local societies, and these can sometimes converge with those of majority societies because of common interests (Wolf 1997:23).

The Saami have, nevertheless, been viewed as a dilemma and as peripheral in Nordic archaeology. There have been both racial and evolutionary overtones in the discussions and, in spite of the social anthropological interpretations regarding the origins of ethnic/cultural identities, the narratives inevitably break down to minority and majority power relations (Eriksen 1993).

## Archaeology and the Welfare State

While the methods of modern archaeology are the same everywhere, there is a fundamental difference between European archaeology and the "archaeology as anthropology" paradigm that characterizes North American archaeology. Anthropological archaeology grew out of the colonial experience of Europeans in North and South America, Africa, Australia and Asia. European archaeology has focused instead on national identities and has had the political goal of asserting the origins and histories of those societies. Social interpretations, particularly since the 1970s, have consequently often been based on European political, economic and sociological theory (cf. Giddens 1977) and especially Neo-Marxism, including World Systems Theory (Wallerstein 1974) and the French Annales School of Historiography (cf. Braudel 1949; Bourdieu 1977). Although I have found these theories very useful in my own research, they have also led many Nordic scholars, in my opinion, to an overemphasis on the explanatory importance of conflicts and crises, a perspective that still dominates interpretations of northern prehistory. Curiously, although northern Sweden has clearly been subjected to internal colonialism (cf. Loeffler 2005), this has manifested itself politically as the victimization of the Swedish settlers, hydroelectric-, forest- and mine workers by the state, and who resent the outflow of capital to Stockholm more than the plight of the Saami.

But, even in its most benign forms, nationalistic archaeology has rendered the rights of minority societies problematic. This was complicated in Sweden by the development of the welfare state system in the 1930s. Racial hygiene (eugenics) and education were among the core principles of this social engineering effort. Sweden had already been the first country in Europe to establish a State Institute of Racial Biology [1921]. The Sterilization Act, implemented in 1941 and affecting some 63,000 Swedish citizens, mostly women, was only discontinued in 1975, 30 years after WWII (Broberg and Roll-Hansen 2005; Broberg and Tydén 2005:77–149).

As early as 1913, special nomadic schools were established for Saami children to help preserve the nomadic lifestyle and perpetuate the stereotype of the Saami as primitive, vulnerable and consequently needing the protection of the state (Lundmark 1998, 2002:40–41). It was believed that the Saami were even physically predisposed for reindeer nomadism. These ideas have been referred to as "a Lapp shall remain a Lapp" policy (Lundmark 2002:63–75). The Germans, while occupying Norway from 1940, seem to have shared this patronizing view, allowing the Saami, for example, to continue with trans-border herding (Lantto 2005). These social goals have had, and still have, major political, economic and cultural consequences. "Real" (nomadic reindeer herding) Saami were put under state protection and Saami land was, and still is, state-owned. The remaining 90% of the Saami in Sweden, the non-reindeer-owners, have been viewed as assimilated (cf. Mörkenstam 1999).

Ironically, in spite of the protectionist ideology for the herders and international solidarity regarding human rights and the support of archaeology in developing countries through the Swedish International Development Agency, the Swedish government still refuses to acknowledge the Saami, including the herders, as indigenous people in accordance with United Nation policies (ILO nr. 169, 1989). Convention 169 comprises the principles, guidelines and obligations for the protection of indigenous peoples, including their institutions, properties, lands and culture. Indigenous people are defined under these provisions as people having their origins in ethnic groups that lived in the country when national borders were formed, and who have wholly or partly retained their social, economic, cultural and political organizations.

The situation has been exacerbated by an unreflective projection of majority culture in Nordic museums (cf. Goodnow and Akman 2008). In her study regarding Saami representations in Swedish and Finnish museums, Janet E. Levy found while Nordic continuities with the Viking past are still presented as an almost foregone conclusion, there is at the same time an earnest desire to "depoliticize" archaeology and to not discuss ethnicity (Levy 2006). Unfortunately, this non-committal position de facto relegates the question of Saami origins to that of a prehistoric wilderness, almost the same attitude toward these people and their "unoccupied" lands as expressed by the Swedish Crown in 1328 (cf. Steckzén 1964:119–128).

Intellectual polarity can go both ways but the majority (master) narrative always has a distinct advantage on the national stage (cf. Zachrisson 2004). This study aims to create a more balanced picture of prehistory. While it should be obvious that one cannot take identities of the present and uncritically apply them to the past, it is equally obvious that these identities have pasts and we have an obligation to understand their origins, particularly when these affect policies today (cf. Ojala 2006).

## The Means to an End

This book is intended to be accessible to a broad professional readership and an international public who have an interest in archaeology, climate change, Nordic prehistory and history, cultural resiliency and northern indigenous issues. One immediate goal has been to publish the original archaeological data from the project, but this is also very much a book of ideas. I have long argued that the Nordic region is one of the best places in the world to study long-term cultural interactions, not only because of the meeting of two great cultural-ecological systems, but because of the socio-economic complexities not often seen this far north (Broadbent 2000).

This is also a highly interdisciplinary study. Like the issue of Saami ethnogenesis itself, it is often at the "borderlands" that the greatest dynamics of systems occur, be they cultural and/or ecological, and where the causes and effects of change are most easily observed and understood (Broadbent 1997). Archaeological data are always fragmentary and to overcome these limitations I have turned to the ecology of lichens, geophysics, chemical analyses, organization of northern church towns, place-name distributions, tax records and so forth in order to fill in the many blanks. From this web of information emerges a picture of the past much like a photograph in a developing tray. This picture is the subject of the book. The narrative is the interpretation of this picture and its origins in 7,000 years of prehistory (cf. Carlsson 1998).

Eric R. Wolf has best described this search for a past:

> *We can no longer be content writing the history of the victorious elites, or with documenting the subjugation of dominated ethnic groups . . . we thus need to uncover the "people without history . . ." (1997:xvi)*

Of course, there are no people without histories of their own, and I trust I have moved us closer toward illuminating the Saami past through this interdisciplinary archaeological effort. The last chapter is a synthesis of the conclusions of the study and offers some perspectives on what we can learn from prehistory about resiliency and the value of cultural diversity in contemporary society.

## Notes

1. The term *circumpolar* refers to the northern lands encompassing the Arctic Ocean and having Arctic and Sub-Arctic climates, plants, animals and cultures.

2. A large iron ring with the oldest Nordic law code written in runes was found spiked to the door of Forsa Church in Hälsingland, northern Sweden. It was probably taken from a pre-Christian cult site or temple in the region ("Ringen från Forsa." Catalogue edited by Jan Lundell and Lars Nylander, Hälsinglands museum-Hudiksvall 2005).

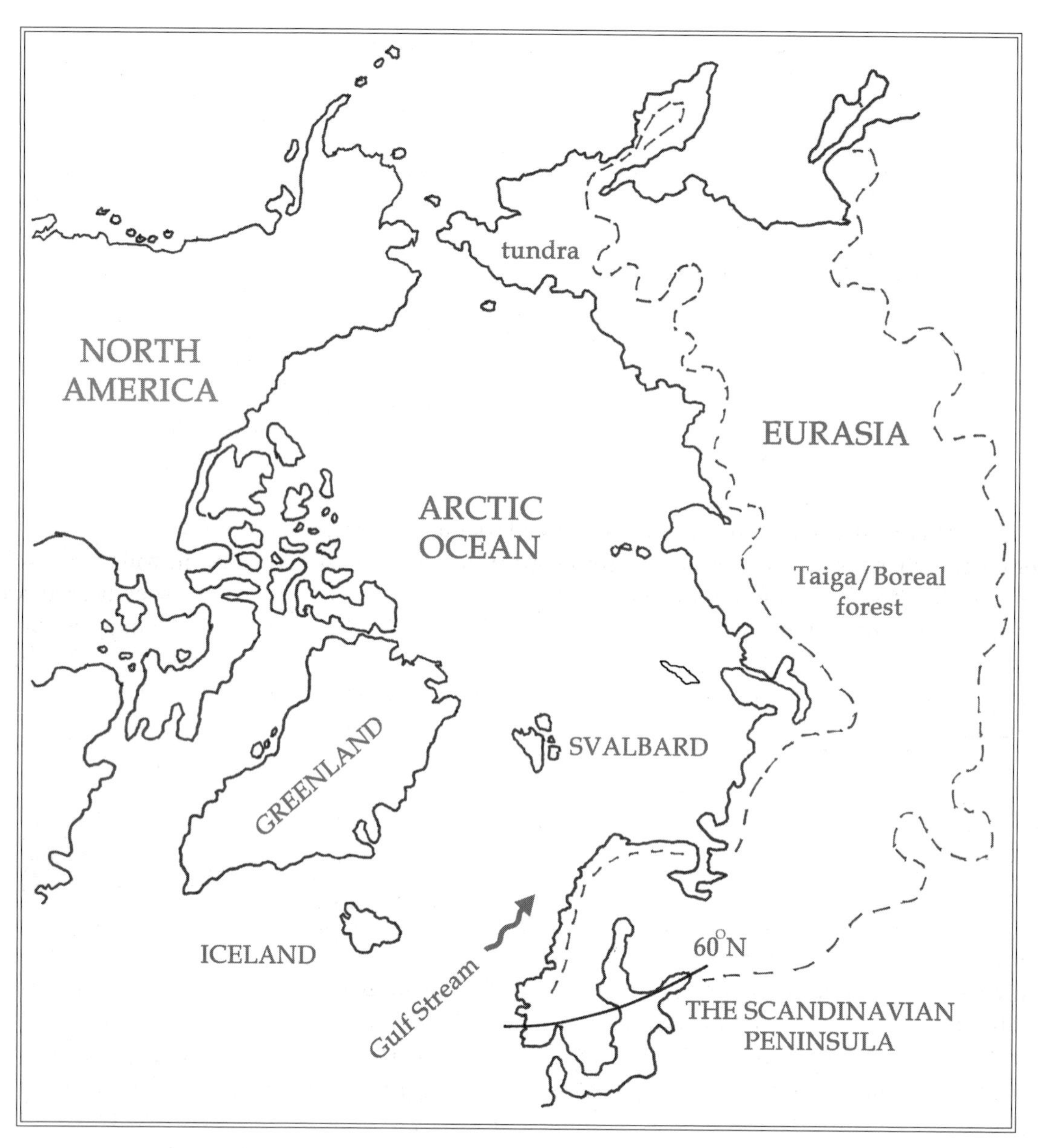


*Figure 4. The Circumpolar Region. The Nordic region is the northwestern corner of the Eurasian continent and a long-term meeting-ground of circumpolar and European plants, animals and peoples. The capital cities of Oslo, Stockholm and Helsinki coincide with the 60th parallel and the ecological boundary between these two worlds.*

# 2

# Culture and Ecology

## The Historical-Ecological Setting

Scandinavia includes the kingdoms of Norway, Sweden and Denmark. The Nordic countries by definition also include Finland, Iceland, Greenland and the Faroe Islands in the North Atlantic. The Nordic region is a meeting ground of two great human-environmental systems: the North European and the circumpolar worlds. The borderland between these two biogeographical regions in Sweden is called *Limes norrlandicus*, the Norrland (North Land) border, and coincides roughly with the Dal River (Dalälven) and the 60th parallel, which runs just north of the capital cities of Oslo and Stockholm and south of Helsinki (Figure 4).

Human history in Sweden and Norway plays out against the background of major environmental changes on land and in the seas within the confines of a ca. 400 km wide peninsula between the North Atlantic and the Baltic Sea. The northern boreal forest (taiga) extends eastward from Norway and Eurasia to the Bering Straits and across Alaska to Canada. The high latitudes and environments make the Nordic North an indisputable part of the circumpolar world. Many indigenous peoples, such as the Saami, developed cultural adaptations and survival strategies that are unique to these northern forest, tundra and maritime environments (Gjessing 1944).

## The Importance of the Coastal Zone

The significance of the Bothnian coast in Saami prehistory has been little discussed in Sweden, even though the idea is not new. Birger Steckzén (1964), an historian and archivist, speculated that the disappearance of the Saami from this coastland was due to brutal taxation by the Birkarls, state-sanctioned tax collectors operating in the fourteenth century. He was well aware of the Iron Age hut sites, but none of this material had been excavated. Gustaf Hallström, who had mapped many of the coastal sites in Västerbotten, had commented on their similarities to the so-called "Stalo huts" in the sub-alpine regions of Sweden (1949:76). In 1965, Skellefteå Museum director Ernst Westerlund rejected the idea of coastal Saami in Västerbotten, rebutting Steckzén (1964), and ascribing the sites to seasonal sealers and fishermen from the south, or even to Swedish settlers (Westerlund 1965). The idea of a "local" culture has also been argued (cf. Rathje 2001). Westerlund's view has been a commonly held opinion (cf. Westin 1962; Norman 1993; Lindström and Olofsson 1993), and there has been little interest, and even an aversion, by any but a handful of Swedish archaeologists in arguing otherwise.

In other respects, the maritime connection has defined Nordic prehistory more than any other single environmental or geographic factor. The Nordic Peninsula is circumscribed by the North Atlantic and Baltic seas, marked by large lake systems and cross-cut by rivers and river valleys. Proximity to water routes was one of the key elements conveying economic advantages in Eurasia and the European Peninsula as a World System (Wolf 1997:31). The Norwegian and the Bothnian coasts were major cultural meeting grounds and coastal waters were the best way to travel to and from the north in both countries; traveling along the shore of the Swedish coast rather than by land made it possible to avoid 12 major river crossings (Figure 5).

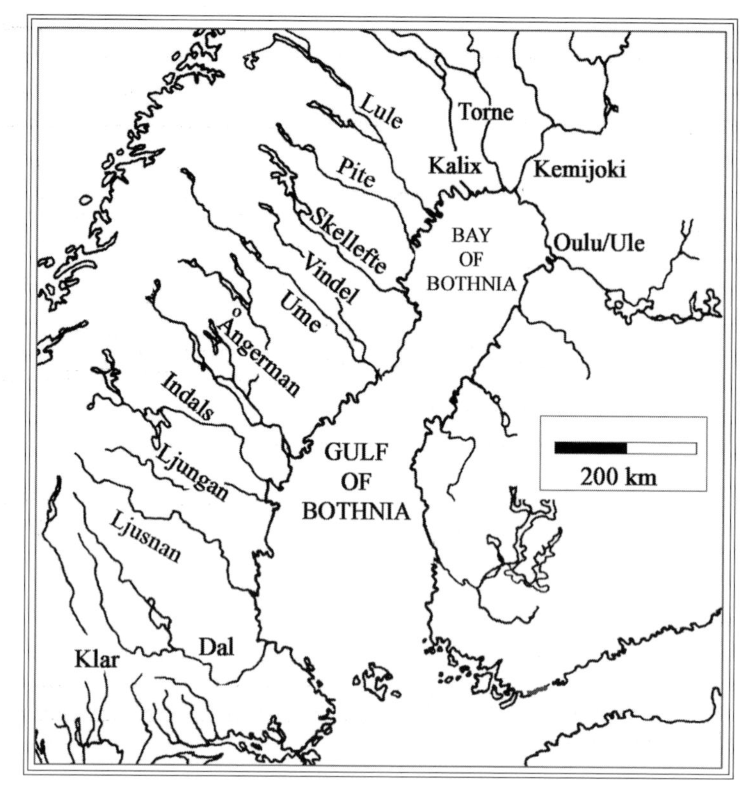


*Figure 5. Main river drainages of Sweden into the Gulf of Bothnia.*

In addition to the direct effects on Nordic climate, marine food resources laid the foundations for larger hunter-gatherer populations and more settled lives that opened the door to cultivation and animal husbandry at these latitudes. Coastal zones were also critically important because of the reliability and accessibility of their resources, including birds, shellfish, fish and fuel that all the members of these communities, including the elderly and the young, could gather on a daily basis.

One of the most fascinating aspects of Bothnian economy is that it involved high arctic ice hunting (cf. Gustafsson 1971, 1988, 1990; Westerberg 1988; Kvist 1987, 1988, 1990; Nyström 1988, 2000; Nilsson 1989; Edlund 1989; Olsson 1990). Seal hunting also has a long history in the region (Ekman 1910:222–260; Hämäläinen 1930; Clark 1946; Forstén 1972; Broadbent 1979; Storå and Lõugas 2005), and there is a rich Swedish vocabulary referring to seals and sea ice (Edlund 1989, 2000). Ice hunting continued into historic times, and for three months of the year a large percentage of the male population of "Norrabotten" (the Mare Botnicum or Bay of Bothnia) was recorded as going out on the ice. As many as 15,000 seals were taken in one year in the sixteenth century (Westin 1962; Tegengren 1965; Kvist 1991). Olaus Magnus, the last Catholic Archbishop of Sweden, illustrated the organized mercantile hunting of seals by northern peasants on his *Carta Marina* map from 1539 (Figure 7).

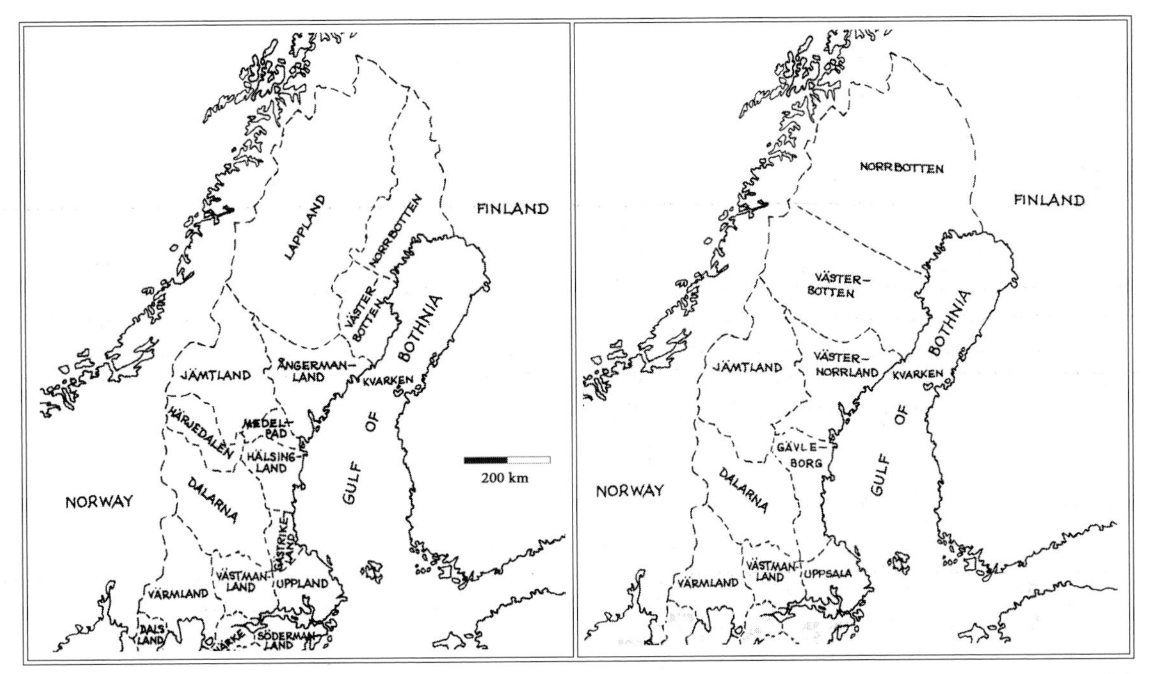


*Figure 6. (left) Provinces of Sweden. (right) Counties of Sweden. The county system (län) was established in 1634 and superseded the older provincial system of administration. The county system is used with reference to archaeological sites, place-names and other data presented in this study.*

## The Saami People

The Saami are the people of *Sápmi* (Saamiland). This name Saami (alt. Sámi) is recorded from the thirteenth century but is probably much older (Zachrisson 1997a:174). The Saami were also called, sometimes derogatively, "Lapps." The name "Saami" occurs in all Saami languages and, whenever possible, this self-designation will be used in this text, although the term "Lapp" is employed concerning administrative areas, place-names or historical documents.

The Saami number approximately 80,000 people today. About 17,000 Saami live in Sweden, of whom 2,000 are involved in reindeer herding. Their ancestors were referred to in the oldest written sources as the *Fenni*, and as *Skrid-finnar* (Ski-Finns). In Norway, Lapland is still referred to as "Finnmark." In 1673 Johannes Schefferus speculated that the Saami had even come from Finland:

> *The Lapps derive without doubt their origin from the Finns, were born among them, but had been driven away and exiled from Finland . . . after leaving their homeland they withdrew as exiles and this is the origin of the name. They did not themselves use this name [Lapp] . . . but that of their former countrymen, the Finns. (1673:40)*

The Roman historian Tacitus had described the Fenni as early as A.D. 98:

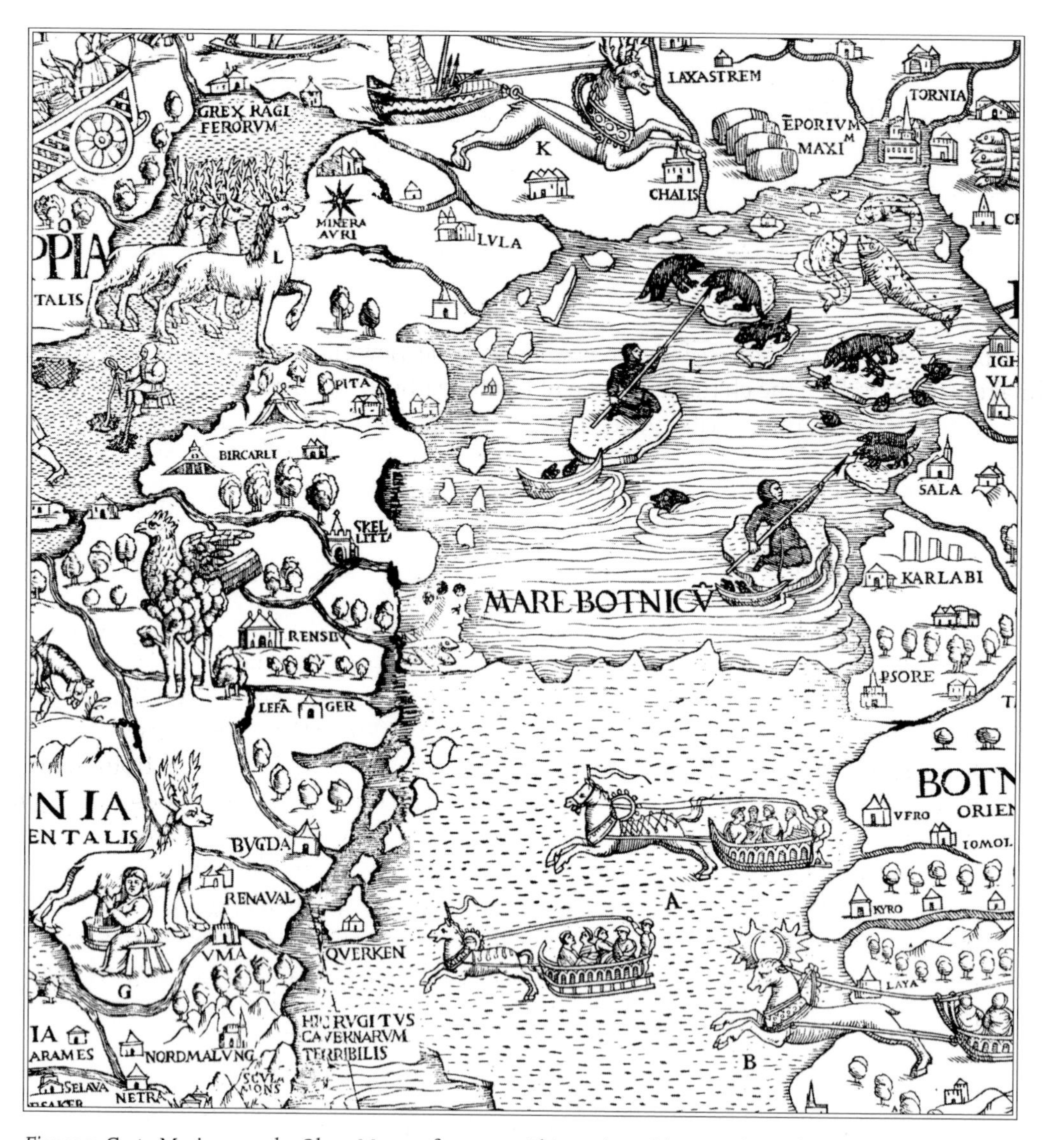


*Figure 7.* Carta Marina *map by Olaus Magnus from 1539. This portion of the map shows the North Bothnian coast, hunters spearing gray seals and sleds pulled by reindeer and horses. A Saami woman north of the Ume River in Västerbotten is milking a reindeer. Original in the Carolina Rediviva Library in Uppsala.*

*The Fenni are astonishingly wild and horribly poor. They have no arms [weapons], no horses, no homes. They eat grass, dress in skins and sleep on the ground. Their only hope is in their arrows, which, for lack of iron, they tip with bone. The same hunt provides food for men and women alike; for the women go everywhere with the men and claim a share in securing the prey. The only way they can protect their babies against wild beasts or foul weather is to hide them under a makeshift network of branches. This is the hovel to which young men come back; this is where the old must die. And yet they count their lot happier than that of others who groan over field labor, sweat over house building, or hazard their own or other men's fortunes in the wild lottery of hope and fear. They care for nobody, man or god, and have gained the ultimate release: they have nothing to pray for. What comes after them is the stuff of fables—Hellusii and Oxiones with the faces and features of men, but the bodies and limbs of animals. On such unverifiable stories I will express no opinion.*

P. Cornelius Tacitus, *Germania*
Translated by H. Mattingly (1948:140)

This account paints a dismal picture and one should view such descriptions with skepticism (Whitaker 1980). In fact, the characterization of hunter-gatherers or nomadic people as wretched is quite common (Sahlins 1972; Cribb 1991). The expression *fattig lapp* "poor Lapp" still has this colloquial meaning in Scandinavia. The ethnonym *Lapp* has an east Nordic origin and probably derives from the Finnish *Lappi* (*Lappalainen* means "Laplander") – or may even derive from the word for a patch of cloth or hide (*lapp*). In Russia, the name *lop* and *lops* is known from chronicles dating to ca. A.D. 1000 (Hansen and Olsen 2004:49–50). According to von Düben (1873:376), the term also has reference to magic and witchcraft.

The ethnonym *Lapp* appears in the *Gesta Danorum* (History of Denmark), written by Saxo Grammaticus in A.D. 1190 (Schefferus 1673:42), and also in the Icelandic Orkneyinga Saga, written down as a revised text in the 1200s (Zachrisson 1997a:159). The place-name *Lappi* has been associated with Saami settlements at more than 575 places all over Finland (Itkonen 1951:33). The term *lappar* was first used in an official Swedish document in the Tälje statutes from September 5, 1328. By my count, there are 1,147 place-names with the prefix Lapp in Sweden, based on the National Land Survey place-name registry (Chapter 9, Figure 195). These place-names have thus far been given little attention in Sweden but are invaluable sources regarding former Saami territory.

The Saami speak nine languages of the Finno-Ugric (Uralic) language family (Collinder 1953; Nickel 1990) (Figure 9), and their mtDNA and Y chromosomes indicate that they are an ancient European population (Beckman 1996: Tambets et al. 2004). The Finno-Ugrian languages probably spread from central Russia and the southern Urals to the Nordic region as early as the Stone Age, and

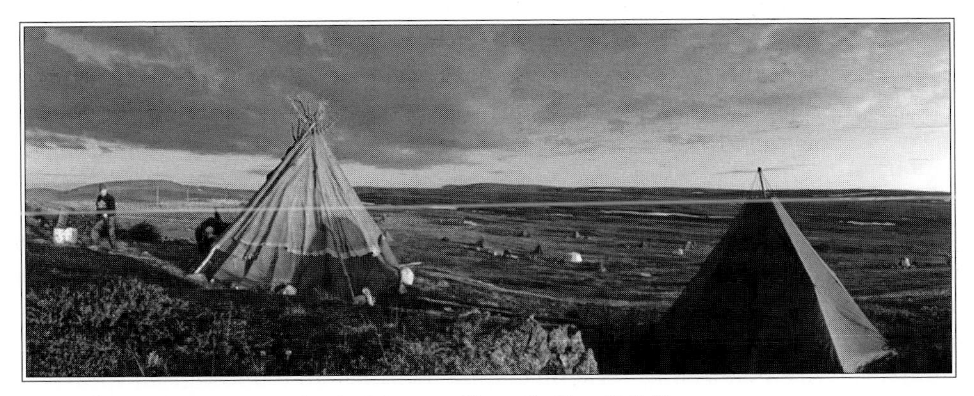

*Figure 8. Saami summer camp in North Norway. Photo: Fred Ivar Utsi Klemetsen.*

the Finnish language developed later through contacts with other Finno-Ugrian speakers from the south Baltic. This linguistic differentiation is believed to have occurred during the Bronze Age/Arctic Bronze Age, some 4,000 years ago (Strade 1997:183; Carpelan et al. 2001). However, on the basis of "Paleo-Lappish substrate" words, such as the word for seal (*morsa*), Aikio (2004) argues for a later date.

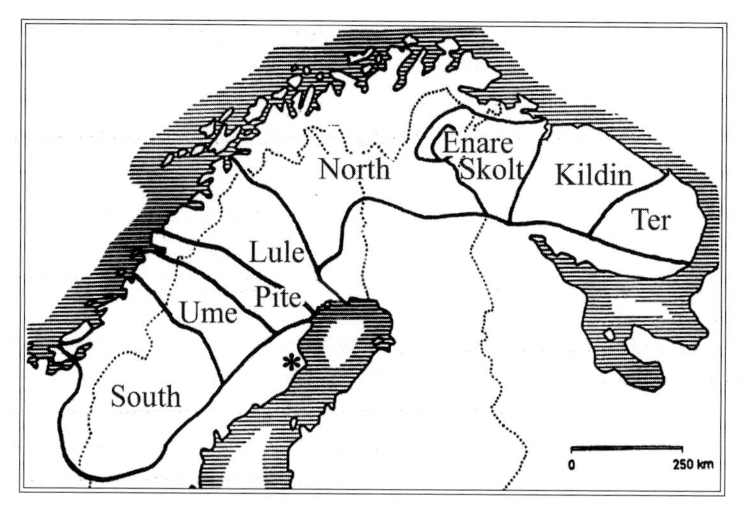


*Figure 9. Present Saami territory and language areas. Asterisk shows the main area of study. Map adapted from Nickel (1990).*

Saami territory in Norway and the Kola Peninsula in Russia extends along a thousand kilometers of northern coasts (Figure 9). According to the Icelandic and Norwegian Sagas from 1100–1200s, the Saami also lived as far south as Hadeland, some 20 km north of Oslo, and throughout southern Norrland and as far south as Svealand in Sweden (Zachrisson 1987:26, 1997a:171). The latter is even implied by mtDNA at the iconic Late Iron Age boat burial site of Tuna in Alsike between Uppsala and Stockholm (Götherström 2001:25–26). The ancestors of the Saami were also known as far south as the Western Dvina (Daugava) River in Latvia (Itkonen 1947; Eidlitz-Kuoljok 1991:32) (Figure 29).

In 1911, Johan Turi, a Swedish Saami reindeer herder and author of one of the first indigenous ethnographies ever written, *Muittalus Samid Birra* (A Book on Lappish Life), wrote the following regarding Saami origins and settlement:

> *It has not been said that the Lapp came from somewhere else. The Lapp was settled all over Lapland and the Lapp lived on the seacoast and there were no other dwellers besides themselves, and that was a good time for the Lapps. And the Lapp also lived everywhere on the Swedish side and there were no settlers anywhere; the Lapps did not know there were other people besides themselves. (1911:2)*

This view is reiterated by most Saami scholars today (cf. Kuoljok 1996; Haetta 2002; Solbakk 2004; Lehtola 2004), although *Sápmi* in Sweden and Finland is invariably shown as coinciding with inland herding areas.

The Germanic speaking groups of Sweden and Norway were referred to as *Svear* and *Nordmenn* in sources such as Adam of Bremen's *History of the Archbishops of Hamburg- Bremen* (ca. A.D. 1081). The Svear settled only as far north as 63°N on the Bothnian coast and as far as Jämtland and Härjedalen in the interior. The Nordmenn occupied the coast of Norway up to Malangen at about 70°N (Odner 1983). Orosius (Othere from Hålogaland), who lived in North Norway in the late ninth century, described the Fenni, Terfenni and the Bjarmi – all Finno-Ugrian speakers – in his account to the English King Alfred the Great (Bosworth 1885). In the *Historia Norvegiae* (A.D. 1195), mention is made of another group, the *Kveni,* who lived on the north Bothnian shores. Egil's Saga, written down in the 1200s, also mentions Kvenland (Paulsson and Edwards 1976). Adam of Bremen referred to these Kveni as "Amazons," but the designation was probably his confusion over *kvenerlandet* (the land of the Kvens) with *kvinderlandet,* which means "the land of the women" in Danish (Lund 1978:68). It has, nevertheless, been speculated that the "Amazon" description related to large-scale sealing expeditions that left Bothnian farming settlements populated by only women and children for three to four months of each year (Tegengren 1965). This curious tale originated among travelers going north who had actually encountered these villages of women (according to Adam). Adam had also written that the people north of the Svear were ruled by a woman. Lillian Rathje (2001) has emphasized the important role that women had in northern agrarian economies while the men were off hunting and fishing.

The Ski-Finns are identified as living south and west of the Amazons and north of the Svear (Figure 10). This description is fairly accurate, and Kvenland could actually thus refer to Finland (Julku 1986). Amazons notwithstanding, there is little doubt that seal hunting was of considerable economic

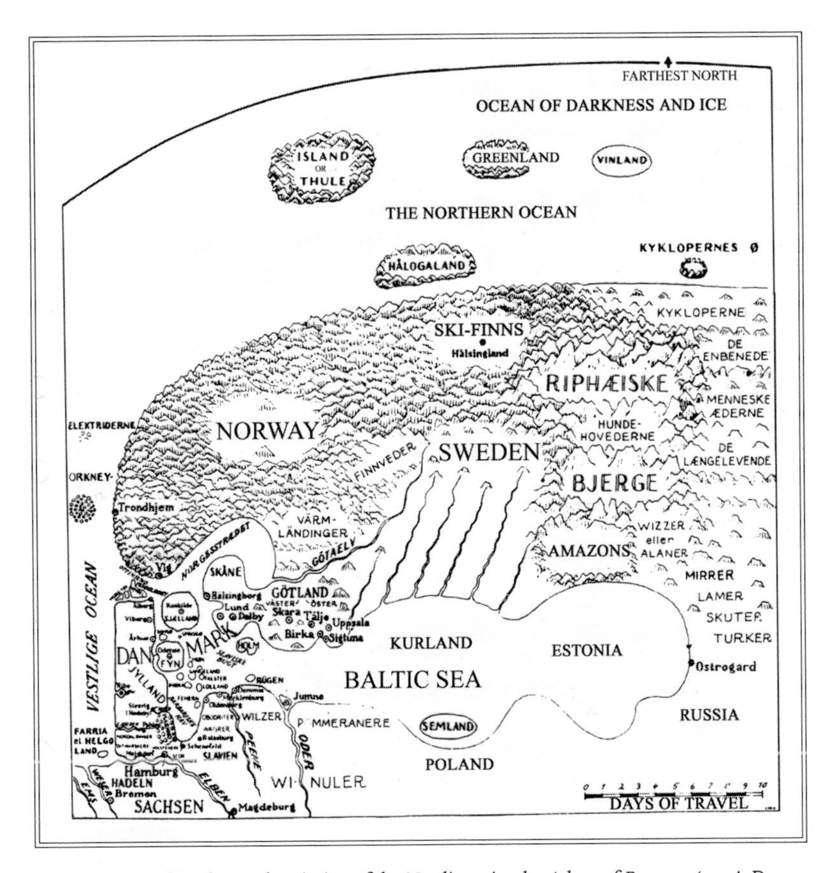


*Figure 10. Map based on a description of the Nordic region by Adam of Bremen (ca. A.D. 1081). The Saami are referred to as Skridfinner (Ski-Finns) and lived in Hälsingland. The "Amazons" lived on the Baltic coast of what was probably Finland. Even Vinland is also mentioned in this early account. Map adapted from Lund (1978).*

importance from the earliest times and into the modern era. Swedish Bothnian sealing sites from the Iron Age have been previously discussed by a number of archaeologists and historians: Hallström (1942, 1949), Varenius (1964, 1978), Westin (1962), Steckzén (1964), Westberg (1964), Westerlund (1965), Nilsson (1989), Norman (1993), and Rathje (2001). Four cultural entities have been considered: the Kvens, the Finns, the Saami (Lapps) and Germanic Iron Age settlers (Scandinavian speakers).

Othere from Hålogaland (ca. A.D. 900), Adam of Bremen (ca. A.D. 1081), the *Historia Norwegiae* (ca. A.D. 1195) and Egil's Saga (ca. A.D. 1200) state that the North Bothnian groups were Finno-Ugric, not Germanic peoples. Adam wrote that Hälsingland was Saami territory. During those times Hälsingland extended around the Bay of Bothnia and down to the Ule River in Finland.

The northern limit of Germanic settlement in Sweden extended only as far as Arnäs in Ångermanland (Figure 12). This is the northernmost limit for Iron Age forts, rune stones, tumulus cemeteries, Nordic long houses and the *ledung* maritime defense system (Westerdahl 1989). Diagnostic Late Iron Age settlement place-names, such as those with the name elements *-sta, -hem* and *vin-*, are not found north of there either (Edlund 1988). Nordic linguists have given considerable attention to these settlement names (Franzén 1939; Holm 1949; Ståhl 1976; Wahlberg 2003). The name *hem* means "home" today, but originally referred to a village settlement and was often a first, or *landnam*, name. The term *landnam* is associated with the first landings by the Norse in Iceland, and this colonization phase usually leaves a distinctive environmental signature on vegetation surrounding northern settlements because of grazing, burning, removal of trees and the introduction of cultivated plants and weeds (cf. Hicks 1988, 1994; Aronsson 1991; Karlsson 2006). *Vin* probably referred to grazing land and also indicates that this was a homestead site. *Sta* originally referred to boat-landing places but was later applied to towns that had developed because there were harbors at these places (*stad* means "town" today). All three names date back to the period A.D. 800 to 1100 in Sweden. These names concentrate in Jämtland, Medelpad and Ångermanland in northern Sweden (Selinge 1997). The name elements *böle* and *mark* are, by contrast, common in northern Västerbotten and are associated with the expansion of Scandinavian farmers starting in the fourteenth century (Holm 1949:94).

In an analysis of the Kven issue regarding potential recognition under ILO 169 (the International Labour Organization's 1989 Indigenous and Tribal Peoples Convention), Swedish historian Lennart Lundmark came to the conclusion that the Kvens were not an indigenous cultural group at all, but were Finnish middlemen for the Novgorod fur trade (Lundmark 2007). They were later formally recognized by the Swedish state as Saami tax collectors, the Birkarls. Thomas Wallerström, a Swedish historian and archaeologist, had earlier reached the same conclusion (1995). Assuming they are right, and I think they are, the Kvens can be discounted as having anything to do with the Iron Age sealing sites. The Kvens seem to have had their operations and farms in the northernmost parts of the Bay of Bothnia and on the Swedish coast only as far south as the Skellefte-Byske Rivers, an area with many Finnish connections (Fjellström 1988). Having eliminated the Kvens from serious consideration, the remaining alternative for these seal hunters is that of an indigenous, but non-Germanic culture.

One complication in all of this is that these two cultural-linguistic entities, the Finno-Ugric and the Germanic, with languages that are as far apart as any on earth, existed side by side for thousands of years. This situation is nothing like North America, where the sudden impacts of European colonialism starting 500 years ago transformed whole continents, and whose diseases, animals and plants almost annihilated indigenous populations (Crosby 1986). In the Nordic region there was, on the contrary, continuous interaction and a slow process of give-and-take. There is considerable evidence that there were mostly peaceful and symbiotic relations between Germanic, Finnish and Saami groups (Mundal 1996; Zachrisson 1997a:221–234; Olsen 2000; Price 2000). Cultures with such a long history of interaction inevitably overlap in numerous ways. It is also likely that these pre-literate people were multilingual. This implies that instead of sharp boundaries between them we are in reality dealing with overlapping cultural and linguistic topographies.

Although people certainly have identities independently of outsiders, this meeting of cultures was itself a potent force of ethnogenesis (Barth 1969, 1994), and a key to the formation of many distinctive Saami ethnic markers as seen by dress, rituals and other practices (cf. Kleppe 1977; Reymert 1980; Baudou 1987; Zachrisson 1987b; Zachrisson 1997a:189–220). Metal artifacts, such as brooches, were produced in many different regions and were readily incorporated into Saami dress. Christian crosses and symbols, as well as decorative styles (e.g., Nordic plaited band designs), were also used by the Saami.

The concept of cultural clines, comparable to population studies, and "seamless cultural topographies" (Caulkins 2001:121), helps conceptualize Saami prehistory as an integrated part of Nordic prehistory. This not only de-marginalizes the narrative, it connects the discourse to the formation of all northern cultural identities. The Early Metal Age, which corresponds to the Scandinavian Bronze Age and the so-called "Arctic Bronze Age" (Tallgren 1949; Bakka 1976), was the period during which Saami ethnicity (as we know it) is believed by many archaeologists to have developed through contacts between "Proto-Saami" and other groups (cf. Carpelan 1975b; Baudou 1987; Olsen 1994).

## Human-Environmental Relations

The Nordic region is situated in the far northwestern corner of the Eurasian continent and stretches some 2,000 km between latitudes 54°N to 72°N, as far north as the North Slope of Alaska, Baffin Island in Canada and northern Siberia. This shoulder of land juts far out into the North Atlantic where it intercepts the warm and salty waters of the Gulf Stream. The climate-mitigating influences of the Gulf Stream have had profound effects on ecology and settlement. Agrarian economies were made possible farther north and earlier than anywhere else in the Arctic and the rich Sub-Arctic waters have been among the most productive fishing regions of the world (Dunbar 1954, 1968). Seals, salmon, whitefish, cod, herring and shellfish have drawn people to these shores from the earliest times, and most Nordic populations still live within 20 km of the coast. The Scandinavian Peninsula is furthermore separated from Finland for most of its length by the Baltic Sea and the Gulf of Bothnia. This body of water cuts deeply into the continent and extends about 1,400 km from north to south. It separates the two regions by 100 km or more of open water today, but had once been twice as wide.

The Baltic has changed from being an ice-dammed freshwater lake 10,000 years ago, to an open arm of the sea, back to a freshwater lake as a result of the many rivers that flow into it, only to once again become a sea (Berglund et al. 1994). Today the Baltic is an intermediate brackish body of water. The most productive fishing-, hunting- and shellfish-collecting periods were when the Baltic was most open to the Atlantic Ocean, and this occurred during the Litorina Period (named after a salt water mollusk) between approximately 5000 B.C. and 1000 B.C. Even today, powerful strokes of saline water into the Baltic have had immediate and positive effects on plankton, shellfish and seal populations lasting for up to five years (cf. Segerstråle 1957:757). Sea level rises due to worldwide oceanic events would have had even longer-term effects.

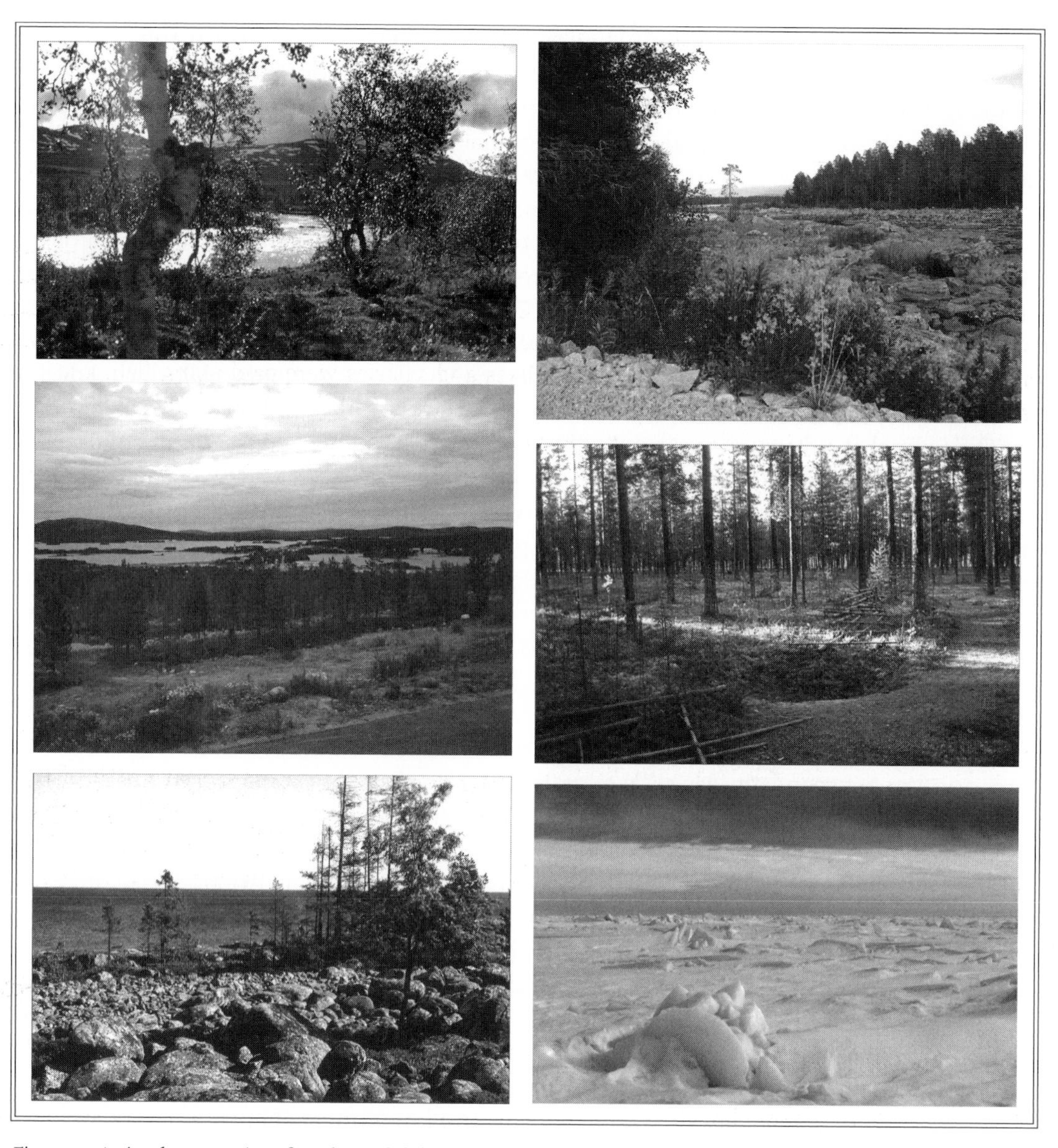

*Figure 11. A visual cross section of north Swedish biogeography. Clockwise from top left: alpine birch forest and mountains, headwaters of the Skellefte River, interior pine heath forest (with trapping pits for moose or reindeer), ice cover on the Bay of Bothnia in April, the Bay of Bothnia with wave-washed moraine beaches, interior lake and esker landscape.*

Most of the vegetation above 60°N in Sweden is classified as northern boreal forest with a sub-alpine birch region in the mountain foothills to the west. The boreal forest environment brought characteristic animals such as bears, moose, beavers, lynxes, wolverines, pine martens, otters, black grouses and hazel hens. During the warm Atlantic climate period, ca. 5000–2500 B.C., there were more deciduous trees such as birch, alder and even elm, and this growth greatly stimulated beaver and moose populations, who fed on their leaves and bark. These are the most commonly found animal bones on archaeological sites in the interior (Ekman and Iregren 1984). The pine forests had changed into a mixture of pine and spruce forests by around 1000 B.C. (Engelmark 1976; Berglund et al. 1994). Black spruce (*Picea abies*) is an eastern hybrid and grows on wetter ground at the expense of alder and birch. Colder and wetter conditions during the Sub-Atlantic period, starting around 2,400 years ago, led to an expansion of reindeer into the southern forests. Bogs increased and covered much greater land areas than earlier.

Although moose, beaver, reindeer and seals were important food resources, freshwater fish were also of great economic value. Salmon, perch, whitefish, pike, burbot (a freshwater cod), trout and char were fished in the rivers and lakes. Starting in the thirteenth century, the Catholic Church asserted ownership of northern salmon rivers. Taxes and salaries were paid using fish, and most parish churches and homesteads in Lapland were established by fish-rich lakes (Campbell 1948). Medieval (Hanseatic) herring fisheries became a basis for many Bothnian coastal villages and towns.

The Gulf of Bothnia is a virtual heat reservoir in the fall that pulls temperature gradients northward into lines parallel with the shorelines. But, unlike the North Atlantic coast, it freezes over in winter and creates a negative temperature anomaly in the spring and summer. The Bothnian coast is ice-bound for up to 200 days per year north of 63°N, which also coincides with a change from a mountainous to a flat coastal topography in Sweden (cf. Ångström 1968; Helmfrid 1994). This was, not surprisingly, the northern limit for Germanic (Iron Age) agrarian settlement in Sweden, and therefore an important cultural-ecological boundary (Figure 12). Although during warmer periods these ice boundaries could have varied, the coastal topography kept the ice locked into the Bay of Bothnia because of the narrow bottleneck of the *Kvarken* between Sweden and Finland. The 100-day ice extended down to the Hornsland Peninsula in Gävleborg County, which is the most prominent peninsula south of Bjuröklubb. Coastal topography was also less broken and with fewer

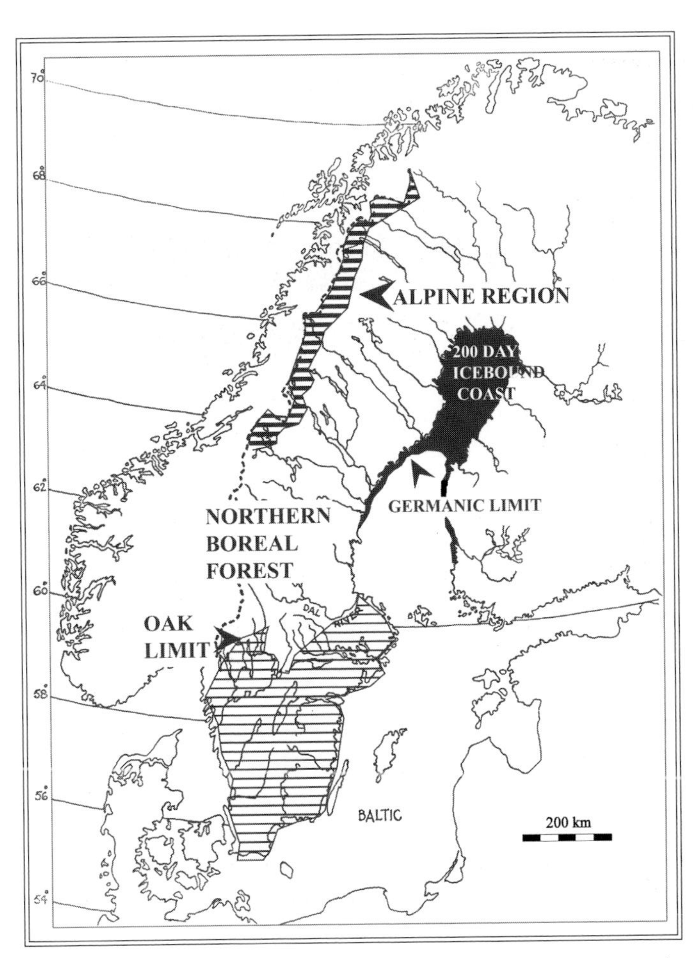

*Figure 12. Map showing the oak limit, alpine and Bothnian ice regions and the northern limit of Germanic Iron Age setttlement.*

islands south of there. Hornslandsudde was therefore an ideally suited place to investigate the southern margins of Saami sealing.

Hunting statistics from 1902 to 1906 (Ekman 1910:262) show the relationship between numbers of seals killed as well as numbers of seals killed per 10 km of Bothnian coast (Figure 13). These figures reflect the relationship between ice conditions and topography. The more broken and island-rich the coastline, the more stable the coastal ice which, together with snow depth, conferred an advantage for ice-breeding seals and the survival of immature seals that could drown if the ice melted before they could swim. Västerbotten was a core area for sealing, and Bjurön, with many Iron Age sites, projects far out into the Bay of Bothnia where it intercepts the counter-clockwise gyre that opens up as a drift-ice channel close to shore. Specialized boat-based seal hunting expeditions from Österbotten in Finland, referred to as the *Fälan* (Cnieff 1757; Gustafsson 1971), sometimes put ashore when the channel was blocked. Many sealers carved their names on the rocks of Svartällviken on Bjurön (Chapter 4, Figure 44).

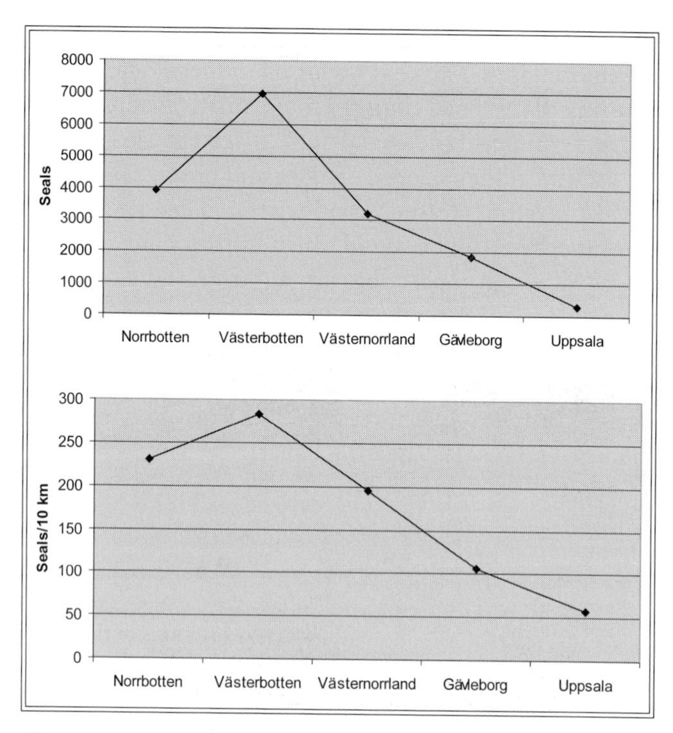


*Figure 13. (top) Numbers of seals taken by county, north to south. (bottom) Numbers of seals taken by length of coastline (based on Ekman 1910:262).*

## Glacial Topography and Settlement

Nordic topography has been sculpted and planed down by the advances and retreats of glacial ice. Sweden and Finland consequently have low rolling landscapes, and Norway, which has a more mountainous topography and softer bedrock, deeply cut fjords. Northern Sweden is also transected by numerous northwest to southeast running rivers, and Finland is speckled by lakes dammed up by a huge terminal moraine that runs north of Helsinki.

Crossing the land in the direction of glacial retreat are long alignments of moraine deposits called "eskers" that mark the courses of former rivers in the ice. Eskers formed natural travel routes for both animals and humans across the lakes and low and boggy expanses of the interior, and are natural connectors between the interior and the coastlands. Most archaeological sites in northern Sweden are found on or near them. Elongated teardrop glacial deposits, called drumlins from the Irish "little hill," formed settlement islands in interior lake and lowland areas, as well as coastal hills and off-shore islands where sealing and fishing could be based.

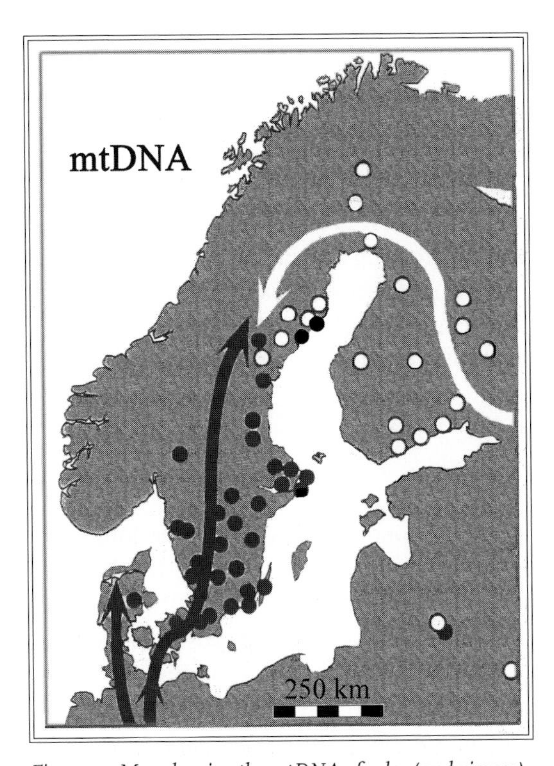


*Figure 14. Map showing the mtDNA of voles (and viruses) in Sweden (Jaarola et al. 1999). The migration of terrestrial animals into the region following deglaciation is a good analogue for human colonization. The cultures, plants and animals of the Nordic North have always been a mixture of these components, one from the south and one from the east, one European and the other circumpolar.*

The Nordic region was de-glaciated starting about 15,000 years ago and by 8,000 years ago northern interior Sweden was completely ice free (Bergström 1968; Bergman et al. 2004). This was one of the last places in Europe to be colonized by humans. The process of glacial melting was so rapid that vast lowland regions of the North European plain were inundated (Björk 1995; Christiansen 1995; Gornitz 2009b). It is likely that many of the western and southern pioneer colonizers of Scandinavia were displaced hunters and gatherers from what is now the bottom of the North Sea between England, the Shetland Islands and the Netherlands (cf. Fischer 1995; Knutsson 2005). This flooding, and related sudden events, seems to have peaked around 6500–6000 B.C. (cf. Björk et al. 1996; Lamb 1977, 1995) and marks a major push into northern Sweden from the south, as seen by the introduction of micro-blade technology (cf. Olofsson 1995, 2003). As the North European hunters and the animals they hunted moved into Scandinavia from the southwest, other human groups and animals moved in from the southeast and east, exploring the newly opened lands before them (cf. Nuñez 1997; Carpelan 2001; Bergman et al. 2004; Knutsson 2005). The mtDNA of everything from voles to bears shows these two groups met up about halfway down in Sweden, or at about latitude 63°N (Jaarola et al. 1999) (Figure 14). Saami mtDNA and Y chromosomes extend southward in an analogous distribution (Tambets et al. 2004).

The crust of the earth was not only flooded, it was depressed by the weight of more than a kilometer of ice and is still compensating following the release of that burden (called isostatic uplift). Land uplift is nearly a meter per century today in Västerbotten (Bergqvist 1977), one of the highest rates in the world, and was perhaps as much as 10 m per year immediately following deglaciation. Shoreline displacement thus provides a unique opportunity for investigating this prehistory (Chapter 4, Figure 34).

## Climate, Ice and Seal Oil

Nordic climate is classified in "Group D" – continental/microthermal – on the Köppen climate classification system, with local maritime influences (Ångström 1968). In winter the region is positioned between high pressure areas in Siberia and Atlantic low pressure centers, resulting in warm southwesterly winds. Inland lakes are frozen from about the beginning of November until the middle of May. The Bay of Bothnia freezes over from the middle of November and usually breaks up by May 20. Snow cover averages 160 to 180 days per year. Precipitation on the outer coast is quite low, but just a few kilometers inland increases to 500 mm per year. During June there is an average of 350 hours of clear sunshine, and in December there are only about 18 hours of sunlight. The average growing season, which corresponds to 3°C, lasts only 160–170 days per year. The total amount of solar energy at 60°N is only a small percentage of what it is farther south, and survival requires taking advantage of food resources during very short growing and breeding seasons. Farmers must keep their livestock alive for six months or more without access to pasturage, and hunters manage on scarce resources during a very long winter and a late spring. Marine mammal oil (seals in the Baltic) was the main source of lighting for circumpolar hunter-gatherers, and seal oil was one of the most important commodities across the Nordic region long before whale oil became commercially important in Europe.

## Periodicity and Settlement Cycles

As defined thus far, three environmental perspectives provide focus in this study: the long-term ecological perspective, the coastal or maritime perspective and the regional perspective. Because of the seasonal fluctuations of both terrestrial and marine resources, northern hunting peoples had to depend on combinations of ecosystems for survival. Depending on geography, this could be done through annual rounds or through sustained uses of particular regions. Economic efforts in northern Sweden, as in most regions of the world, were concentrated during times of maximum productivity, including spawning, breeding and growing seasons (cf. Ekman 1910:455; Campbell 1948:81–211). Hunter-gatherer/fisher societies were also dependent on longer-term resource fluctuations. It is now generally accepted, however, that far from always living in perfect harmony with the environment even these societies could over-exploit and even wipe out game, particularly when engaged in extensive trade. Over-exploitation is considered by some historians as having been a factor in the transition to nomadic reindeer herding and farming, and over-grazing is still a problem in the interior (cf. Hultblad 1968; Lundmark 1982).

Long-term human-environmental dependencies can be analyzed at the landscape level using the concept of historical ecology (Crumley 1994); this relates large-scale environmental changes to the level of human interaction and impacts on local ecosystems. Interactions on much larger scales have been discussed by archaeologists through World Systems Theory, which encompasses global climate change (Kristiansen 1994; Chase-Dunn and Hall 1997; Kardulius 1999; Hornberg and Crumley 2007).

## World Systems and Northern Ecology

The Circumpolar Region has not generally been discussed as a World System, and yet it is one of the great cultural and ecological regions in which vast trading networks, as well as even more integrated economic systems, were operating. One of the first great world industries was the Russian fur trade (Wolf 1997:158–194; Crowell 1997). This is also a region in which early bronze and iron metallurgy developed (Chernykh 1992; Hjärthner-Holdar 1993; Khlobystin 2005; Kuz'minykh 2006). Trade had always played a part in Nordic prehistory but was operating on a Eurasian scale from at least the Bronze Age/Early Metal Age and reached a culmination during the Viking Period around A.D. 1000 (cf. Fedorova 2002). World Systems Theory emphasizes the redistribution of resources, such as furs for metal, between a periphery and a core. The "exporting" and the "receiving" societies underwent recurring periods of expansion and regression due to environmental as well as economic cycles (Wallerstein 1974; Modelski and Thompson 1999). Pulses of these kinds are particularly common in arctic regions, especially when there was heavy exploitation of resources through over-hunting, or when agriculture had been carried out at the limits of its sustainability (cf. Martin 1982; McGovern 1988).

The brackish Gulf of Bothnia is a relatively species-poor marine system, although influxes of ocean water through global warming and worldwide sea level rises probably dramatically raised productivity. These warm periods are indirectly measurable through shoreline transgressions (flooding) in the south and are seen as increased beach erosion in the north. But they are also seen through settlement accumulations at these levels, hunters taking advantage of increases in seal and fish populations, and by agrarians expanding their settlements northward. These fluctuations are very pronounced on the Västerbotten coast (Chapter 3, Figure 16).

It is well known that Bothnian ice conditions were critical for the hunting of ice-breeding seals, particularly the ringed seal (Ekman 1910; Gustafsson 1990). Hunting statistics (Svensson 1904; Hult 1943; Söderberg 1974a, b) and tax lists from the sixteenth century (Kvist 1988, 1990, 1991), suggest that heavy ice conditions led to fewer hunting bounties being paid out and diminished profits in the seal oil trade. In general, the ringed seals were more widely distributed and harder to find when ice cover was widespread, and the other seal species moved southward. Warmer winter conditions seem to have had the opposite effect. Less ice meant that the seals were more concentrated in the north and sought out the stable ice of archipelagos. The seals came to the hunters. This circumstance is described in Chukotka in Russia (Krupnik 1993), eastern Canada (McLaren 1958) and Greenland (Vibe 1970). Reduced ice cover and rises in temperatures at these latitudes also had major effects on terrestrial growing periods, as seen by tree pollen, insects and macrofossils on the North Bothnian coast (Broadbent 1979:158–169). The most common response by hunter-gatherers to major fluctuations of these kinds has been settlement mobility, with moves to coastal regions and then back to inland territories when conditions changed. Whole regions could be largely abandoned for up to a generation between periods of bounty (cf. Minc and Smith 1989). Igor Krupnik has also described this reciprocal settlement phenomenon, involving reindeer hunting and herding in the interior and whaling on the coasts in the Eurasian Arctic (Krupnik 1993:194–197). Shoreline erosion data from the seal hunting sites of the Lundfors complex in Västerbotten indicate, for example, that these sites were only occupied over a 35-year period, or about one generation, and then abandoned (Broadbent 1979:30). The same phenomenon could also be true of interior settlements in northern Sweden, as moose were also subject to natural population swings and were highly vulnerable to predation (cf. Ekman 1910:30–38; Markgren 1974; Peterson et al. 2003). Boreal mammals generally benefit from cold and dry winters that limit parasites, ground ice and snow depth (Sugden 1982:114–127; Pruit 1978). This implies that there could have been a negative correlation between peaks in moose populations in the interior and the accessibility of seals on the coast. This possibility has considerable consequences for interpreting how the region may have been used by hunter-gatherers, but even more so regarding the role that animal husbandry played in adapting to environmental and cultural changes during subsequent periods. Husbandry offered a viable alternative to both natural and human-caused declines in resources as well as changes in territorial accessibility.

## Punctuated Sedentism

It is known that the Saami took precautions to maintain fishing waters by shifting to different lakes every few years (Ekman 1910:460–462), but longer-term regional shifts in settlement could have been forced on by the combined effects of ecological changes and over-hunting (cf. Krupnik 1993:156–159). Abandonment of the interior for up to a generation would have also helped keep moose, beaver and fish populations viable by allowing them to recover from predation. As shown by historic accounts, moose and beaver had almost been completely wiped out by north Swedish settlers within a few centuries (Hülphers 1789). Trapping pits were made illegal in 1864 in an effort to restore moose stocks, and beaver had to be reintroduced from Canada. I have described this long-term coast plus interior settlement model as "punctuated sedentism" (Broadbent 2004) (Figure 15). A system of periodic or generational depopulations of the interior may have been the very reason why moose and beaver populations survived thousands of years of predation within this narrow peninsula of boreal forest. Rich coastal hunting resources offered an alternative, but also underwent cycles, and rapid landscape changes due to shoreline displacement may have necessitated decadal reorganizations. For a semi-sedentary regional system of this kind to work, however, these groups would have needed access to both coastal and interior regions. When access to either one of them was blocked by other groups for any length of time, it would no longer be possible to fall back on these alternative sources of livelihood. That is probably one reason why reindeer and sheep/goat pastoralism was so readily adopted by these northern hunter-gatherers. Obviously fishing was of great importance, but there was fierce competition for fishing waters in the interior as well. Most northern strife recorded by the courts related to fishing waters (cf. Campbell 1948:231–236).

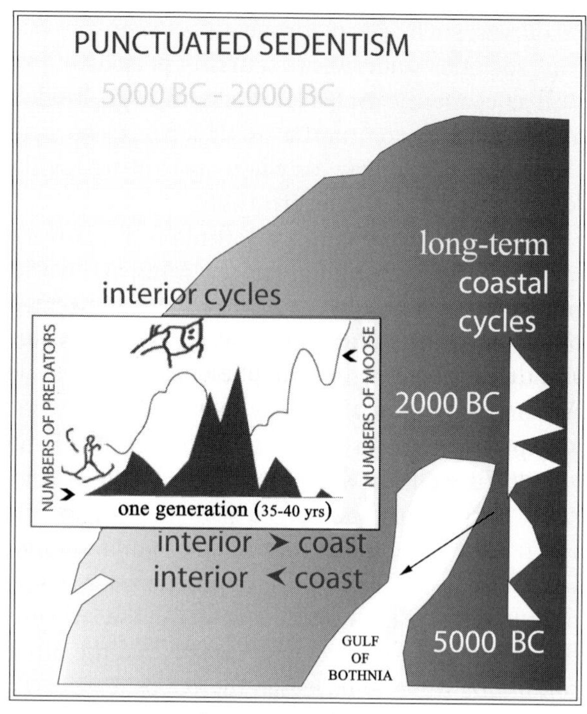


*Figure 15. Cycles of moose populations in the taiga, and long-term cycles of settlement on the Bothnian coast. Moose/predator figures cover a 40 year period (Peterson et al. 2003).*

## Resilience Theory

Successful long-term adaptive strategies, as proposed here, can be characterized using the concept of resilience, the amount of change a system can withstand and still retain its structure. Resiliency builds on a system's ability to maintain diversity, flexibility and opportunity under changing conditions (Redman and Kinzig 2003:13). Cultural heterogeneity is the equivalent of species diversity, and the loss of diversity, while often increasing efficiency, also leads to vulnerabilities. Resilience theory (Holling et al. 2002; Holling and Gunderson 2002; Redman and Kinzig 2003) encompasses many themes of interest in this study: the diversity of "Saaminess," the pulses observed in coastal settlements and, perhaps most important, the fact that the Saami have survived as a viable cultural and economic presence for thousands of years in northern Sweden. The persistence and survival of indigenous societies is starting to be recognized, as is the fact that indigenous cultures have greatly influenced settler societies (Murray 2004:1–16).

The now-classic book *Finns and Ter-Finns, Ethnic Processes in Northernmost Fenno-Scandinavia* (translated title) by Knut Odner (1983) builds on Fredrik Barth's interpretations in which Saami ethnic identity is essentially defined as a process created through contacts with others (Barth 1969). This definition, and the dynamic concept of adaptive change through resiliency, can be extended to the idea of cultures as clines or seamless topographies, rather than entities with sharp boundaries or as patchworks of cultures (Caulkins 2001). Clines are also a way of mapping cultural landscapes, and this approach will be applied to artifacts, sealers' huts and place-names throughout this book. As already noted, cultural and environmental change tends to be episodic and punctuated in time and space rather than incremental. Adaptive change occurs in two social dimensions according to resilience theory, one based on the amount of stored "capital" or energy and the second on the degree of connectedness of social systems (Holling and Gunderson 2002; Holling et al. 2002). The more complex, more specialized, larger and more connected a system, the more brittle and less resilient to major ecological or economic changes it becomes. In theory, all systems nevertheless eventually reorganize. This release of capital, social as well as economic, is followed by a new growth period. When applied to the archaeological material presented here, one can readily identify some of these trends. Starting in the Early Metal Age/Bronze Age, there was a major reorganization of northern hunter-gatherer societies. This process accelerated during the Late Metal Age/Iron Age. Northern trade networks evolved into economic dependencies on the scale of World Systems and were finally absorbed into state-level systems during the Early Medieval Period. These trends and the character of Saami resiliency as seen in the Bothnian coastal zone are major themes of interest. As an overall starting point, five hypotheses have been formulated to structure my analysis.

## Five Hypotheses

1) The Saami are an indigenous people with roots going back at least 7,000 years in northern coastal Västerbotten.
2) There are two major cultural-ecological regions in Sweden, the Circumpolar and the European. During the Iron Age the Germanic agrarian settlement boundary coincided with the 63rd parallel on the Bothnian coast.
3) Proto-Saami, Proto-Finnish and Proto-Germanic societies (for lack of better terms) had been in close contact for thousands of years and were heterogeneous and overlapping.
4) Coastal and interior settlement during the Stone Age in northern Sweden occurred in semi-sedentary cycles relating to peaks and declines in terrestrial and marine resources. Animal husbandry changed this pattern and contributed to sedentism as well as to nomadism.
5) Northern Sweden was part of a World System of trade and information exchange that had roots going back to the Stone Age.

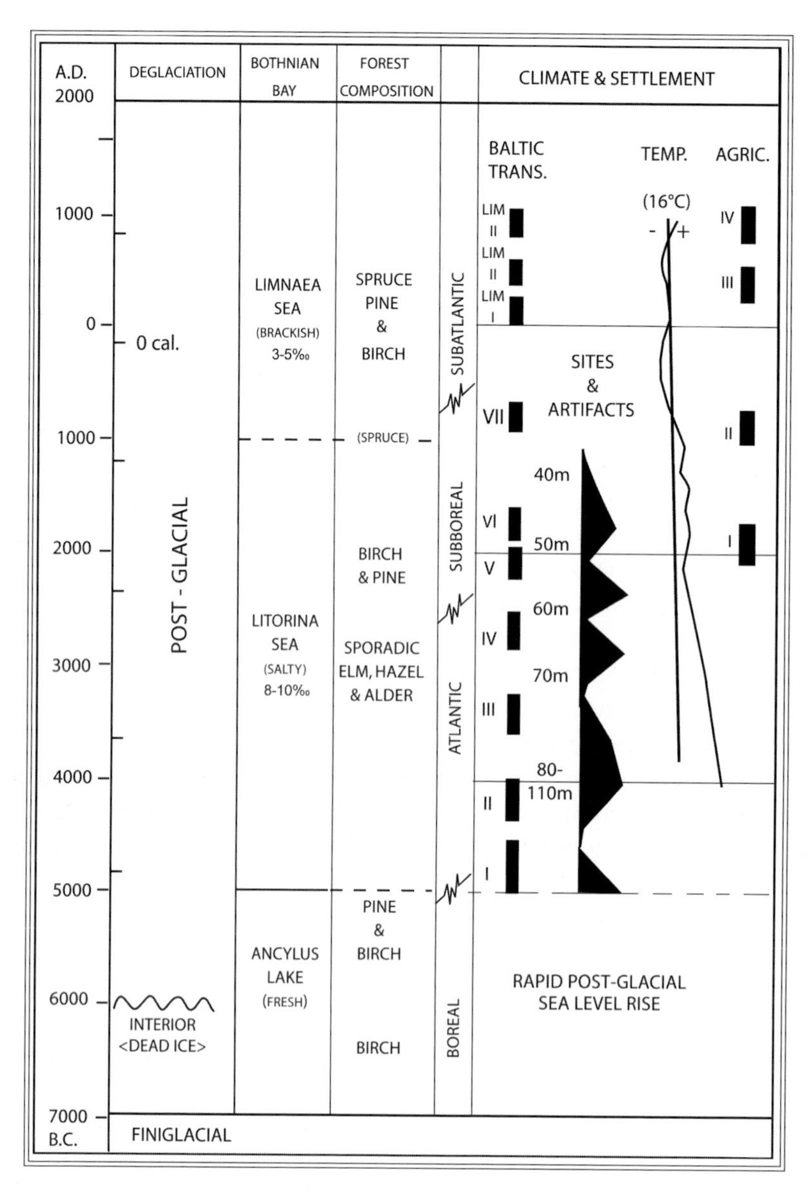


*Figure 16. Diagram of environmental changes, stray finds, site aggregations and agrarian indications in Västerbotten. Peaks and settlement cycles on the coast appear to coincide with warm periods as reflected by Baltic transgressions (Fairbridge 1963; Berglund 1964; Digerfeldt 1975; Miller 1979). A warmer climate would have encouraged northern agrarian expansion, and sealing and agriculture have gone hand in hand in the region since at least 2000/2534 B.C. There are at least five horizons in Västerbotten during which coastal settlement concentrated (uncal/cal): 5000/5900, 3400/4300, 2700/3470, 2000/2534, and 1000/1230 B.C. There are also four periods of agrarian expansion: 2000/2534 B.C., 1000/1230 B.C., A.D. 400/635 and A.D. 1000/1039. Climate data in Northern Europe indicate warm periods between 2600–1900 B.C., 1500–500 B.C., A.D. 0–550 and A.D. 900–1300. Cold and cool periods are recorded for 1900–1500 B.C., 500 B.C.–0, A.D. 550–900 and A.D. 1300–1850.*

# 3

# Prehistoric Foundations

## The Early and Late Stone Ages

This overview characterizes the long-term adaptive strategies of local societies as well as the environmental and cultural influences that have affected change in coastal Västerbotten. The general prehistory of the region is described by Broadbent (1979, 1982), and of the Metal Ages by Serning (1960), Forsberg (1999), Rathje (2001) and Liedgren and Johansson (2005). Environmental changes following de-glaciation, including temperatures and forest succession, salinity and evidence of agriculture, are summarized in Figure 16.

Nordic prehistory has been divided into three periods since first proposed in 1836: the Stone-, Bronze- and Iron Ages (Stenberger 1964; Burenhult 1999). A somewhat different terminology is used in North Norway and Finland (cf. Carpelan 1975b; Olsen 1994) that is particularly useful because it encompasses the concept of the Saami Iron Age (dates according to Olsen 1994:14). The dates of the Saami Iron Age (1–1500 A.D.) coincide with the material in this study and are therefore referred to as the Late Metal Age in this text, unless referring to a specific Iron Age period (Table 1). Calibrated dates in the text are listed together with uncalibrated dates (uncal/cal).

The salty Litorina Sea (ca. 5000/5600–2000/2400 B.C.) was a time of maximum productivity in the Baltic. The Atlantic climate was 3–5°C warmer than today; there was a greater overall terrestrial biomass in the north with more deciduous trees and the animals that feed on them, such as moose and beaver (Berglund et al. 1994:12–17). Specialized adaptations to coastal and inland resources developed with larger and more permanent settlements, increasing social and cultural complexity and new symbolic expressions and exchange networks. Sedentism and semi-sedentism were the hallmarks of most of the Eurasian world during this time (cf. Hall 1999:8). This was an era of demographic and social consolidation and the establishment of the regional societies that were the foundation of many cultures throughout Eurasia.

The *Flurkmark* site (ca. 5000–2500 B.C.) near Umeå in Västerbotten is a huge settlement area that extends over 300 m on several sandy terraces about 95 m above current sea level on what was once an inlet of the Litorina Sea (Lundberg and Ylinen 1997; Sjögren 1997; Lundgren 2001; Storå 2002; Broadbent 2003). The site was connected by an esker to the Vindel River valley. This site is a superb example of the early, sustained and intensive use of the Bothnian coast and the natural routes that connected the coast to the interior and other regions. Raw materials used for tool-making include Baltic flint, basalt, quartzite, quartz, jasper and other stone types from widespread western, southern and eastern sources. Red ocher, which was used in both graves and rock art in northern

Table 1. Chronological periods in Sweden and Norway (uncalibrated).

| SWEDEN | | NORTH NORWAY | |
|---|---|---|---|
| Mesolithic | 13,000–4500 B.C. | Early Stone Age | 10,000–4500 B.C. |
| Neolithic | 4500–1800 B.C. | Late Stone Age | 4500–1800 B.C. |
| Bronze Age | 1800–400 B.C. | Early Metal Age | 1800 B.C.–1 A.D. |
| Early Iron Age | 400 B.C.– 400 A.D. | Late Metal Age (Saami Iron Age) | 1–1500 A.D. |
| Late Iron Age | 400–1100 A.D. | | |
| Medieval Period | 1100–1500 A.D. | | |

Sweden and Finland, was found in thick deposits on the site. The animal bones include those of ringed- and possibly gray seals, moose, beaver and a variety of small mammals, fish and birds (Storå 2002). Ringed seals were the most common species, followed by beaver. Pike was the most common fish, and ducks the most abundant of birds. Spring, summer, fall and winter are indicated by this material. Several trapping pits had been dug on the site in much later times. (The site was discovered because a transverse-based arrowhead of Early Metal Age type was found there.) This is still good area for moose hunting. Large settlements of these types are found in considerable numbers at similarly high elevations along the Bothnian shores, from Norrbotten County in the north to the Stockholm region in the south (cf. Lindgren 2004).

The *Lundfors Site* (3400/4200 B.C.) is about 100 km north of Flurkmark and lies at 78 m above current sea level. It consists of seven separate settlement concentrations on an inlet south of the Skellefte River estuary (Figures 18). This site exemplifies the collective hunting strategies that were widely employed on the coast and in the interior to catch terrestrial and maritime animals (Broadbent 1979:174–198).

The Lundfors economy was based on the capture of ringed seals using long net systems, known to be the most effective during the dark fall months (cf. Hämäläinen 1930). Ringed seals would enter these bays and swim up rivers, gorging on fish in the fall; their blubber and pelts were at their maximum at this time of year (Ekman 1910:252; Holm 1921; Helle 1974; Broadbent 1979:187). The use of nets to catch ringed seals – other species are usually too large to be caught this way – was still the main sealing method in Västerbotten in the sixteenth century (Kvist 1991). The same wide-meshed nets could be used to catch salmon and beaver (Ekman 1910:218). In addition to seals, bones of moose, beaver, small game, fish and shellfish were identified and these show that local islands, inlets and valleys were also exploited. A perforated digging stick weight (otherwise typical of Finland) was also found (Figure 17), indicating plant (especially root) collection (Broadbent 1986; Broadbent 1979:171–173). The seal nets were probably made of braided roots, willow or other plant fibers, although only the net weights have survived. Huge Stone Age net systems for both seals and salmon have been found preserved in Finland at the Pori site (Luho 1954) and at Kierikki (Koivonen and Makkonen 1998).

Stone technology at Lundfors was based on quartz that was quarried locally, ground schist adzes of Finnish types, and slate knives and projectiles, some of which were made of red slate from the Swedish alpine regions. Red ochre was found in clumps and produced by burning on the site (Broadbent

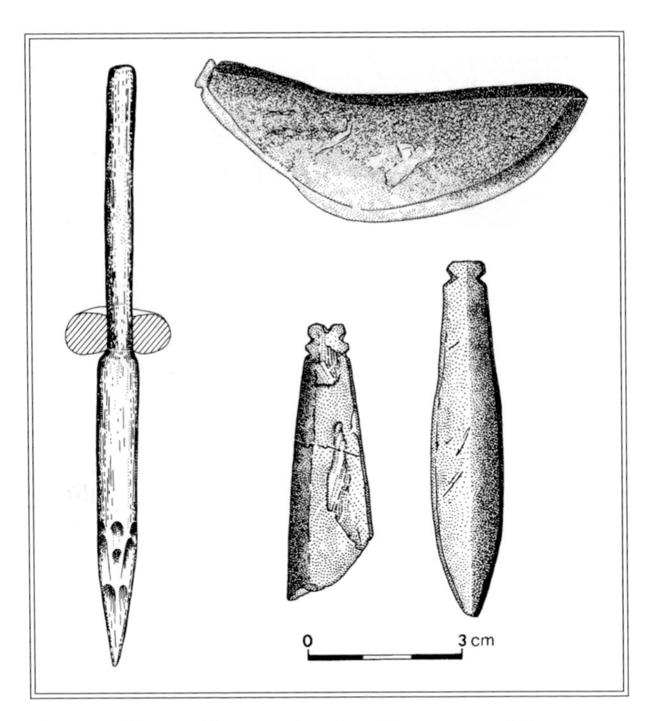


*Figure 17. Stone artifact types from Lundfors (not to scale): a perforated digging stick weight, a ground slate knife for butchering seals and two slate pendants.*

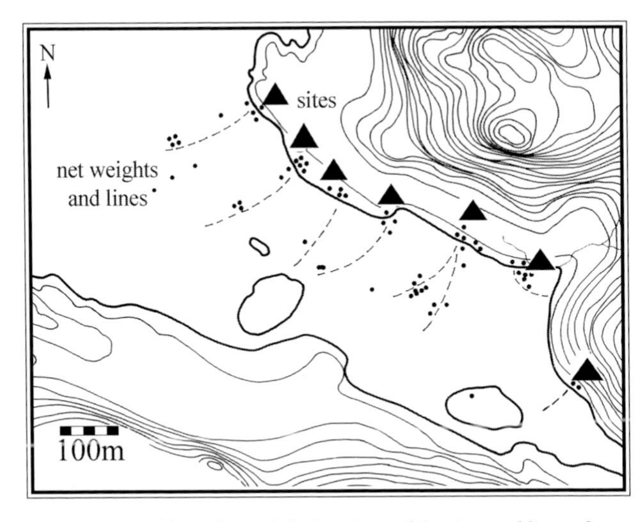


*Figure 18. Lundfors inlet and the locations of the sites and lines of nets that were used to catch ringed seals in the fall. Hundreds of net weights were found on the site and on the bottom of the former inlet that now lies 78 m above sea level.*

1979:134–135). A rock painting of a moose is recorded behind the site but has never been relocated. Massive amounts of fire-cracked stones link this settlement to the indigenous boiling stone (and non-ceramic) technology of interior northern Sweden, where dwellings were built up by mounds of fire-cracked rocks (Lundberg 1997). The Lundfors settlement area covers 12,000 $m^2$ and was almost certainly semi-sedentary. A detailed analysis of beach erosion shows, nevertheless, that the whole complex was used over only a 35-year period, or one generation (Broadbent 1979:30).

A comparative analysis of 13 sites from both coastal and interior Norrland, dating to the period 7000 B.C. to A.D. 1, challenges the idea that these types of sites were only temporary "aggregation camps" (Käck 2009). The Lundfors settlement model repeats itself even at the great rock art site at Nämforsen in coastal Ångermanland, which dates to the Late Neolithic-Bronze Age. Some 590 transverse-based projectiles, 6 kg of asbestos-tempered and textile-impressed ceramics, grooved stone clubs, large amounts of slag and even part of an iron furnace, were found at the adjacent Ställverk settlement site (Käck 2009:50–94). The rock art was produced by a local population with widespread social networks (Käck 2009:154–184), and this artifact material is closely associated with the most formative period of Saami ethnogenesis throughout the Nordic region.

## Rock Art

Moose remained the central icon in rock art and represented the core of indigenous identity in both coastal and interior northern Sweden until the end of the rock art period about 600–400 B.C. The moose as a symbol, especially in the South Saami region, harkens back to the roots of these societies in the boreal forest zone and was widespread in northern Eurasia (Hultkrantz 1964; Ramqvist 1992; Zachrisson 1997a; Fandén 2002). The brown bear also persisted as an important symbol and was one of the most significant wild animals in the Saami pantheon (Bäckman and Hultkrantz 1978; Helskog 1988; Edsman 1994; Mebius 2003). The largest rock art site on the Västerbotten coast is at Stornorrfors on the Ume River (Ramqvist et al. 1985). Moose figures dominate, including "x-ray" images (Figure 19), which are also seen at the aforementioned rock art site at Nämforsen (Hallström 1960).

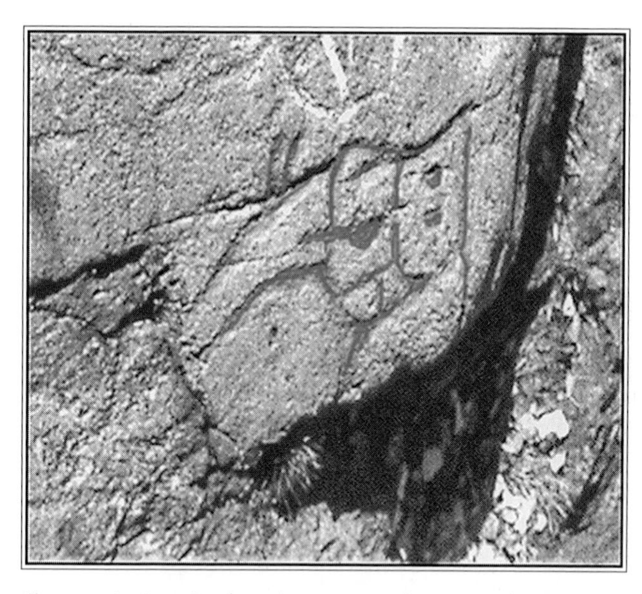

*Figure 19. An "x-ray" rock carving at Stornorrfors in coastal Västerbotten. The image shows a life-line or a spear, the sectioning of the body, and two points perhaps representing the testicles of an immature bull.*

## New Ideologies, New Technologies

The Late Middle Neolithic (1800/2250 B.C.) has been identified as a climate optimum in northern Europe that led to an expansion of agriculture and husbandry northward throughout the Nordic region (cf. Gräslund 1980; Sjøvold 1982). The Sub-Boreal Period, 2400–400 B.C., was a time of extreme dryness in western Eurasia (Mayewski et al. 1993; Mayewski and White 2002). The desertification of the Russian steppes led, among other things, to the northern and western expansion of herders and herding technologies into the boreal forest zone (cf. Toynbee 1934; Gimbutas 1965; Frachetti 2008). These societies introduced new burial practices, religious and social ideologies and, equally important, metal technologies (Chernykh 1992).

The *Bjurselet* site (1900/2400 B.C.) is one of 10 locales in coastal Västerbotten characterized by caches of thick-butted flint adzes of Baltic types, useful for working wood but also kept as grave goods (Christiansson and Knutsson 1989). Over 295 adzes have been found, 175 from Bjurselet alone (Figure 20). This technology is associated with the spread of the Boat Axe (Battle Axe) Culture, also referred to as the Single Grave or Corded Ware cultures in Sweden, Denmark and Finland and the Fatjanovo culture in Russia (cf. Malmer 2002).

The largest find locales in Västerbotten are by rivers and estuaries, and the smaller concentrations are in coastal valleys. Pollen analysis has indicated that barley was cultivated and some sheep/goats were kept (Königsson 1968), but ringed seal bones are by far the most common animal bones found at Bjurselet, and net weights like those at Lundfors were found at the Kusmark site (Lepiksaar 1975; Broadbent 1982). A thick-butted flint axe was even found in a grave cairn in Västerbotten (Huggert 2001) and the Battle Axe Culture people are known to have cremated their dead. There is a continuation of these burial practices into the Early Metal Age. As regards metallurgy, early copper finds have been found in northern Sweden and Finland dating to as early as 3900 B.P. (Huggert 1996). This was, in other words, a major turning point in north Swedish prehistory and established the foundation for subsequent cultural development.

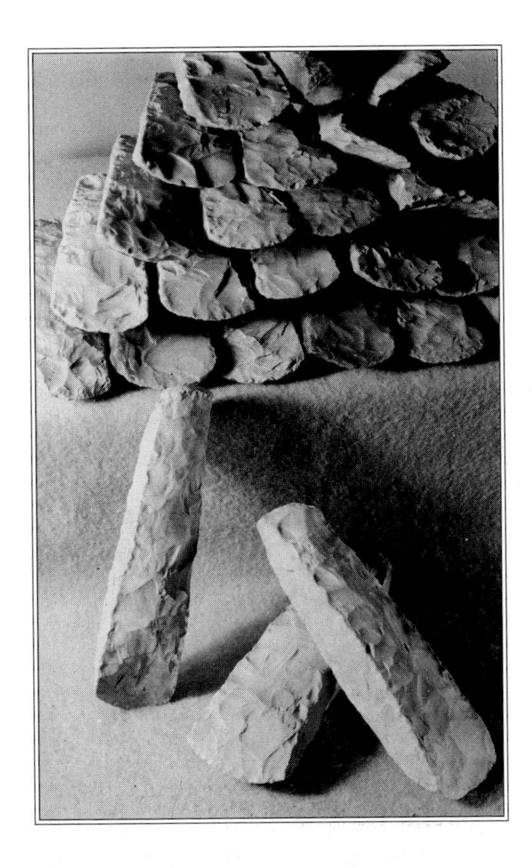

*Figure 20. Unused thick-butted flint adzes from the Bjurselet site in Västerbotten. Courtesy Antikvariskt-topografiska arkivet, the National Heritage Board, Stockholm.*

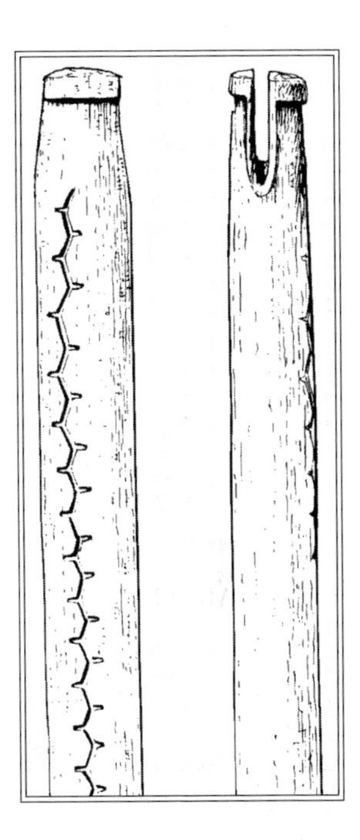

*Figure 21. A notched wooden spear shaft from Östra Åbyn in Bygdeå Parish, coastal Västerbotten, was pollen dated to the Bronze Age (Westin 1962). The pattern looks like stitching and is uncannily similar to Saami pewter wire designs on cloth and leather (courtesy Antikvariskt-topografiska arkivet, the National Heritage Board, Stockholm).*

## The Early and Late Metal Ages

The Early Metal Age of the Nordic North, during which there was an intensification of eastern influences, is characterized by asbestos-tempered and textile-impressed pottery, transverse-based projectiles, grooved stone hammers and Russian "Ananino" bronze artifacts and molds (Carpelan 1975a; Bakka 1976; Chernykh 1992; Olsen 1994; Hjärthner-Holdar and Risberg 2001) (refer Figure 22).

Transverse-based projectiles, also called straight-based, originated in the southern steppe regions of Russia and have been found in Proto-Scythian Timber Grave burials in the Lower Volga basin (Gimbutas 1965:544). They are associated with the spread of powerful, probably composite, bows. The projectiles date to approximately 1700–500 B.C. in Sweden (Baudou 1992:43), but finds have been made in North Norway dating to as early as ca. 2200 B.C. (Helskog Thrash 1983).

Asbestos fiber-tempered clay vessels may have functioned as portable furnaces for metal working (Hulthén 1991). The grooved clubs were probably used as sledge hammers and are also found in South and Middle Russia (Indreko 1956:58–59). Asbestos (chrysotil) deposits have been found far upstream on the Skellefte River at Ruopsok near Lake Hornavan in northern interior Sweden (Hulthén 1991:14) and in East Finland. This metallurgy, which also has many shamanistic aspects, is central to the development of Saami culture (cf. Carpelan 1975a; Jørgensen and Olsen 1988).

Whole complexes of pits in coastal Norrbotten were used for the rendering of seal oil (Lundin 1992). They have also been documented in coastal Västerbotten (Forsberg 1999) and date to the

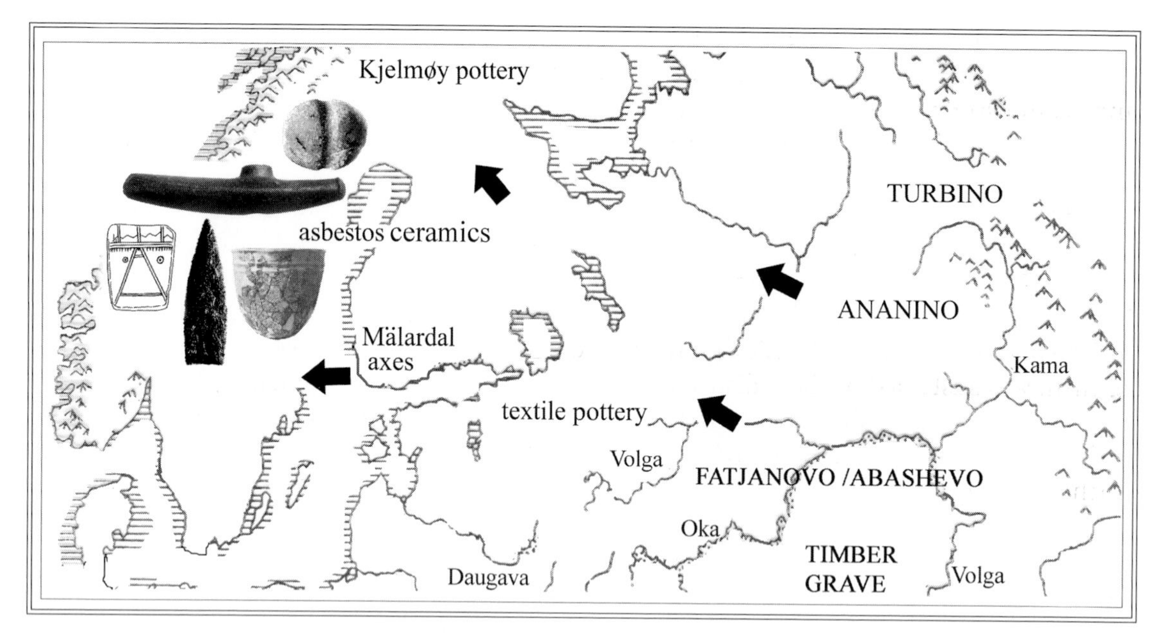


*Figure 22. Map showing the spread of related technologies into the Nordic region from the Russian steppes and the Ural Mountains, Late Stone Age/Early Metal Age.*

Late Bronze Age/Early Metal Age. The intensification of sealing and processing, together with large numbers of trapping pits in the interior during the Late Metal Age/Saami Iron Age, is undoubtedly connected to intensified trade (cf. Selinge 1974; Spång 1997). North Swedish hunter-gatherers were becoming part of a large-scale trading network that would reach its maximum during the Viking Period.

The *Fahlmark* site in northern Västerbotten lies at 39 m above sea level, dates to ca. 1300 B.C., and has three finished and 35 rough-outs of quartzite and basalt projectiles (Arwill 1975). A bundled cache of similarly worked projectiles was found at Vännäs near the confluence of the Ume and Vindel rivers. A fragment of a point made of Baltic flint, a grooved stone club, and a red slate projectile of Sunderøy type, a contemporary artifact type first described in North Norway (Gjessing 1942:172; Baudou 1977:30–31; Olsen 1994:106), was found at the Kåddis settlement at the 40 m elevation near Umeå (Broadbent 1984). There are some 16 additional projectile finds in this Swedish coastal region, including one made of Russian flint at Bjurselet (Huggert 1984) and another at the Flurkmark site. A bifacial projectile or knife of this type was even found on the Lundfors site (Broadbent 1979:237).

*Prästsjödiket* is a stone grave setting that had been placed on an island near the Kåddis settlement during the Early Metal Age. The grave goods consist of a quartz knife, transverse-based arrowheads of Baltic flint, Russian flint, basalt and quartz, and a bronze spear. The cremated bones of two young individuals were found (Lundberg 2001). Like Flurkmark, which is dated 3,000 years earlier, this find reflects a diverse mixture of raw materials and the far-reaching networks that connected this region to the outside world.

There are almost 600 whole or fragmentary arrowheads with transverse-bases at the rock art site of Nämforsen in coastal Ångermanland (Forsberg 2001; Käck 2001, 2009). The sheer numbers of these characteristic artifacts in these coastal contexts imply that these people were no different from the cairn builders (cf. Bolin 1999 for the same conclusion regarding Ångermanland). A transverse-based arrowhead of quartzite was actually found in a Bronze Age cairn grave in Ångermanland (Baudou 1968), and this funerary association is paralleled by the Prästsjödiket grave in Västerbotten.

Bronze is an alloy of copper and tin and required access to these two rare metals. Nearly all of it had to be brought in as raw materials, or as finished products. There are two primary European sources of these metals, one in the Ural Mountains of Russia and the other in central Europe. Copper, tin and gold helped solidify the power of a social hierarchy that had started to take form in the Late Middle Neolithic in Sweden (Malmer 2002). A hierarchical social system, with chiefs and big men, was sustained by the redistribution of metals for agricultural products, furs, hides and amber (Welinder 1977). Vast trade networks and alliances were reinforced and validated by religious symbols as seen in south Scandinavian rock art, such as sun disks, weapons and boats, some of which have been found at Nämforsen, as well as grave rituals and sacrificial practices (Kristiansen 1994; Larsson 1999).

## Cairn Graves

There are more than 550 grave cairns in coastal Västerbotten. Most large cairns (38%) are at the 35 m elevation, corresponding to the Bronze Age shoreline, and smaller cairns are found at Iron Age levels, or 10–20 m above sea level (Figure 23). Most of the cairns occupy coastal headlands and islands, but others lie in inner fjords where settlements were located (Bergvall and Salander 1996; Forsberg 1999). Baudou (1968) noted that the cairns in Ångermanland seem to divide the coast into segments 5–15 km in length, probably corresponding to social territories or clans. I have proposed the same clustering (Broadbent 1982:117–121), as did Bergvall and Salander (1996) in northern Västerbotten. The cairn graves probably also mimicked their circular and oval house forms. These northern graves had been built by local populations who had taken up southern Scandinavian rituals, including cremation, but can hardly have been building monuments to Bronze Age chiefs, as often argued in southern Scandinavia (Broadbent 1983).

One of the oldest theories about the end of this large cairn building era is that climate deterioration had caused the Scandinavians to withdraw, and that this vacuum was filled by the Saami (Hallström 1929). The Sub-Atlantic Period, starting at 650 B.C, was indeed a period of climate deterioration, with lower average temperatures and increased precipitation (Lamb 1977, 1995). Granlund (1932) first recognized these changes in northern Sweden through water-logged levels in bogs called “recurrence” surfaces. There were drops in tree lines and glacial advances (Nesje and

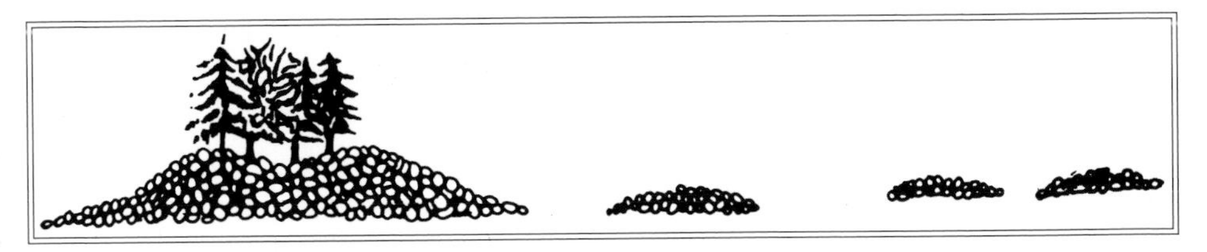

*Figure 23. Sketch of both large and small grave cairns in Västerbotten by A. F. Ekdahl, 1827.*

Kvamme 1989). Cultivation completely disappeared on the northern Västerbotten coast at this time (Engelmark 1976).

These changes in Bothnian coastal settlement are best seen as an overall adaptive response by indigenous populations that took the form of greater mobility, a pattern that occurred at exactly the same time in northern interior Sweden (Forsberg 1985; Mulk 1994:229–251). Olsen described this same phenomenon in northern Norway, with a greater focus on interior and alpine regions and an increase in reindeer hunting. These changes dated from ca. 900 B.C. to A.D. 1 and coincided with the Kjelmøy ceramic phase (Olsen 1994:106–124).

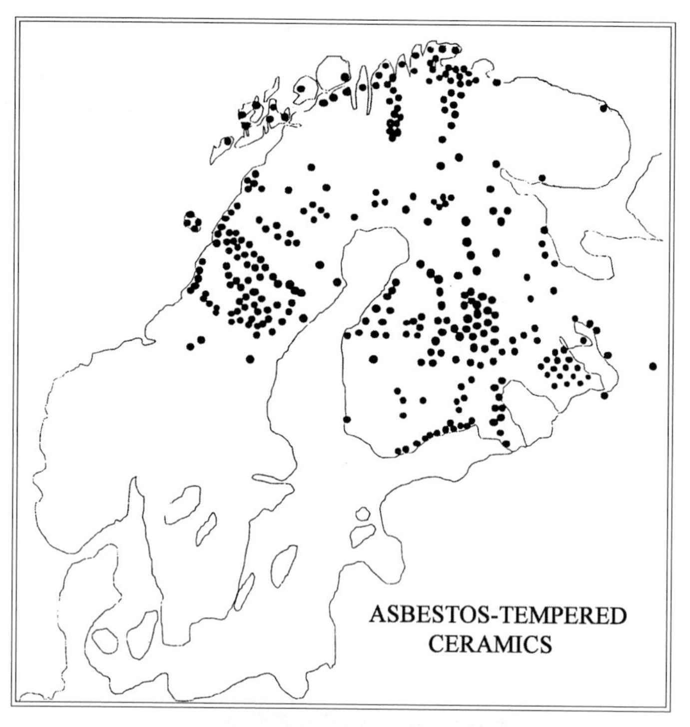


*Figure 24. The distribution of asbestos-tempered vessels (after Baudou 1995 with additional points). Arctic Bronze Age artifacts and the Bothnian ski, a probable forerunner of the Saami ski, have almost identical distributions (Broadbent 1982:143,146).*

## Iron

Iron deposits are formed as precipitates in lakes and in bogs and could be easily scooped up into boats or through the ice in winter. The widespread availability of iron ore in Sweden thus completely side-stepped the old bronze redistribution system. Eva Hjärthner-Holdar (1993) has described the introduction of iron technology into the Sweden and Finland as closely associated with the boreal forest and as "the first great egalitarian movement in Europe" (Hjärthner-Holdar, pers. comm. 2006).

*Harrsjöbacken* and *Hamptjärn* near Bureå in Västerbotten are good examples of this pattern. Textile-impressed and asbestos-tempered Kjelmøy type pottery was found, as well as iron slag, in a forging pit at Harrsjöbacken. Hamptjärn is a nearby small cairn cemetery, as is the site of Nedre Bäck, with one grave containing bear phalanges. An oval cooking pit at Harrsjöbacken was radiocarbon-dated to A.D. 79–245 (Sundqvist et al. 1992). Testing of the soils for lipids shows that seal oil had been rendered there as well. Asbestos-tempered pottery of Kjelmøy type and textile-stamped pottery, with flakes characteristic of the production of transverse-based arrowheads, were also found at the Sävar site, which has been interpreted as a semi-sedentary sealing settlement (Sandén 1995).

## Animal Husbandry and Cultivation

Pollen diagrams from northern coastal Sweden indicate sporadic cultivation during the Late Middle Neolithic or around 2000/2400 B.C. and from 600 to 400 B.C. (Königsson 1968; Huttunen

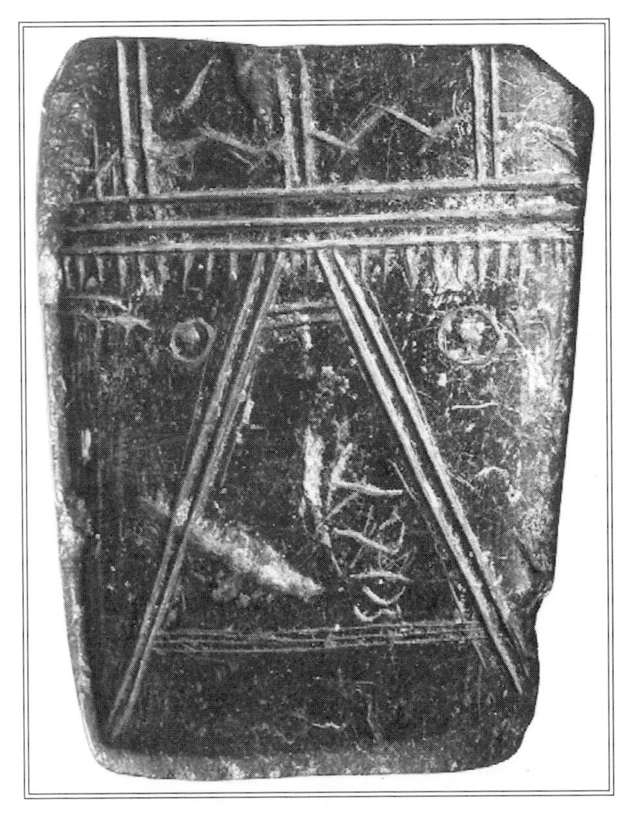

*Figure 25. A soapstone mold for a socketed axe of Russian Ananino type. Courtesy Antikvariskt-topografiska arkivet, the National Heritage Board, Stockholm.*

and Tolonen 1972; Engelmark 1976; Wallin 1994). Sheep/goat bones have been found at Bjurselet, Kåddis and Fahlmark (Lepiksaar 1975; Broadbent 1984). There is a 900-year gap in the agrarian footprint in Västerbotten from ca. 400 B.C. to 500 A.D., however, followed by yet another gap in the seventh century, particularly on the Lule and Torne rivers. Wallin (1995) interprets the agrarian discontinuities as a result of frequent shifts in the small coastal field systems, but they were also undoubtedly due to climate deterioration during the Sub-Atlantic Period and a worldwide climate deterioration in the seventh century (Lamb 1977; Nesje and Kvamme 1989; Roberts 2009).

When conditions were favorable and cereals or livestock could be obtained, cultivation and animal husbandry were undoubtedly part of a northern indigenous economic strategy during the Early Metal Age and continuing through the Saami/Late Iron Age. Asbestos pottery of Kjelmøy type was found with some charred barley in northern Ångermanland (Lindkvist 1994:98), and hair-tempered textile ceramics have been found at the Bjurselet site (Sandén 1995).

Textile-impressed ceramics, which arose between the Oka and Middle Volga, accompanied early metallurgy and possibly agriculture to Karelia and eastern Finland (Lavento 2001). Bones of domestic animals, especially sheep and goats, have been identified at Hälla, Rå-Inget and Ställverket by Nämforsen in Ångermanland, and this evidence shows that animal husbandry and even cultivation were part of the "package" of both Proto-Saami and later Saami culture in northern Sweden. Early Saami Iron Age cultivation has likewise been documented in Norway (Bergstøl 2008).

## Artifacts in Context

Although we don't have any iron implements from this earliest period, there are some 25 Iron Age artifacts from the coastal area under study. One remarkable archaeological find was a bundle of decorative bronze pins and brooches, dating to ca. A.D. 350, at Storkåge. They derived from the South Baltic Finno-Ugric region (Estonia) (Hjärne 1917; Serning 1960:21–24). These items were brought to the north, only to be buried on a small coastal river bank. This find resembles the Saami metal offerings of later times in which valuable, and especially exotic, ornaments were put into bogs or lakes.

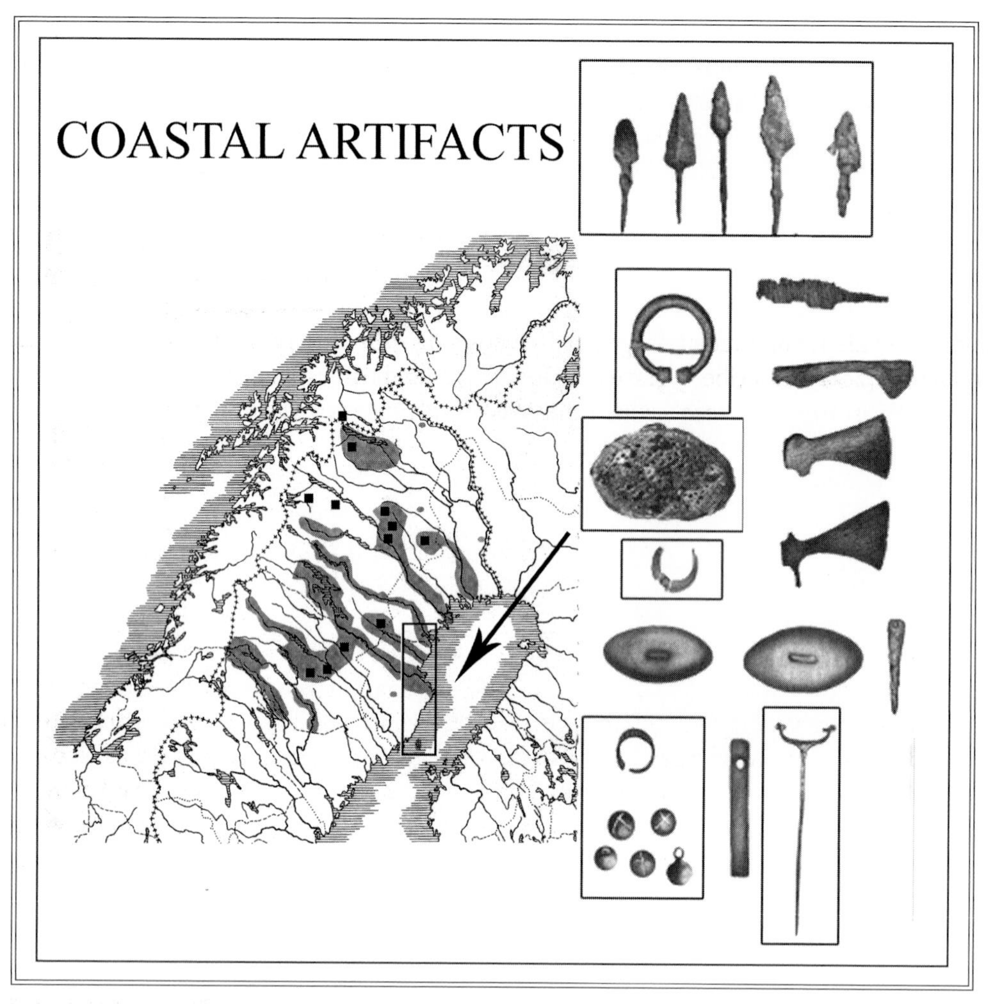


*Figure 26. Iron Age artifacts from coastal Västerbotten with parallels at Saami offer sites (boxes). Metal artifact distributions in interior indicated by shaded areas.*

Fifty percent of the coastal metal artifacts have parallels at Saami offer sites in the interior. Among these are iron arrowheads and oval and horseshoe-shaped brooches (Serning 1960; Fossum 2006) (Figure 26). Bronze bells and a silver ring from the Island of Stora Fjäderägg, some 14 km offshore, have parallels at the Saami offer sites, as does a crescent-shaped earring from Tåme in Byske parish (Serning 1960:36–49). An odd fork-like object, possibly for shamanistic divination, was found at Skråmträsk, near Lundfors, and has a parallel at the offer site of Gråträsk (Serning 1960:147). A decorated knife from Karelia was found at Kåtaselet on the Byske River (Broadbent 1982:170). Archaeological investigations of sacrificial/offer sites in the interior, which were known from oral traditions, have sometimes rendered great numbers of finds (Serning 1956; Zachrisson 1984). The most common artifacts derive from Finland, Russia and the Baltic, but many coins witness contacts with Norway, Germany and Britain. The objects consist of brooches, pendants, clasps, buckles of pewter, bronze and silver, silver coins and iron arrowheads. The finds date to A.D. 700–1400, with most sites dating to A.D. 900–1100 (Zachrisson 1984; Wallerström 2000; Mulk and Bayless-Smith 2006).

Seven metal artifacts (28%) from the coastal region are from small grave cairns. These cremations are parallels to the so-called "inland lake graves," "forest graves" or "hunting ground graves" found in Jämtland and Härjedalen in Southern Lapland. In evaluations of the evidence regarding the hunting ground graves in Jämtland and Härjedalen, and Tröndelag in Norway, Sundström (1997:21–27), Gollwitzer (1997:27–33), Zachrisson (1997a: 195–200) and Bergstøl (2008) argue that these inland graves are of Saami origin. In the case of the Vivallen cemetery there is, however, physical anthropological evidence of intermarriage (Iregren 1997:84–98; Alexandersen 1997:99–116). Liedgren and Johansson (2005) describe 15 graves in Upper Norrland that can date to the Early Iron Age. Most graves are known from the coast, where there is no evidence whatsoever of Germanic settlement. These authors state, somewhat ambiguously, that the "burial customs" were probably not of Saami origin, and that the metal artifacts in Lapland were due to the Saami dependency on trade for iron objects. As will be discussed in Chapter 9, there is ample evidence that the Saami were themselves able iron metallurgists and, except for arrowheads, most Lapland finds are non-utilitarian.

It is very likely that many Swedish Saami groups practiced cremation in the first centuries A.D. (cf. Zachrisson 1997a:195–197) and this pattern is certainly seen at the large cemeteries at Smalnäset and Krankmårtenhögen in Härjedalen in southern Lapland (Ambrosiani et al. 1984). These cremation graves, including triangular stone settings, are Germanic in form, but offerings of reindeer, moose and bear, in addition to their locations far outside any known Germanic settlement areas, indicate that they are the graves of what has been circumspectly described as "local hunting cultures." With some individual exceptions, the northern coastal graves should be interpreted in the same light as the other "hunters' graves," as those of local populations (cf. Forsberg 1999:251–285; Rathje 2001:91–118; Fossum 2006:89–99). Albeit in close contact with their neighbors, these societies could logically only have been Saami in origin.

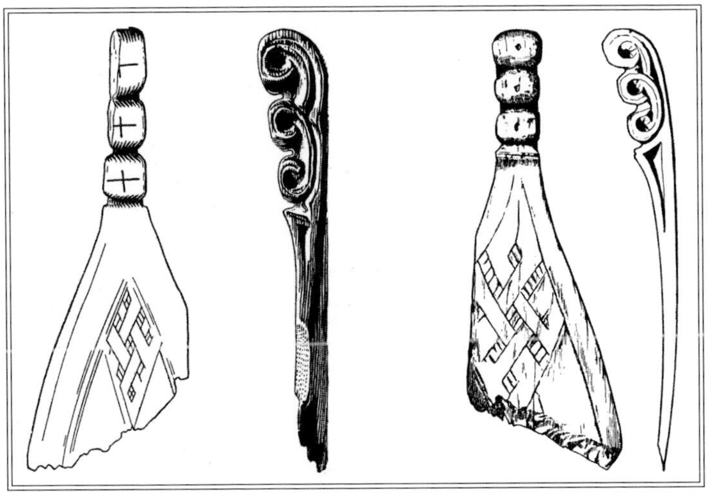

Wooden artifacts shed some additional light on the identities of these people in coastal Västerbotten, including two nearly identically decorated skis from Klöverfors and Bygdeträsk (Serning 1960:62) (Figure 27). Both have Viking Period pollen dates, substantiated by C-14 (Åström and Norberg 1984). Their plaited-band and ribbon ornamentation is typical of Southern Saami decorative styles (Holmqvist 1936). Västerbotten is, in fact, the core area of the Bothnian ski type, which is

*Figure 27. Two decorated Viking Age Saami skis from Västerbotten (after Serning 1960:280,278).*

the basis of the Saami ski (Manker 1971; Åström and Norberg 1984). These ski types, as pointed out by Manker (1968), together with finds of sewn boats (Westerdahl 1988), are evidence of a long-standing Saami presence in the North Bothnian region, as do trapping pits with Lapp place-names (Broadbent 1982:90-97).

## Summary

On the basis of this overview, the following generalizations can be formulated with respect to continuity on the northern Västerbotten coast:

### Economy

1) Sealing was a major activity during all periods. Subsistence sealing was combined with terrestrial hunting, fishing and gathering and with animal husbandry/farming from ca. 1900/2340 B.C. Moose-hunting, beaver-hunting and seal-hunting were organized collectively through the use of trapping and netting systems. Hunting took on an almost mercantile focus starting in the Early Metal Age, as seen by boiling pit complexes and trapping pit systems, and this was intensified during the Late Metal Age. A special form of seal oil rendering pit, more trench-like, but also containing fire-cracked rocks, has been described by Rathje (2001:134–136) and dates to the seventh century A.D.
2) Mixed hunting and herding societies established territories that divided the coast into socio-economic units encompassing bays and islands in 5–15 km wide segments.
3) Trade was extensive during all periods. Both raw materials and artifacts of stone, bronze and iron were regularly circulated within an area extending from Norway in the west, the Urals in the east, and to southernmost Scandinavia, Finland and the Baltic region. This can be seen as part of a World System of information and object-exchanges with roots going back to the Early Stone Age.

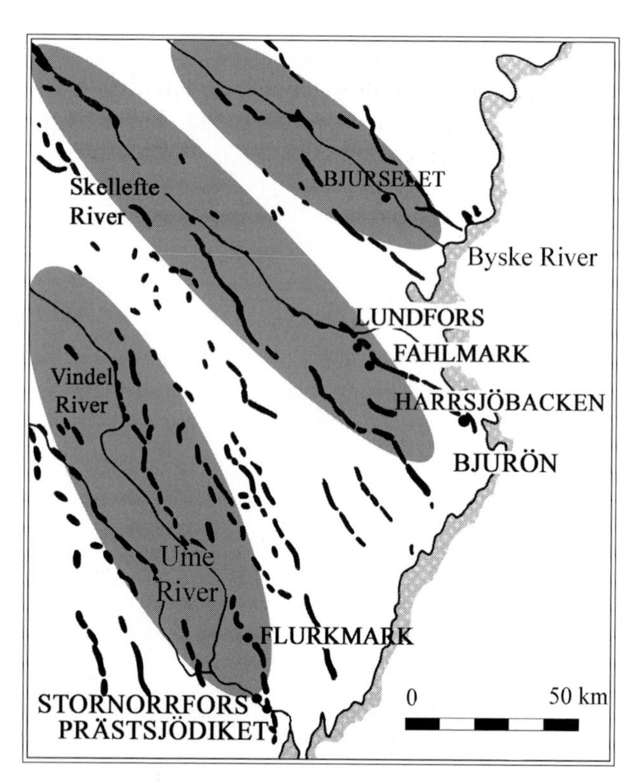


*Figure 28. Eskers, sites mentioned in the text, and the economic zones that connected the coastlands with the interior.*

### Settlement

1) Most coastal sites align with the larger eskers and river valleys. The important archaeological sites of Fahlmark, Harrsjöbacken, Lundfors and many other sites are found along natural inland travel routes.

2) Larger and more permanent coastal settlements concentrated in inner fjords and bays where there was the best micro-climate and, in the case of husbandry, grazing-lands.

**Technology**

1) Quartz/slate and boiling stone technology was identical on the coast and interior ca. 5000 B.C.–2000 B.C.
2) A "stimulus package" of new technological knowledge (including metallurgy) reached the northern coast ca. 2400–1800 B.C.
3) Transverse-based projectiles of quartz, quartzite, flint, and fluted slate projectile types, asbestos-tempered ceramics, Ananino bronzes and iron technology were associated with sealing, animal husbandry and even cultivation on the Bothnian coast during the period 1600 B.C.–A.D. 100.
4) Iron working was being practiced from the late first century A.D. This world was served by mobility and the exploitation of new ecological niches. New cultural identities were being formed in an ever-widening circle that came to encompass most of northern Scandinavia and Finland.

**Ideology and Religion**

1) The iconography of coastal and interior rock art reflects circumpolar cosmologies that involved mediation with the northern animal world, especially moose and bears. Shamanism was also manifested through transformative technologies, especially metal working.
2) New burial rites, including cremations, and offer practices were introduced to the Bothnian coast from the south and east. Cairn graves were built by local people to mark their coastal territories during the Early Metal Age and continued until the influences of Christianity took hold in the late Viking Period.

## Conclusions

These data demonstrate that all the social, economic, technological and symbolic components associated with the process of Saami ethnogenesis were present in coastal Västerbotten, and there is little difference in these respects from North Norway, interior Sweden or Finnish Lapland (cf. Carpelan 1975a; Forsberg 1992; Hansen and Olsen 2004:36–42).

In nearly all regards, there is a congruence of cultural characteristics, artifacts and landscape geography, beginning in the deep past and continuing into later prehistory. This is a historical trajectory, as conceived of by Wolf (1997:3–24), that defines adaptive strategies at the local level, the regional level and the super-regional (World System) level. The coast was intimately connected to the interior by natural west–east travel routes, by social interdependencies, and through the exploitation of combined terrestrial and maritime resources. These patterns were strongly manifested during the Early Metal Age. These criteria set the stage for and regionally contextualize the narrative of coastal settlement during the Late Metal (Iron) Age and Medieval Periods. This material offers an alternative to the interpretation of northern cultures as the results of continuous population incursions. The focus is shifted to indigenous societies undergoing transformations through frequent interactions with the outside world. The ethnogenesis of the coastal Saami is part of this process within a framework of the meeting of eastern and southern networks at cultural-ecological borderlands.

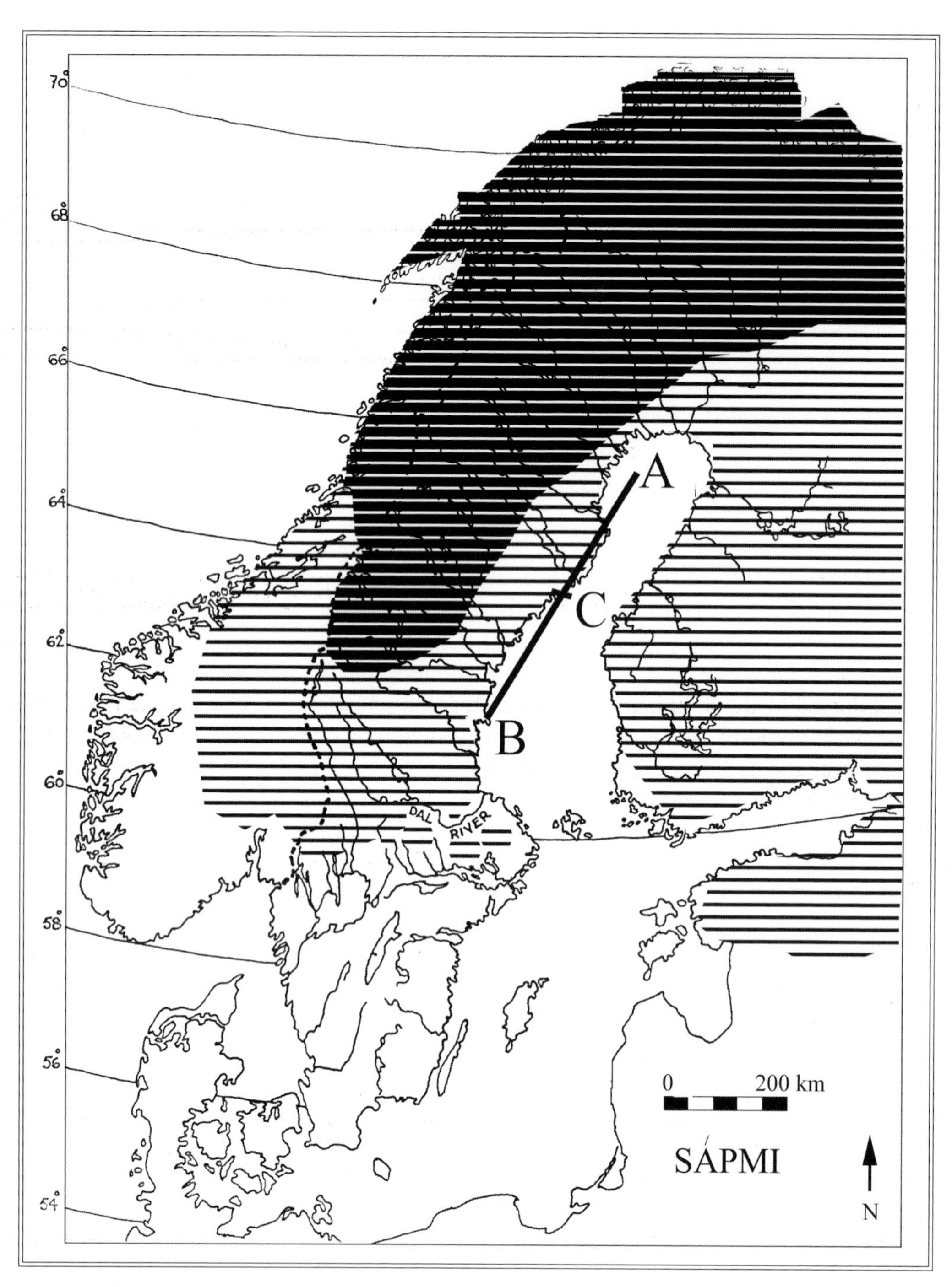


*Figure 29. The north to south transect along the Bothnian coast: (A) Stor-Rebben, (B) Hornslandsudde, (C) The northern limit of Germanic settlement. The dark shaded area marks current Saami territory, and the lighter shaded area is the probable former extent of Saami territory.*

# 4

# The Research Strategy

This section presents the methods, surveys, excavations and results obtained during the project. Each site is presented individually and includes artifacts, radiocarbon and AMS dates, archaeo-zoological and botanical analyses, soil-chemical and other results. Archaeological investigations were carried out at nine locales. Thirty-one huts at 12 elevations between 3 and 20 m above sea level were excavated. A glossary of the main types of archaeological features provides an overview of these and other constructions. The core area of Bjurön is presented first, followed by the sites of Stora Fjäderägg, Snöan, Stor-Rebben and Hornslandsudde.

## Surveys

Surveys conducted by the Swedish National Heritage Board list numerous Bothnian locales lower than 20 m above sea level. There are two principal contexts: sites on raised beaches more than 10 m above sea level and harbor sites less than 10 m above sea level. Both types of locales were investigated to determine their chronological relationships and to address questions regarding continuity from the Iron Age into medieval times. Seal hunting sites were closely associated with islands and promontories where hunters could establish camps, oversee nets or kill seals on land, in the water and on the ice. Lower-lying hut foundations were associated with fishing locales, especially harbor basins (Norman 1993). Similar sites with temporary huts and shelters have been documented in southern and western coastal areas of Sweden and Norway (Magnus 1974; Atterman 1977). Excavations of the North Bothnian sites were first carried out by the author in 1987–1988, with follow-up excavations and analysis in 2004–2006. The excavations at Hornslandsudde were made possible by Britta Wennstedt Edvinger and Kjell Edvinger (Arkeologicentrum i Skandinavien AB).

It has long been recognized that hut foundations found between 10 and 20 m above sea level were associated with Iron Age shorelines (Hallström 1942, 1949; Westin 1962; Varenius 1964, 1978; Westberg 1964; Steckzén 1964; Westerlund 1965). According to the national survey, there are 497 of these huts: 74 huts (14%) in Norrbotten, 219 huts (44%) in Västerbotten, 136 huts (27%) in Västernorrland and 68 huts (14%) in Gävleborg County (Norman 1993:194–195). Sixty percent are found in the two northernmost counties, of which 75% are in Västerbotten County.

## Site Investigations

The first goal of the project was to obtain as representative a sample of sites, features and artifacts as possible. The second goal was twofold: to investigate sites at different elevations above sea level and to sample sites along a north–south transect. This approach facilitated comparisons of different time periods within different regions and constituted a form of horizontal stratigraphy and chorology.

The northernmost investigations were carried out on Stor-Rebben Island, Piteå Municipality, in Norrbotten County at 65° 11′ N, 21° 56′ E. This site complex is the largest of its kind this far north. Bjuröklubb is located about 80 km south of Stor-Rebben and is 200 km north of Arnäs in Ångermanland County, the northern limit for Germanic Iron Age settlement and settlement place-names. The southernmost excavations were carried out at Hornslandsudde in Hälsingland at 61° 37′ N, 17° 29′ E. Hornslandsudde is ca. 460 km south of Stor-Rebben as the bird flies, and 300 km north of Stockholm. This is the largest site of its kind this far south and is comparable in size to Grundskatan and Stora Fjäderägg in Västerbotten and Stor-Rebben in Norrbotten. The association of this site with "Lapp" place-names and its oral history make this locale of special interest to the project. Surveys of Saami settlements in Hälsingland were previously carried out by Wennstedt Edvinger and Ulfhjelm (2004). The Hornslandsudde site is otherwise within a region of well-known Germanic Iron Age settlement (cf. Liedgren 1992).

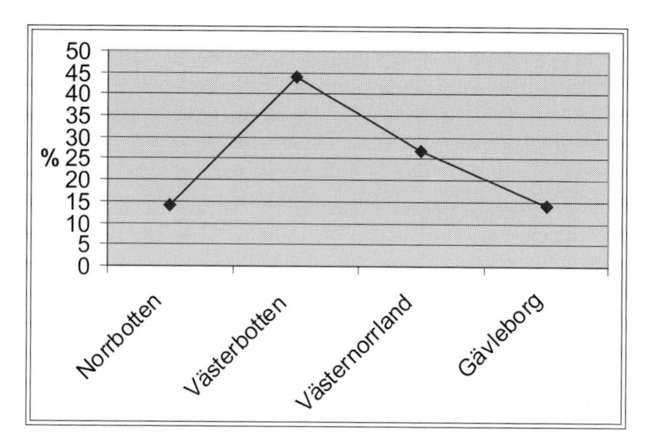


*Figure 30. Distribution of Iron Age huts along the Bothnian coast, from Norrbotten County in the north to Gävleborg County in the south (total: 497).*

Some of the largest sites are located near Bjuröklubb on Bjurön Island in Lövånger parish in Västerbotten. This is a poor region as far as salmon fishing, or even agriculture, are concerned and the parish is not associated with any larger river systems. This contrasts with what is known regarding typical Germanic settlement areas in southern and middle Norrland.

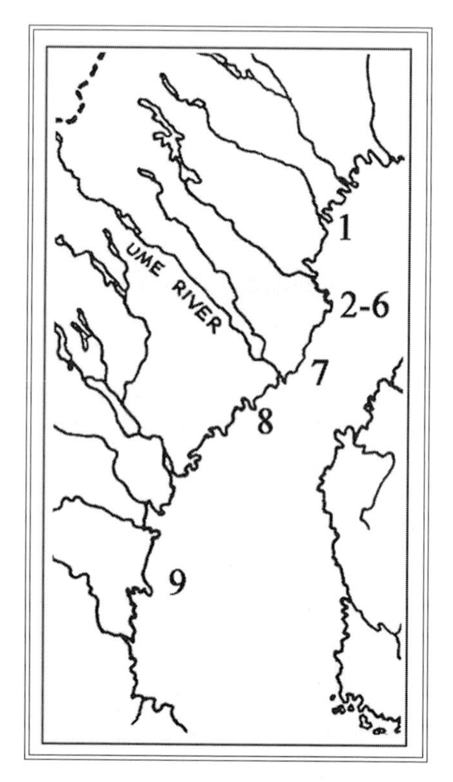


*Figure 31. Detail of Gulf of Bothnia and river drainages showing the locations of Iron Age sites excavated within the project: (1) Stor-Rebben, (2) Bjuröklubb and Bjurön, (3) Jungfruhamn, (4–6) Grundskatan, (7) Stora Fjäderägg, (8) Snöan, (9) Hornslandsudde.*

## Elevations

One of the most important aspects of the project has been the determination of accurate elevations of features and beach levels. This was accomplished through the use of on-site surveying equipment, including laser total stations. Daily sea levels were obtained by automatic "mariographic" stations. Handheld sighting levels were also used to determine elevations above mean sea level.

Table 2. Investigated sites, the distances between site areas, elevations sampled at each site and numbers of radiocarbon dates from each site.

| SITES (N–S) | INTER-SITE DISTANCES (KM) | SAMPLE ELEVATIONS (M) | DATES |
|---|---|---|---|
| Stor-Rebben | 0 | 16, 13, 12, 7 | 4 |
| Bjuröklubb (67) | 75 | 17 | 1 |
| Site 70, Jungfruhamn (138, 139) | 2.4 | 12, 15, 16 | 4 |
| Grundskatan | 2.4 | 16, 15, 14, 13, 12 | 15 |
| Stora Fjäderägg | 76 | 20, 19, 15, 13, 8 | 6 |
| Snöan | 73 | 15, 5, 3 | 6 |
| Hornslandsudde | 172 | 20, 18, 16, 13 | 7 |

Because of the effects of land rise, the harbor basins were short-lived and boat houses and cottages had to be moved numerous times. When possible, historical records were used for dating such sites, but when these were uncertain, harbor basin thresholds were determined. Excavations were also carried out on any huts or related features by these basins in order to obtain radiocarbon dates. Threshold levels for harbors were determined at Jungfruhamn on Bjurön, at Gamla Hamnen

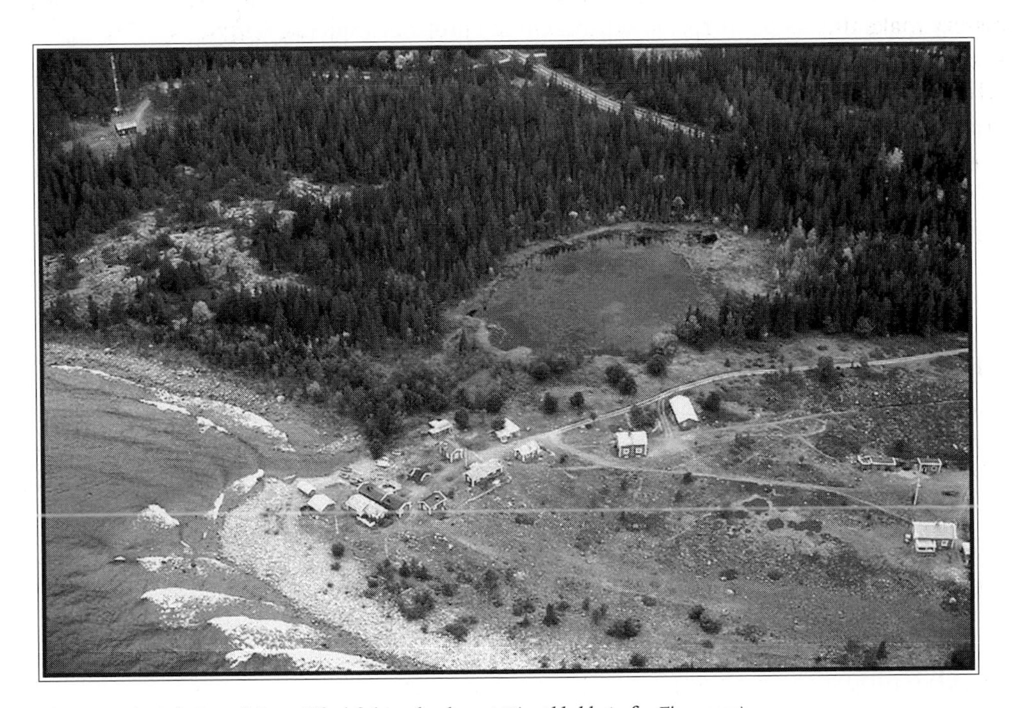

*Figure 32. Aerial view of the uplifted fishing harbor at Bjuröklubb (refer Figure 50).*

on Stora Fjäderägg Island and at two harbors on Snöan Island. In addition to survey information provided by the Swedish National Heritage Board and local county authorities, independent surveys were conducted at all site areas, resulting in a greatly expanded corpus of archaeological features.

## Excavations

The outer coastal landscape is characterized by exposed bedrock, wave-washed moraine and shallow soils. Preservation of organic material is poor. Excavations were therefore most often directed toward hearths, which were usually the only preserved cultural deposits. On the positive side, it is rare that one has so many visible architectural features. The use of beach cobbles for construction resulted in a rich inventory of often intact and fully exposed dwellings, stone alignments, cairns and other features.

Although the find elevations provide a chronological foothold, since features cannot be older than their contemporary shorelines, many constructions could have been built long afterward. Because of this source-critical problem, considerable efforts were put into additional ways of dating them. Radiocarbon dates were obtained from hearths, but for most other categories of constructions there is nothing to date but the stones themselves. Our application of lichenometry (lichen growth measurement) was intended to overcome this problem. These methods have always been used in combination with shoreline displacement dates (maximum ages), radiocarbon chronology of adjacent features and historical data. Lichen dates are always considered as *minimum* ages. Rock weathering made it possible to determine if stones had been overturned during construction, thus reducing the risk that lichens had only been moved from beaches as opposed to colonizing a newly exposed surface, although lichens don't normally survive being moved (Benedict 1985). Rock-weathering was quantified using the Schmidt Test Hammer (Sjöberg 1987).

## Sampling

Excavation was based on a sampling strategy intended to recover charcoal, macrofossils, animal bones and artifacts from different elevations above sea level. Hearths and different hut forms were chosen at different elevations, from the highest-lying to the lowest-lying, at each given site. Hearths were first tested using a soil auger and subsequently chosen for excavation based on the presence or absence of organic materials. All soils were screened using 4 mm mesh or less, and sometimes whole hearths were removed for flotation in the lab.

## Soil Chemistry

Phosphate enrichment of site soils, due to human or animal defecation and urination and animal carcasses, was analyzed using laboratory methods by Johan Linderholm at the Environmental Archaeology Laboratory at Umeå University. Later comparative field tests were conducted by the author using the La Motte Soil kit. Phosphate analysis ($P^{o}$) is based on the extraction of organic phosphates from soil samples using a weak (2%) solution of citric acid and measured colorimetrically. Phosphate content is defined as mg/$P^2O_5$/100 g dry soil. The La Motte system is based on a colorimetric scale indicating Low, Medium or High levels of soil enrichment.

## Animal Osteology

All animal bones from the project were analyzed by Dr. Jan Storå of the Osteological Research Laboratory of Stockholm University (Storå 2002, 2005, 2008). When possible, bone fragments were identified as to class, species, bone or bone fragment and side. Because of fragmentation, only a few metrics were possible. The identified fragments were individually counted and weighed, while unidentified fragments were only counted. Quantification was based on the numbers of individual fragments (NISP, or numbers of identified specimens). Refitted fragments were counted as single specimens, as were fragments found together. The reference collection is the comparative collection of the Osteological Research Laboratory at Stockholm University.

### Charcoal Analysis

Charcoal from hearths was analyzed by Dr. Imogen Poole in association with the National Herbarium Nederland, Universiteit Utrecht Branch, the Netherlands, and by Mr. David Black, M.A. University of Western Michigan.

### Macrofossils

Macrofossils were analyzed by Karin Viklund, Environmental Archaeology Laboratory at Umeå University.

### Radiocarbon Dates

Radiocarbon and AMS dates were processed at three laboratories: Stockholm (St), Uppsala (Ua) and Beta-analytic (Beta). Dates were calibrated using OxCal 3.10 and 4.0. The uncalibrated dates are listed together with calibrated dates (uncal/cal). All dates are listed in Appendix 2.

### Metallurgy

Analysis of slag and residues from hearths relating to iron working was conducted by the Geoarchaeology Laboratory (GAL) of the National Heritage Board, under the direction of Dr. Eva Hjärthner-Holdar. Analysis was carried out by Eva Grandin, Eva Hjärthner-Holdar, Emma Grönberg and David Andersson.

### Shoreline Displacement

The starting points for uplift curves are old watermarks that had been carved by students of Carl von Linné (Linnaeus) in the 1700s (Broadbent 1979:199–201; Nordlund 2001). The theory at that time was that the sea was evaporating, not that the land was rising. It was believed that Earth goes through three stages: one of flooding (the Biblical Flood), the intermediate stage we are experiencing today, followed by conflagration, when all the seas have evaporated. Although these scholars were unaware of the idea of glaciation, their watermarks are an invaluable contribution to geophysics and archaeology.

Stone Age sites in northern Sweden are found on old beaches that have been uplifted 120 m or more. Settlements are distributed in time at different elevations like steps in a stairwell. Because of the flatness of north Swedish topography, however, several meters of difference between site elevations can lead to a kilometer or more of horizontal separation between them. Coastal archaeological sites in northern Sweden therefore have little overlap and chronological resolution is exceptional. Increases and decreases in worldwide sea levels due to climate changes have either accelerated the effects of land-rise by lowering sea levels or stabilized the shorelines by keeping pace with the uplift. During warm periods, prehistoric settlements and artifacts tended to collect in greater numbers at stabilized levels because of slowdowns in displacement. During cold periods,

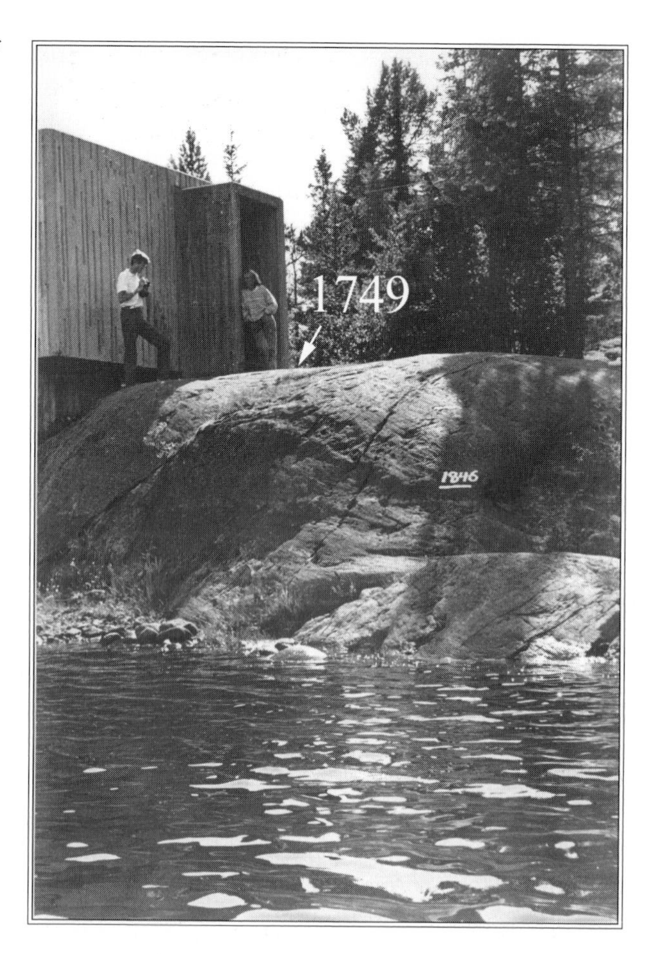


*Figure 33. Watermark at Ratan, 40 km north of the Umeå. The oldest mark was carved by Anders Chydenius, a student of Carl Linnaeus, in 1749. An automatic sea level (mariographic) station is housed in the concrete building.*

the opposite took place and sites and artifacts were more widely spread across the landscape. These patterns are particularly evident during the Litorina Period when sea level rises were greatest.

The shoreline displacement curve for Västerbotten is based on a watermark from 1749, radiocarbon dates, archaeological finds and pollen zones (Broadbent 1979:204–211). These points were fitted in a least squares curve-fitting analysis using an exponential model simulating crustal rebound. (The physical model is that of a steel spring releasing and contracting in a viscous solution.) The resulting shoreline displacement model for the past 2,000 years has been verified by counting annual lake sediments (varves) in uplifted lake basins in coastal Västerbotten (Segerström and Renberg 1986).

This shoreline curve is illustrated in Figure 34 and includes four new points from the current study. The highest rates are in the north near Storkåge, and somewhat lower rates occur to the south of there. This downward tilt (slowing) toward the south can be seen by the calibrated radiocarbon dates from Stora Fjäderägg and Snöan. Estimated sea level fluctuations (based on Miller and Robertsson 1979) are shown as a dashed line.

It should be remembered that dates of settlements and place-names using elevations are *maximum* possible ages; that is to say, they cannot be older than their contemporary shorelines (have been under

Table 3. Calculated rates of shoreline displacement in Västerbotten County.

| YEARS (UNCAL/CAL) | ELEVATIONS (M) | UPLIFT RATES (M/YR) |
|---|---|---|
| 5000/6100 B.C. | 119 | 2.9/2.4 |
| 4000/4900 B.C. | 92 | 2.4/1.9 |
| 3000/3800 B.C. | 70 | 2.0/1.7 |
| 2000/2600 B.C. | 51 | 1.8/1.5 |
| 1000/1450 B.C. | 35 | 1.6/1.3 |
| 0/–200 A.D. | 20 | 1.4/1.1 |
| 500/300 A.D. | 15 | 1.2/0.98 |
| 1000/950 A.D. | 9.6 | 1.1/0.93 |
| 1500/1400 AD | 4.5 | 0.98/0.87 |
| 1900–Present | 0.67 | 0.92/0.81 |

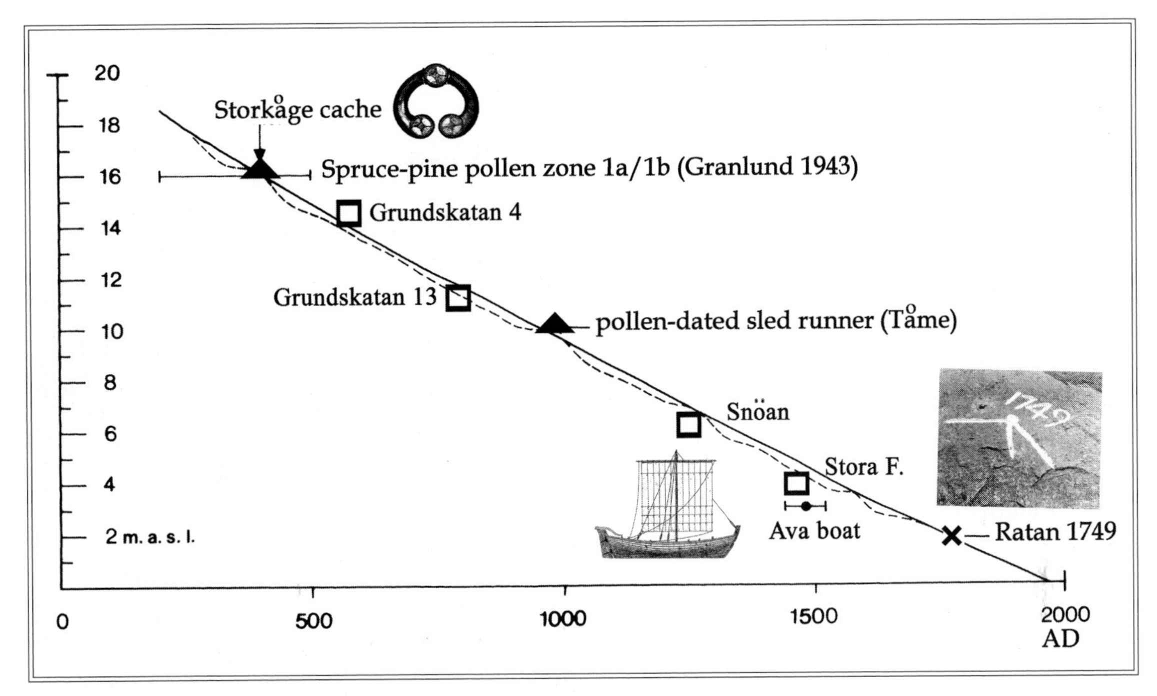


*Figure 34. Shoreline displacement curve for Västerbotten. Dashed line shows eustatic (sea level) fluctuations. Squares indicate radiocarbon dates from Iron Age huts.*

water). Because of the rapidity of uplift in Västerbotten there was no extended inundation of sites although some could have been temporarily flooded during storms. Exceptions to this are shipwrecks, such as the Ava boat in Lövånger (Jansson 1981).

## Lichen Growth on Uplifted Beaches

One of the most daunting challenges of the project has been the fact that most constructions consist of exposed piles of rocks. Only dwellings with hearths could be radiocarbon-dated, and shoreline dates provide only maximum possible ages. This means that labyrinths and other constructions were essentially undatable. Following a suggestion by ecological botanist Christer Nilsson, I pursued the idea of using lichen growth on stones for dating cultural features on uplifted beaches.

The lichenometric method was developed in the 1950s and has been mostly used in mountain environments for the dating of glacial moraine (Beschel 1950; Benedict 1967, 1985; Locke et al. 1980; Karlén 1975; Topham 1977). The most often used species is the gray-green crustose group *Rhizocarpon geographicum* and *R. alpicola*. Crustose lichens grow symmetrically, and thallas (lichen body) diameters can be used to estimate age once their growth rate has been determined. Thallus diameters can vary on the same specimen because of competition or other impediments to growth, but a maximum diameter where there are no impediments always corresponds to the maximum age of the lichen. Age can be calculated indirectly through lichen colonization on previously dated surfaces, such as headstones, and in the Bothnian region on rocks on uplifted shores (Figure 35). Using the previously calculated rates of shoreline displacement and an analysis of headstones at Bygdeå cemetery, it was possible to calculate growth rates for this coastal region. Lichen growth proceeds in two phases, a short period of very rapid growth, the so-called great period, during which the surface is colonized, and thereafter a constant rate of linear growth. The rapid colonization rate for this region was determined at Bygdeå (Broadbent 1987a), and linear growth rates at Grundskatan, Bjuröklubb, Stora Fjäderägg and Snöan (Broadbent 1987c) (Figure 36).

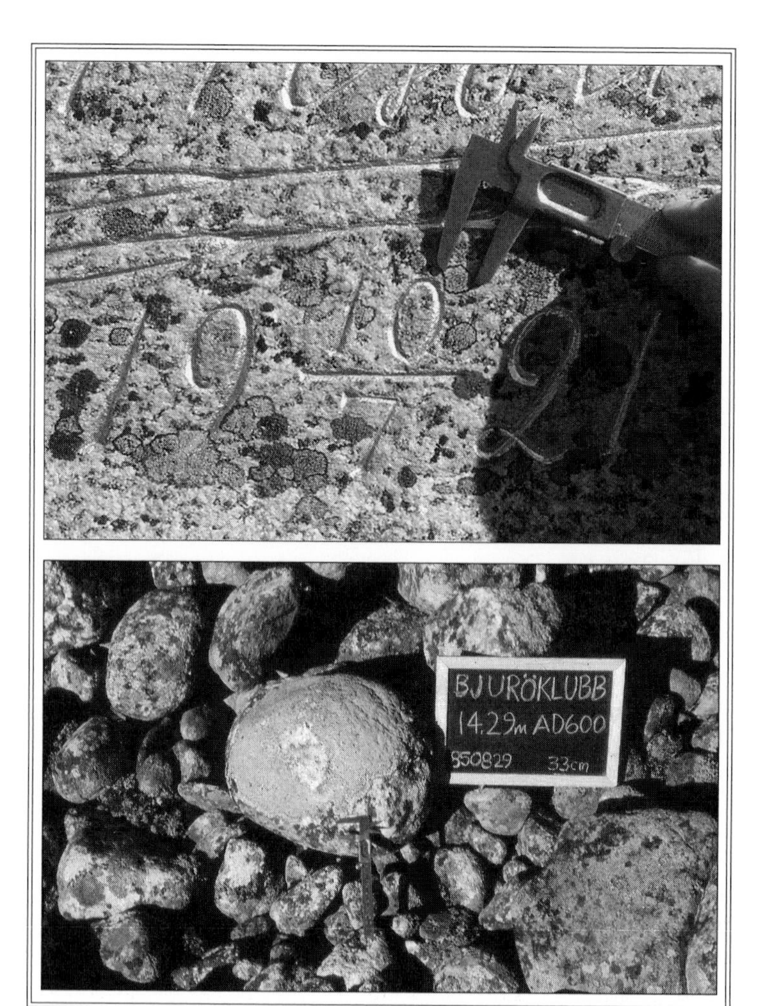


*Figure 35.* Rhizocarpon geographicum *lichens growing on a monument by Lövånger Church and a 33 cm diameter lichen growing on a beach boulder at an elevation of 14.29 m above sea level at Bjuröklubb.*

The hypothesis behind this approach is that following colonization of uplifted beaches, lichen sizes will correlate with their elevations above sea level. For every meter above sea level, the original colonizers will have added approximately a century of growth (Broadbent and Bergqvist 1986; Broadbent 1987c). The largest (oldest) lichens at every meter above sea level were measured at numerous sites including those mentioned above. Bjuröklubb is, for example, characterized by eight fairly straight exposed cobble terraces extending up to 15 m above sea level. Lichens were measured at 14 levels starting at colonization, which was observed at the 1.28 m level. The largest (oldest) lichens ranged in diameter from 19 mm at the lowest level to 358 mm at 14.29 m above sea level. The correlation coefficient between elevations and maximum diameters was 0.99 at this site, 0.98 at Grundskatan and Stora Fjäderägg, and 0.94 on Snöan Island. On the basis of this data, individual linear regression equations were calculated for each site.

The growth equation for estimating lichen age, based on the combined data from Bjuröklubb and Grundskatan (22 points), is: Y (age) = 152 + 3.47 × (diameter in mm). This means that a lichen diameter of 100 mm is 152 + 347, or 499 years old. The standard deviation is 31 years, so the range

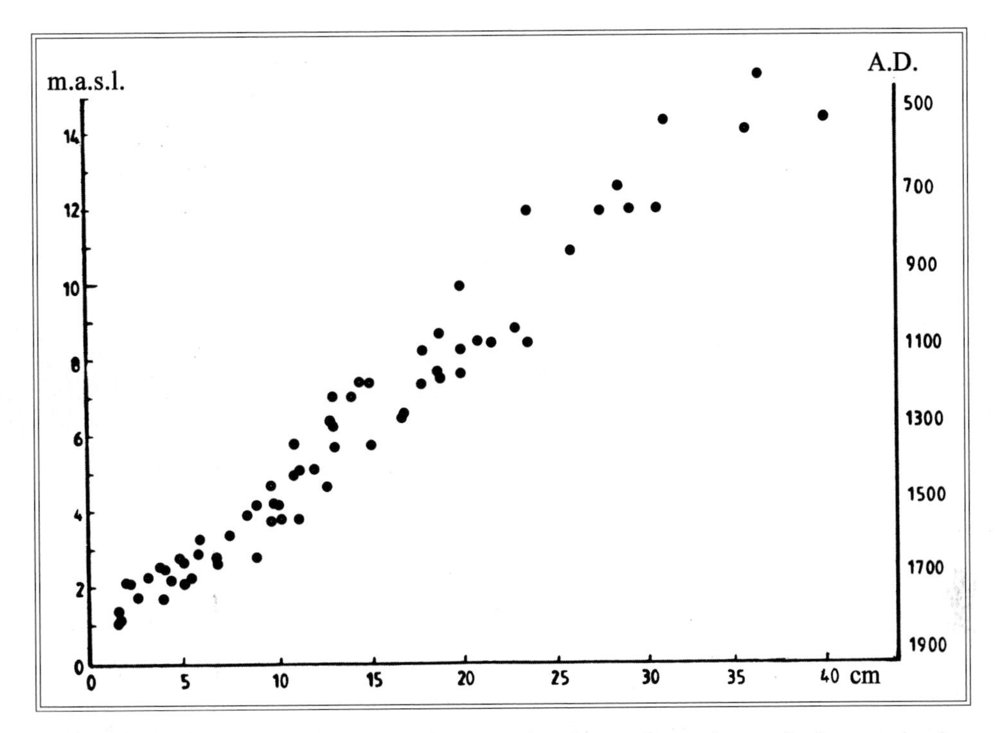


*Figure 36. Maximum diameters of* R. geographicum *at elevations up to 15 m above sea level on seven beaches between latitudes 63° N–65° N (uplift between 8.3–9.1 mm year). Linear growth was observed at all sites.*

with one standard deviation is 468–530 years, or A.D. 1478–1540. Equations were calculated for each individual site, but varied only slightly along the Bothnian coast, which indicates that there were minimal micro-environmental differences between locales.

A lichen date is a minimum age, which means that an archaeological feature, such as a labyrinth, is at least as old as the lichens growing on it. Its elevation above sea level provides a maximum age, so there is a means for bracketing the feature in time. Lichen growth also makes it possible to determine relative differences in construction periods as some surfaces may have large lichens growing on them, whereas other areas that may have been built later or were disturbed, will have smaller ones. The best approach in using lichenometry is to combine all the chronological information about a site, including the overall find context (cf. Broadbent 1987d:43–45). Historical data, elevations above sea level, rock-weathering and proximity to other dated features were used to evaluate the results.

## A Glossary of Archaeological Features

A number of characteristic stone constructions have been documented within the project. They were made using dry-wall methods and, although sometimes chinked using pebbles and often incorporating boulders, neither mortar nor bricks were used to build them. Each site has been designated by a number assigned by the National Heritage Board (*Riksantikvarieämbetet* or *Raä*). Because of the variety of constructions at each site, these are referred to as "Archaeological Features" or as "Features" (*anläggningar* or *anl.*), and identified by a number or letter corresponding to the order in which they were investigated.

### Huts

Bothnian huts (Swedish *tomtningar)* are shelters or foundations consisting of low cobble walls, usually less than 30 cm in height, with cleared and level floor surfaces (Figure 37). Their walls are ca. 0.3–1.0 m in thickness. There can be one or more entrances. The foundations can be open-sided, but most doorways measure less than a meter in width and were often well set, sometimes with sills. Average floor size is 3 × 4 m, although some floors are smaller and some are over 6 m in length and 4 m in width. The foundations usually occur in clusters of two to nine constructions and can be built in rows with shared curved or straight walls. Most are rounded-rectangular in shape, although oval and rectilinear shapes are found at nearly all levels. Secondary features include internal chambers with rounded walls, small cairns built into walls, small well-built pits in floors, and external wall lines that could have served as parts of enclosures. There is no certain evidence of internal roof supports, such as postholes or post supports, and it can be assumed that the roofs were supported by wooden frames embedded in or braced against the cobble walls. Most huts had central hearths, and these normally measure 1 m in diameter and are recognizable from traces of charcoal, fire-cracked rocks and burned bones. Most lack stone rings, although many have one or several larger stones by them. Hearths in dwellings were possibly bordered by wooden frames that are no longer preserved. Hearth deposits are shallow, 10–20 cm in thickness, but can have lenses indicating multiple uses. Other bowl-shaped hearths associated with iron working were found near the rear walls of huts. Hearths are also found adjacent to and in front of huts and are often identifiable by vegetation and lichen growth on the otherwise sterile cobble surfaces.

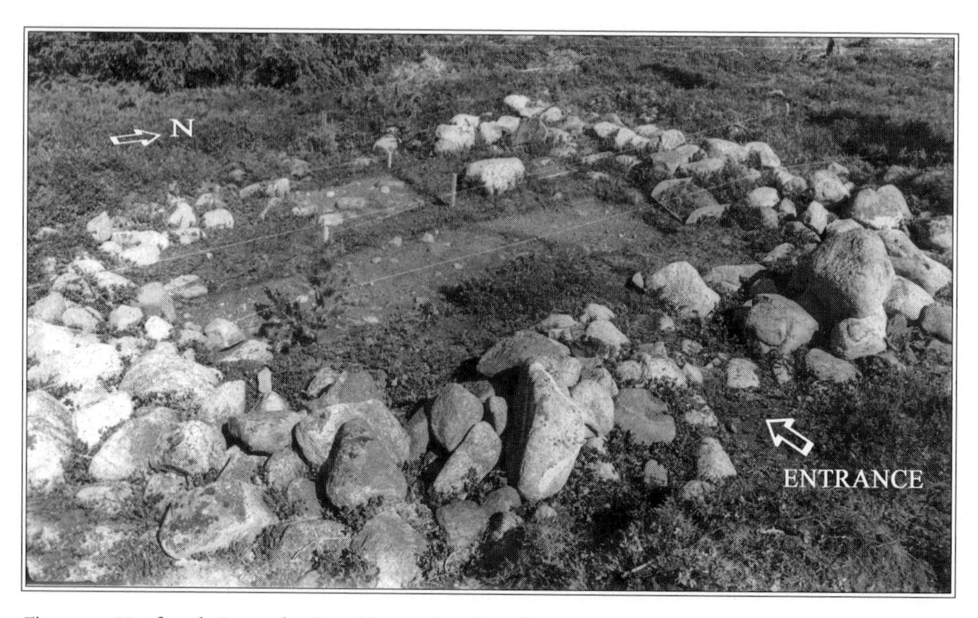


*Figure 37. Hut foundation at the Grundskatan site (Site 78, Hut 3).*

### Cairns

Cairns can be roughly divided into stone constructions of less than 1 meter in diameter and those that are greater in size, usually 3 m to 4 m in diameter. The largest cairns can be graves, sea markers or food storage caches. Cairns can occur singly or, in the case of the smaller cairns, in tight groups or in lines. These small cairns frequently occur as "fields" of post-supports by fishing sites and harbors and were used in connection with the drying and repairing of nets (Swedish *gistgård*) (refer Figure 112).

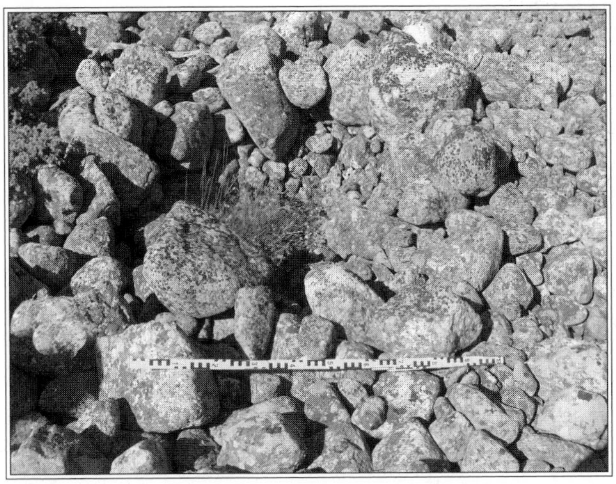

*Figure 38. Small cache beside a hut on Stora Fjäderägg Island (Sites 31–32).*

### Caches

Caches are storage places for perishable items and lack any traces of burning or burned bones. They consist of cairns or subsurface stone chambers of different sizes. They often occur near, or even in, huts and are often found in open boulder fields. They were frequently built next to boulders and bedrock outcrops (Figure 38).

### Alignments

Alignments are lines of stones that are not dwelling constructions or net-drying post supports. Some are probably associated with enclosures for livestock. These kinds of alignments are documented elsewhere in Scandinavia (*stensträngar*) (Lindqvist 1968; Myhre 1972; Carlsson 1979). Other alignments occur in long parallel lines with spaced openings and were probably used for snaring birds, as seems to have been the case at the site of Hornslandsudde (Figure 144). Some parallel stone alignments are set at right angles to former shorelines and mark boat-landing places.

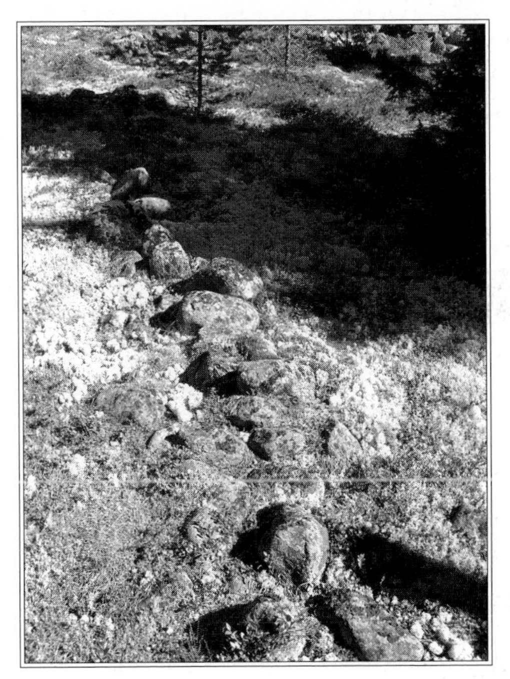

*Figure 39. Stone alignment at the Grundskatan site.*

### Circles

These features have been described regarding Saami sacrificial sites (Vorren 1985, 1987; Vorren and Eriksen 1993; Wennstedt Edvinger and Broabent 2006). They consist of a single circle, concentric rings of stones or a wall enclosure, and often have a central cairn. Single circles can also be tent rings, distinguishable by their hearths and entrances (refer to Figures 109, 187).

### Labyrinths

These are spiraling stone constructions made up of single lines of stones forming walkways toward a center point (Figure 40). Bothnian labyrinths normally emanate from a central cross (refer to Chapter 10). They are most often associated with fishing sites (Kraft 1977).

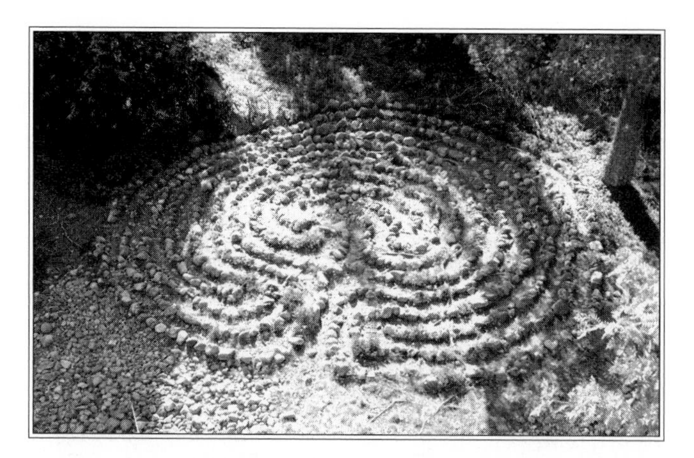

*Figure 40. Labyrinth at Ratan in coastal Västerbotten.*

### Compass Roses

These elegant features are small stone settings with eight arms and N–S and E–W alignments. They were built to afford compass bearings on land and were probably practical ways to orient fishing and sailing activities (Figure 41).

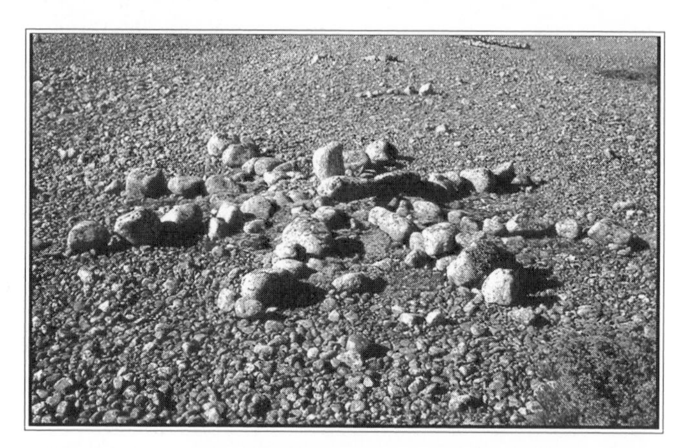

*Figure 41. Compass rose on Snöan Island.*

### "Russian" Ovens

These features are free-standing stone chambers with openings toward the front. They sometimes have a lintel stone. During the eighteenth and nineteenth centuries, they were used by the Russian Navy for baking bread on shore, and are therefore frequently referred to as Russian Ovens (Figure 42).

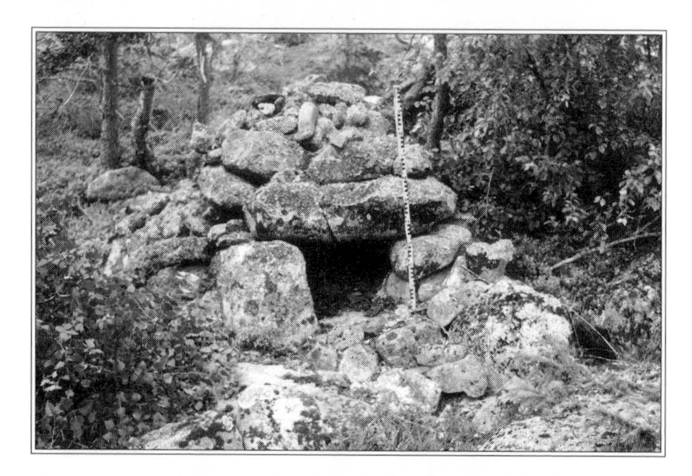

*Figure 42. Large intact Russian Oven in Österbotten, Finland.*

### Shooting Blinds

These blinds (Swedish *jaktskåror* or *gömslen*) consist of short lines or piles of stones on beaches or by ponds where hunters could hide themselves. They are associated with firearms and the shooting of seals or birds.

### Engravings

Engravings have been recorded at numerous places and consist of watermarks carved during the eighteenth and nineteenth centuries as well as names, dates and ownership marks carved by seal hunters and fishermen. A large number of engravings dating between 1797 and 1915 were documented at Svarthällviken on Bjurön in Västerbotten (Figure 44).

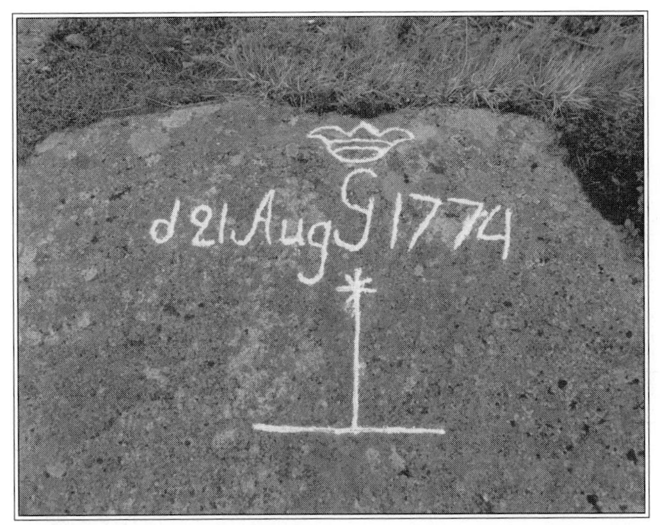


*Figure 43. Watermark at Ratan in Västerbotten carved during the reign of Gustav III.*

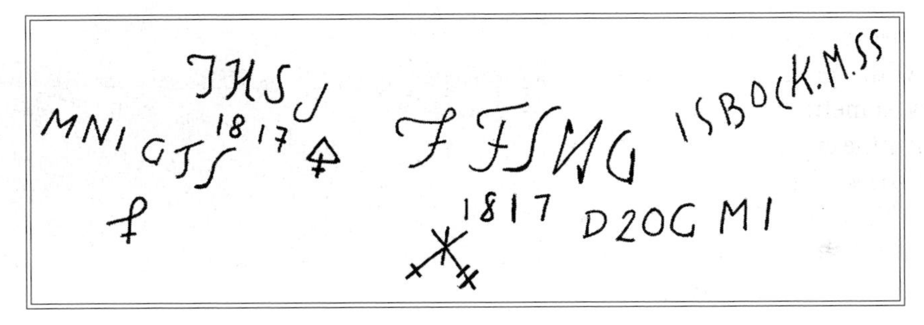


*Figure 44. Engraved names, ownership marks and dates carved by sealers from Österbotten in Finland at Svarthällviken near Bjuröklubb.*

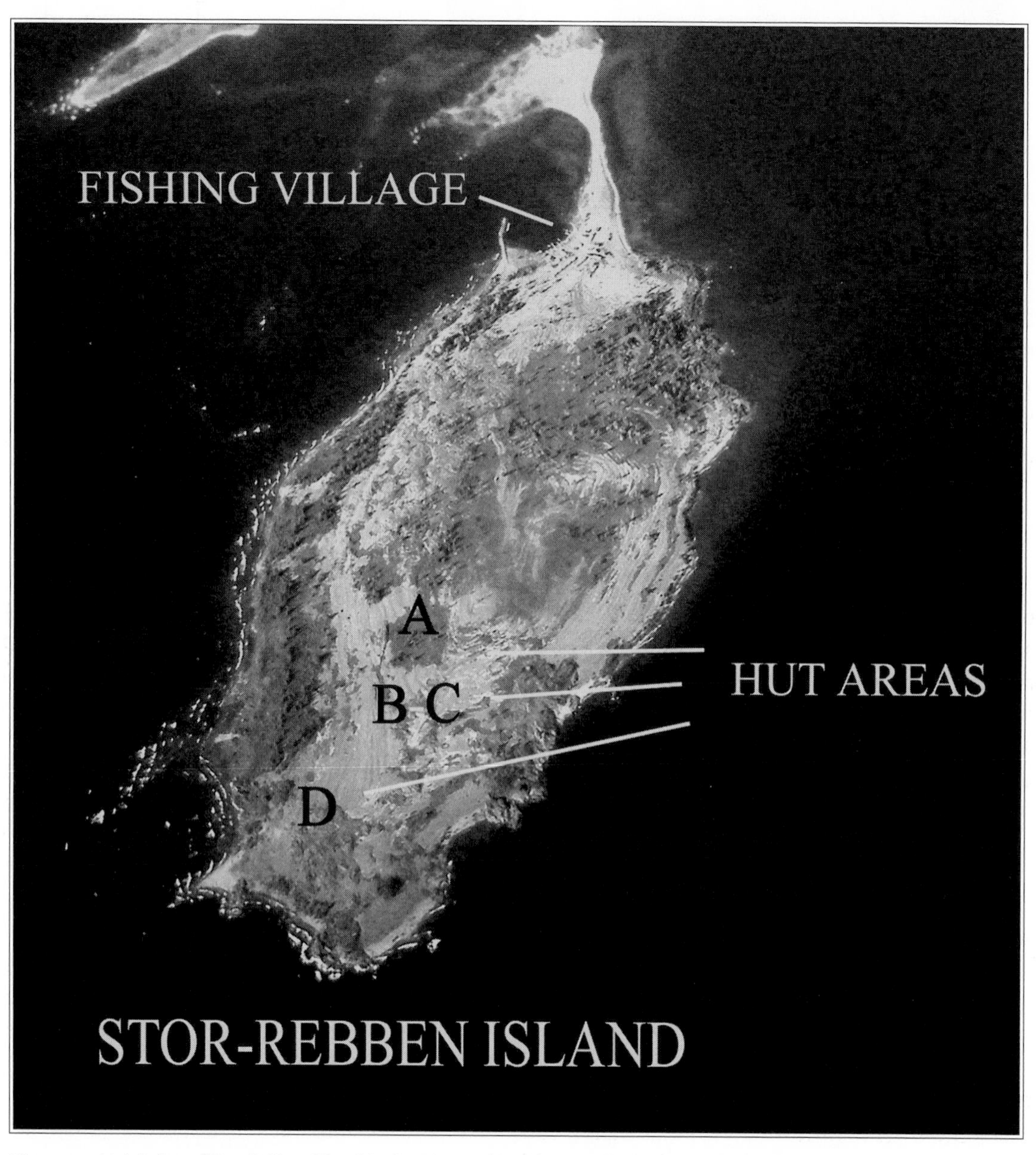


*Figure 45. Aerial view of Stor-Rebben Island in the Piteå archipelago, Norrbotten County. Locations of investigated huts indicated.*

# 5

# Excavations and Analyses

## Regional History

The main region of the study is Skellefteå Municipality in Västerbotten County and Skellefteå and Lövånger parishes. The name "Västerbotten" dates to 1454 and refers to the western (*väster*) side of the basin (*botten*) of the Bay of Bothnia (Ågren 1969:45) (Figure 47). Coastal Västerbotten is characterized by a plain with elevations of less than 50 m with some undulating hilly country of 50 to 100 m elevations. The area south of the Skellefte River, especially the Lövånger region, has numerous old fault lines forming more rectilinear relief with low fjords and narrow bays.

In the Telje statutes of September 5, 1328, Knut Jonsson wrote that the northernmost parts of Helsingland up to the Ule River in Finland should be settled and cultivated, but that the Lapps should not be prevented from hunting there. The first official mention of the "Lappmarks" (Laplands) is from 1340. King Magnus Eriksson's government declared that this area was *bona vacantia* (wilderness), "not known to be occupied by many people," and was now subject to the Helsinge Law. The land was made available for settlement to Christian folk and to those who would convert, and land-title would be granted to them (Sommarström 1966). The eastern boundaries of Lapland in Västerbotten, about 100 km inland, were established as late as 1752. This boundary was strengthened in 1865 as the so-called Agricultural Limit, intended to separate Saami territories from Swedish and Finnish agrarian expansion. The use of "Lapland" as the demarcation of *Sápmi* is therefore misleading for archeological as well as linguistic purposes. Lapland, as shown on maps in most sources, is best viewed as state-mandated territory.

Johannes Schefferus stated that although Lappish (Saami) territory did not in his time encompass the Bothnian coasts, it did so before the time of Damianus á Goes (1502 –1574). He also quotes Olaus Petri Niurenius, a priest and rector in Umeå in Västerbotten (1580–1645), who stated: "the Lapps formerly had their camps on the Bothnian coast but had been driven away from there" (Schefferus 1673:50).

Swedish colonization of the northern coasts was almost certainly underway in the late thirteenth century and by 1316 Uppsala Cathedral had claimed ownership of salmon fisheries on the Ume River (Olofsson 1962). This is about the same time that Norwegian settlement expanded in Finnmark (1307) and Sweden tried, unsuccessfully, to gain control of these territories as well (cf. Odner 1983; Urbańczyk 1992).

The vagueness of the new boundary with Russia through the Treaty of Oreshek/Nöteborg in 1323 made it imperative for Sweden to occupy the north Bothnian coastlands. These northern peoples were already taxed differently than Swedish settlers to the south, in Medelpad and Ångermanland. Under the Hälsingelagen, the old Provincial legal system, Swedish peasants were expected to pay taxes and support the *ledung*, the ship-based defense system. People living to the north of Ångermanland were, by contrast, to pay two skins for every bow (a taxable adult who could span a bow and thereby hunt), and were not expected to contribute to the *ledung*. In addition to this policy, the Birkarlar, Bothnian merchants of Finnish extraction, were given special privileges to tax the Saami on behalf of the Crown, especially the fur trade (Steckzén 1964:119–128). King Magnus Eriksson's Municipal Law furthermore designated Stockholm as the market for all surpluses, which effectively put a lid on independent mercantile activities in the North. The city of Stockholm was fully established by Birger Jarl in about 1300 and thereafter became the capital of Swedish commerce.

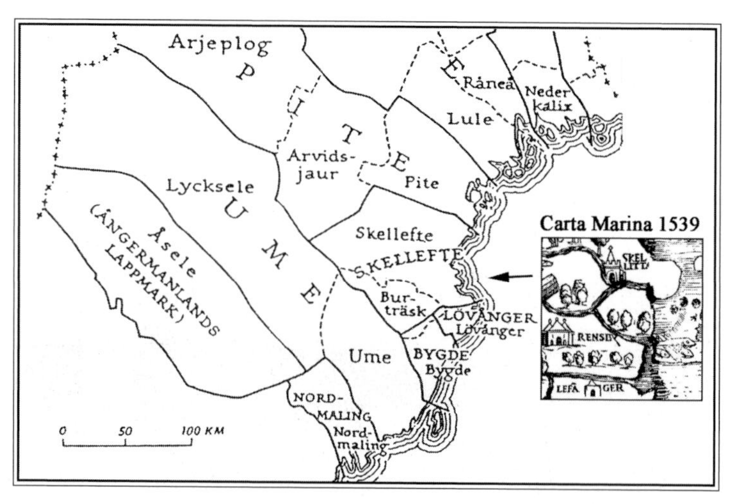


*Figure 46. The Ume and Pite Lappmarks and Skellefte and Lövånger parishes in the Province of Västerbotten in the fifteenth century. The Ume and Pite designations refer to the two Saami languages that align with these rivers. Inset from Figure 7.*

The Saami in interior Västerbotten, speakers of the Ume Saami language, were evidently taxed differently than other Saami under the Birkarl system. According to the *Lundii Ädiscriptio Lapponiae* (1670), the Uhmålappar (Ume Lapps) and the Nårrlappar (North Lapps) were quite different. Fjellström (1987) postulated that taxation of the Ume Saami was more directly tied to the Swedish Crown because they were *konungslappar* (the King's Lapps). This suggests that they had been "appropriated" by the Crown at a very early stage. They had probably already been forced out of the coastal areas which were so important for medieval maritime communications, fishing and trade. This appropriation of territory was logically paralleled by a special tax burden, both as a part of the process of displacement and a means for controlling future settlement and economic activity. Colonization continued throughout the fifteenth century, and by 1519 Bjuröklubb had become a major center for the Swedish herring fisheries (Magnus 1555; Olofsson 1962). Eight medieval churches (Umeå, Bygdeå, Lövånger, Skellefteå, Piteå, Luleå, Kalix and Torneå) were established. Of these, only Bygdeå and Lövånger were not situated by larger rivers.

Skellefteå and Lövånger parishes were first established under the Archbishop in Uppsala, Jakob Ulfsson, in 1340 (*Skellopt cum capella Lavanger*). The present stone church at Lövånger dates in all probability to 1507 and was dedicated to Saint Anna, but the church town could be much older (Figures 47, 194). Historical sources indicate that there had been competition for the church

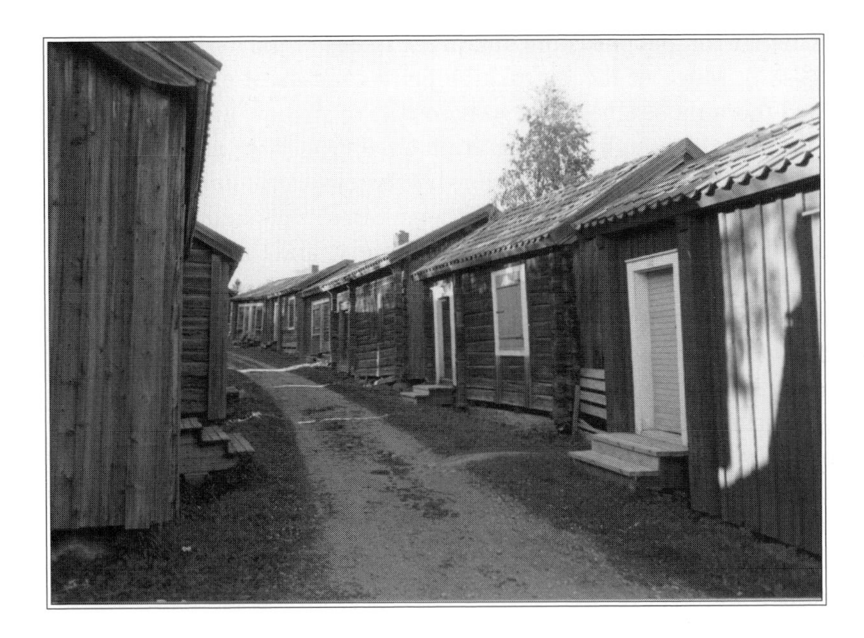

*Figure 47. Lövånger church town. Each cabin along this street belonged to a household from the same village, and the street points in the direction of the village. The church town was a microcosm of regional demography.*

site between the villages of Lövånger and Mångbyn (Hedquist 1949:276–277). The area of Mångbyn/Broänge is interesting because it contains archaeological remains dating to the Late Iron Age (Broadbent and Rathje 2001), and church sites of these kinds usually piggy-backed on already established market places.

## Bjuröklubb and Bjurön

Bjuröklubb point on Bjurön, at latitude 64° 28′ N, longitude 21° 34′ E, rises 47 m above sea level and is best known from an account published by Olaus Magnus in 1555 (Figure 48). He had visited the area in 1519 and described the point as "a cliff in the sea, of local people called *Bjuraklubb*, whose high prominent crown appears from a distance to sailors as consisting of a crown with three points." He goes on to describe this vision as leading sailors to safe harbor. Once closer, one could observe great quantities of fish drying on the black rocks along the shore [Swedish *Svarthällorna*]. These fish, according to Magnus, were consumed locally, traded for cereals since local crops rarely ripened because of the cold, or "as delicacies for those who lived in

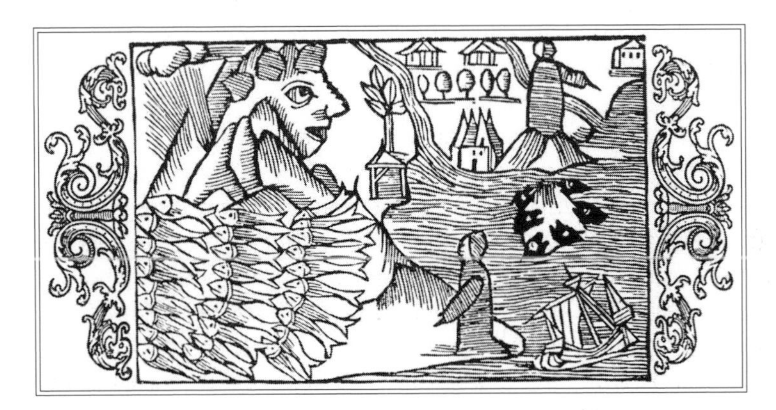

*Figure 48. Woodcut of Bjuröklubb from 1555. The image shows herring drying on the rocks at Svarthällviken, the rocky point with three crowns, a medieval ship and seals in the Bay of Bothnia (Olaus Magnus 1555, Book II:88).*

the interior, and through an exchange for fish one could obtain the riches of the forest in the form of expensive furs" (Book II: 88–89). Much of the Bjuröklubb point consists of exposed granite, gneiss bedrock and wave-washed moraine beaches. The soils consist of shallow gravel and sandy sediments with weak podsolic profiles although in some areas on Bjurön large sand dunes are found. Vegetation consists primarily of pine heaths with dry blueberry (*vaccinium*) type ground cover and lichen vegetation is abundant, especially reindeer lichens. Birch, alder and spruce woods predominate on marshy and low-lying ground. The area is a nature reserve and there are rare plants of mountain *fjäll* type.

The name Bjuröklubb, which literally means "beaver island point," derives from the name of this former island (and beaver hunting areas) and the historic harbor and point. The oldest harbor basin on the island, and adjacent to Svarthällorna, is Jungfruhamn. Its threshold was determined to be 2.59 m, meaning that it had to have been abandoned by 1656 (Broadbent 1989b:26). The harbor and chapel at Bjuröklubb dates to 1658 and was thereafter used into the twentieth century (Figure 32). Even the name Jungfruhamn was probably secondary, however, and derives from what may have been the original name of Bjuröklubb, which was Jungfrun (The Virgin) (Wennstedt 1988:25). The Jungfru name was often used to describe dangerous coasts and rocks and was probably a taboo word referring to the female demons that caused shipwrecks and other mischief. The name also referred to the narrow vaginal shape of Jungfruhamn harbor and was an obscene reference, according to one source quoted by Wennstedt (1988:25). The name Jungfrun was, in any case, to be avoided in everyday conversation, as was the case in many taboos, and was therefore probably replaced with the neutral administrative name it has today, Bjuröklubb (Wennstedt 1988:26).

Against this background, the so-called Jungfrugraven (The Virgin's Grave), two boulder walls enclosing a cairn, becomes interesting as a potentially pre-Christian construction. Although the lichens on its stones date it to A.D. 1532–1604 at the latest, its elevation (10 m) associates it with the Viking Period. We have interpreted this feature as a sacrificial site and contemporary with other circular sacrificial sites on Bjurön that are discussed in Chapter 8 (cf. Wennstedt Edvinger and Broadbent 2006). The name Jungfru suggests the place was menacing. This was perhaps due in equal measure to the dangers for mariners as to the many highly visible pre-Christian constructions in the area. Excavations in the vicinity of Bjuröklubb were conducted at Site 67 (Bjuröklubb), Site 70, Site 78 (Grundskatan), Sites 138 and 139 (near Jungfruhamn) and Site 144 on Lappsandberget. Soil samples were additionally collected at Site 79 (Jungfrugraven) and mapping was carried out at Sites 64, 65 and 68 (Figures 49, 50).

### Jungfrugraven, Site 79

This construction consists of a ca. 13 m wide and 17.5 m long oval enclosure encompassing a stone cairn (Figures 51, 52). The walls are 1–1.5 m wide and 0.75 m high. One straight wall runs parallel with the inlet and a curved wall 21 m in length connects with it, leaving 1 m wide entrances at its south and north ends. A 7 × 8 m horseshoe-shaped cairn is situated at the north end of the enclosure. A small pile of stones with an upright and engraved cross lies in its center. The largest lichens on the walls and the elevation above sea level bracket this construction to the time period A.D. 950–1604. Phosphate mapping was carried out within and around the enclosure and revealed no enrichment, as would be expected at a fishing harbor. Lichen growth on the central cairn displays two patterns: the innermost area has relatively large lichens, while the outermost lichens are very small (Figure 52).

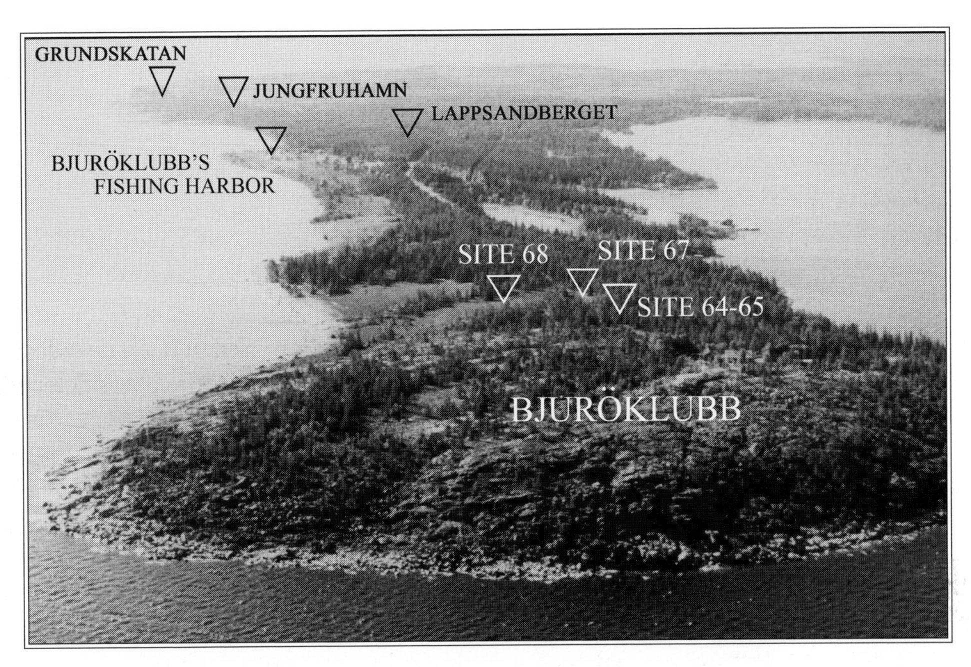


*Figure 49. Aerial view of Bjuröklubb facing south. Sites mentioned in text shown.*

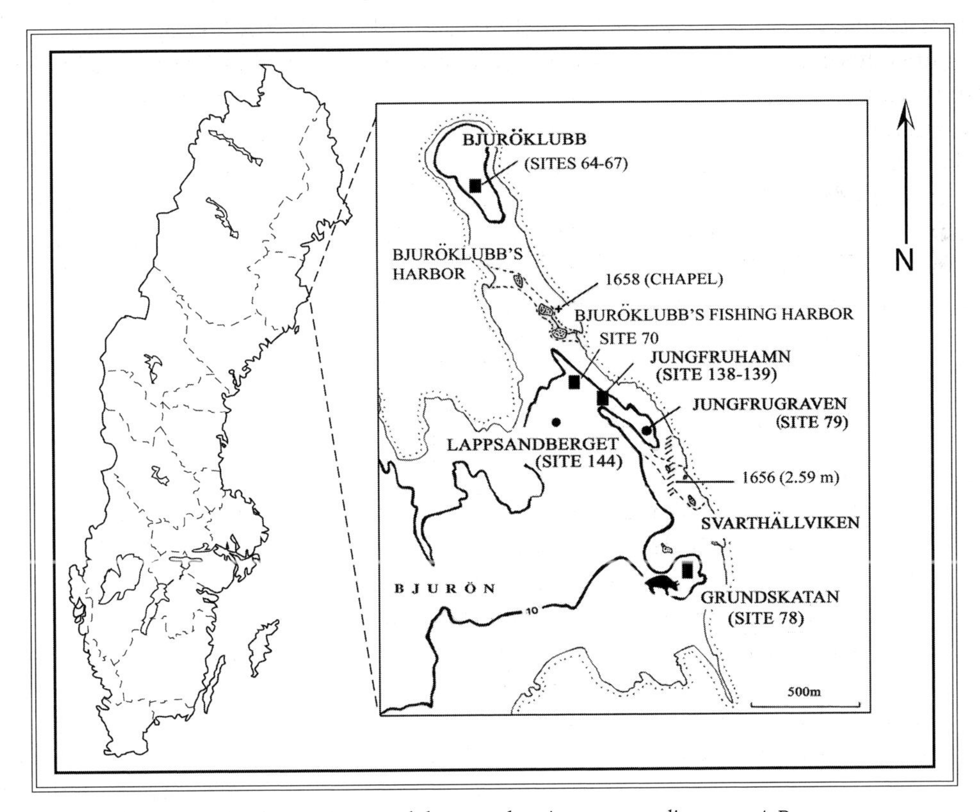


*Figure 50. Map of site locales on Bjurön and the 10 m elevation corresponding to ca. A.D. 950.*

Figure 51. Photo of Inga-Maria Mulk and Tim Bayliss-Smith in the Jungfrugraven enclosure.

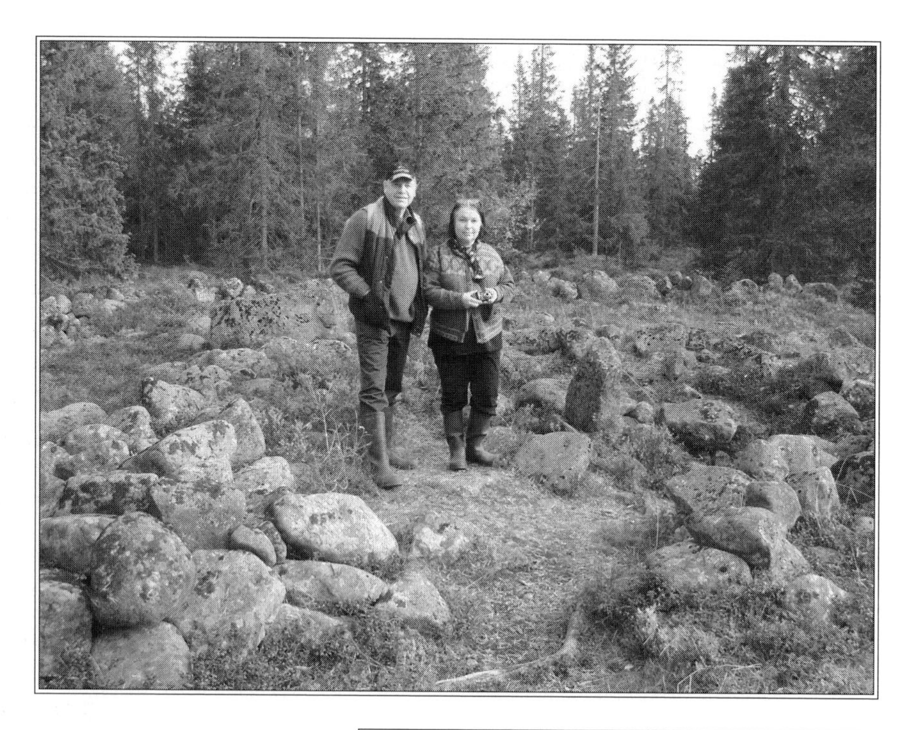

This indicates that the horseshoe-shaped cairn is relatively recent, and that the stones in its outer ring had been taken from the center of the cairn. This horseshoe shape is shown in A. F. Ekdahl's documentation from 1827, but the small pile of stones with the engraved cross is not shown in this drawing. Lichen growth confirms that the small cairn and cross had been set up in the early twentieth century.

Cemetery enclosures of this type are known from the Medieval Period, for instance on Holmön Island. What distinguishes Jungfrugraven is its cairn, which was not the foundation of a chapel, but something more akin to Saami offer sites in North Norway. These cairns and enclosures are associated with hunting and fishing sites (Vorren and Eriksen 1993). Although the Jungfrugraven enclosure is larger than the Norwegian sites, it coincides by form, location and chronology to this material and, most significantly, to the cultural context of the Iron Age huts adjacent to it (refer to discussion in Chapter 8).

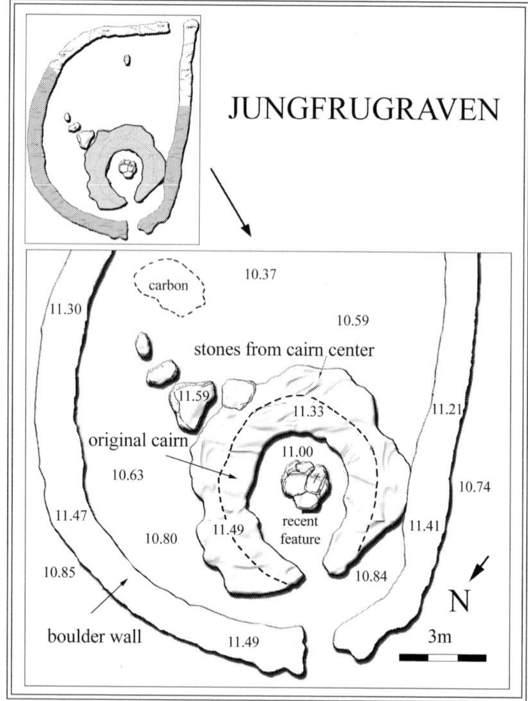


Figure 52. Map showing the wall lines and displaced cairn stones at Jungfrugraven. The original cairn could have had supported an idol.

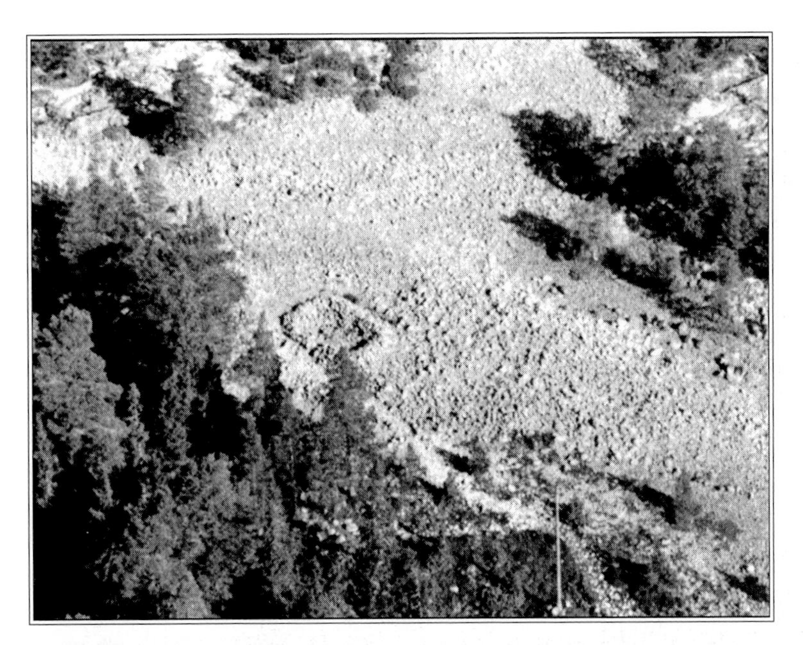

*Figure 53. Aerial view of Site 64.*

## Site 64

Site 64 is a large reconstructed 7 × 5.5 m rectangular hut with walls measuring 90 cm in height and up to 1.5 m in width (Figure 53). The floor measures ca. 5.5 m in length and 4 m in width. A doorway faces southwest toward the mainland. This large dwelling lies higher than Site 65, ca. 17 m above sea level, and was probably contemporary with Site 67, or A.D. 450–650.

## Site 65

Site 65 is a cluster of four huts in a well-protected depression at 14–15 m above sea level (Figure 54). Three huts lie within 3 m of each other and a fourth hut stands 37.4 m to the southeast on the edge of a steep waterlogged ravine. Three of the huts have hearths that are mostly overgrown. The floors measure 4 × 4.5 m, 4 × 4 m and 3 × 2.8 m respectively. The smallest hut lacks a hearth and may have been used for storage. A second small round foundation measuring 3 × 3 m is located within 35 m of this complex and could have been a "goat hut" (refer to Chapter 7). No excavations were undertaken at this site, but these huts are interpreted as analogous to and contemporary with the hut groups at Grundskatan, Site 78. They probably date to A.D. 700–1000.

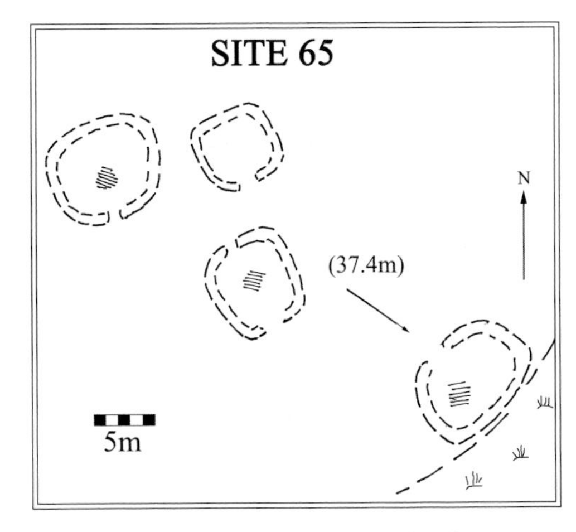


*Figure 54. Sketch map of Site 65 with three huts in a cluster, and a fourth hut on the edge of a ravine 37.4 m to the southwest.*

## Site 67

Site 67 is a solitary construction and lies on a 17 m high saddle of land with access to both sides of the island (Figure 55). The hut is kidney shaped and measures 6 × 5 m with a floor area of 4.5 × 2.6 m. A 75 cm wide entranceway runs through its southwest wall. Nine soil phosphate samples were collected from the floor and range from 30 P° to 194 P°, which is relatively high. Small amounts of burned and unburned bones were also obtained. One fragment was identified as a seal humerus. A 3 cm thick deposit of sooty soil was found adjacent to the back (north) wall. The burned area extended into the wall and into an opening that appears to be a chimney or vent of some kind (Figures

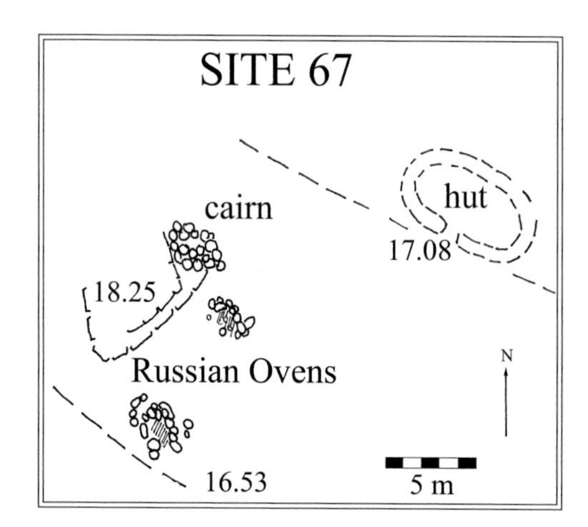


*Figure 55. Sketch map of Site 67 with associated features. An oval hearth lies about 100 m to the south and downslope from these features.*

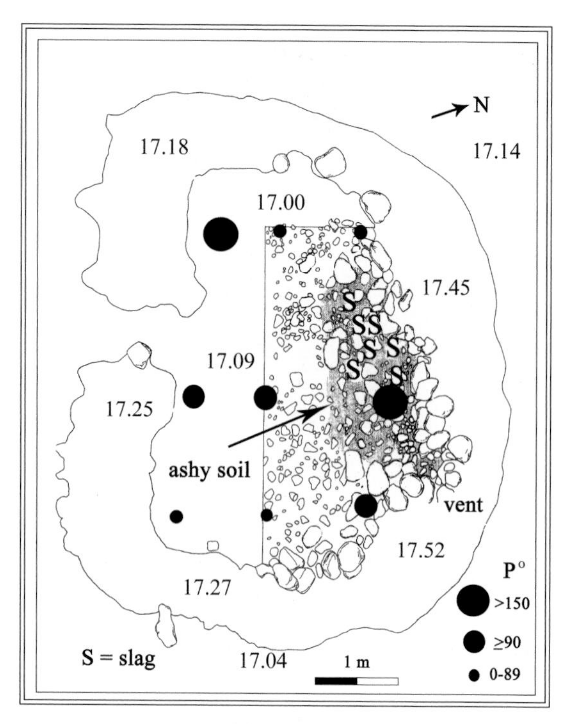


*Figure 56. Plan of excavation of Hut, Site 67.*

56, 173). This arrangement is unlike most dwellings, but has close parallels to huts at Grundskatan (Hut 11) and at Hornslandsudde (Hut 12). In all three cases, the hearths were associated with iron slag and furnaces.

*Finds*
22 pieces of slag (207 g)

The slag from the Hut 67 was analyzed by the Geoarkeologiska Laboratoriet. (GAL) in Uppsala and determined to be the by-products of forging (Grandin et al. 2005). This material is discussed in detail in Chapter 7. One radiocarbon date was obtained from this site: (1485±70 B.P.), which calibrates to A.D. 467–648. The structure stood just under the top of the rise and had some protection from westerly winds, but its elevation also provided a good draft for a furnace. Phosphate enrichment and seal bone suggests that this was also a dwelling. This hut was probably associated with nearby dwellings, Sites 65 and 68, but these have not been dated. The age of this site makes it contemporary with the oldest phase of the Grundskatan settlement on the opposite end of Bjurön. Three additional features were recorded within 15 m of the hut. A small cairn, possibly a cache, lies on a rock outcrop, and two stone constructions, one fairly recognizable as a Russian Oven, stand parallel with each other below the outcrop. Both ovens have traces of charcoal in them and can be assumed to date to the Russian invasions of the early 1700s.

Table 4. Hut 67: Osteological finds.

| ANATOMY | SEAL? | UNIDENTIFIED | TOTAL |
|---|---|---|---|
| Humerus | 1 | | 1 |
| Ossa longa | | 4 | 4 |
| Indeterminate | | 7 | 7 |
| Total | 1 | 11 | 12 |

A small hearth was also discovered partly exposed in the pathway leading up to Site 67 (Figure 57). It is roughly oval in shape and consists of a selection of stones 20–30 cm in size, with one larger flat stone measuring 50 cm across. The surrounding sandy soil was stone free and

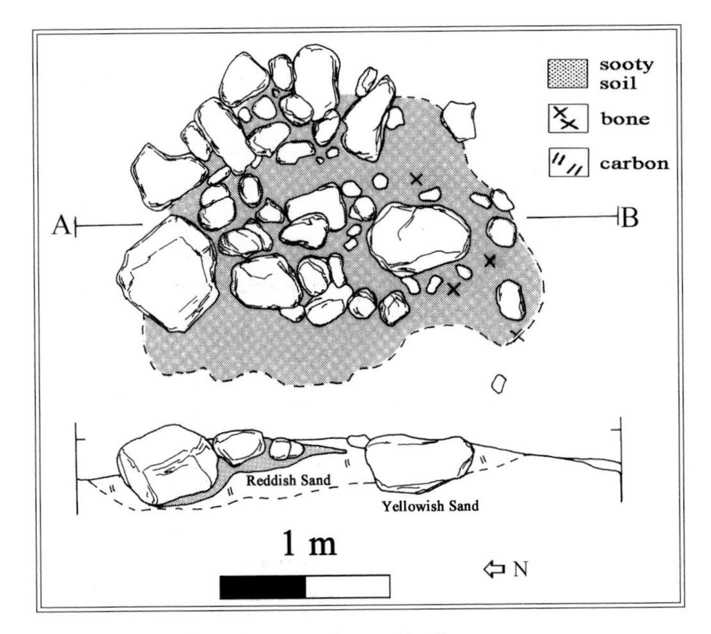


*Figure 57. Plan of hearth excavated near Site 67.*

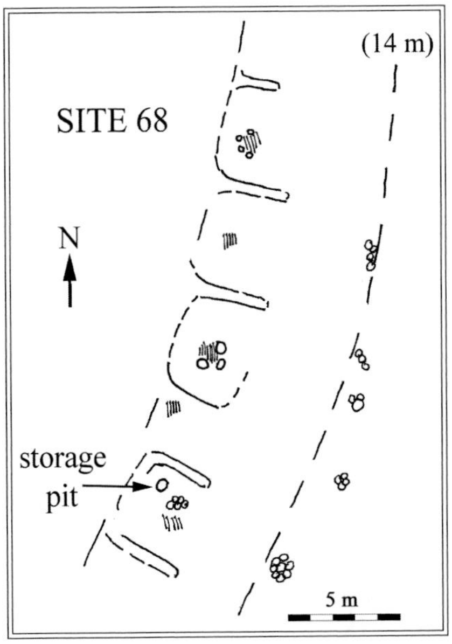

*Figure 58. Sketch map of hut row, Site 68.*

red-burned. Some 6.8 g of burned and unburned bones were found, and a radiocarbon date of the charcoal (Beta 191232) rendered an age of: 230±40 (A.D. cal. 1641–1953). The bone is from a large ungulate, probably a reindeer, suggesting the hearth was connected with Saami in the area, as is noted in historic accounts of Bjuröklubb (cf. Wennstedt 1988).

### Site 68

This site is in an area of completely exposed wave-washed moraine beaches lying to the east of the previous site. A row of five disturbed floors with six dividing walls lies on a terrace at the 14 m level (Figure 58). Traces of four, possibly five, hearths are indicated by fire-cracked rocks. One hut has a small storage pit that is identical to that observed in a group of row houses at Grundskatan Site 67, Hut 1. As the row huts at both sites are similar in appearance, and are at the same elevations above sea level, it can be assumed that they were contemporary. The radiocarbon date from Hut 1 at Grundskatan is: 1160±70 B.P. or A.D. cal. 779–968.

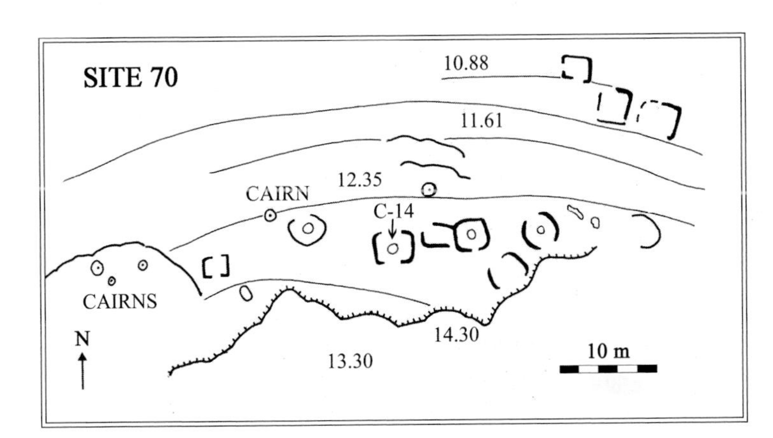


*Figure 59. Map of Site 70 and three adjacent huts and wall alignments.*

### Site 70

Site 70, at 64° 27′ N, 21° 35′ E, consists of a group of 10 hut foundations between ca. 10 and 13 m above sea level (Figure 59). This complex was situated on the north shore of Bjurön Island and faces Bjuröklubb. A charcoal sample was obtained from a hearth in the middle of the complex, as well as 4.6 g of seal bone. The charcoal was dated to: 1020±60 B.P. (A.D. cal. 902–1149) (Beta-196485) and this is consistent with the elevation of the site. Foundations of three huts with adjoining wall alignments were mapped in an area near Site 70 and at a somewhat higher elevation (Figure 170). These features had not been previously registered and were very overgrown, so much so they could barely be relocated in 2005. There are two adjoined huts with floors measuring 3 × 4 m and 3 × 3.5 m, and a third simpler construction measuring 3 × 3.5 m. What makes these huts especially interesting are the stone alignments/walls that measure up to 10 m in length. Based on their elevation and proximity to Site 70, these features date sometime between A.D. 900 and 1150.

## Jungfruhamn, Sites 138–139

### *Huts A, B and C*

Two huts (Hut A and Hut B) were sampled at Site 138 (Figures 60–61). Their elevation above sea level is 15 m. A third hut (C) was shovel tested, but not excavated. It lies in the woods some 20 m away (Site 139) and radiocarbon-dated to: 1710±125 (A.D. cal. 139–526) (St. 11909). Hut A is rectangular and measures ca. 7.5 × 5.5 m. The hut has two entrances on the opposite walls facing north and south. The floor area measures 5 × 3 m. A 1 m² test pit was excavated to sample the hearth. A diagonal profile was drawn through the pit showing a layer of 10–20 cm burned soil with bone and charcoal (Figure 62). Two dates were obtained: (St. 11176) 985±70 B.P. (A.D. cal. 990–1155), and (Beta 196490) 1210±50 B.P. (A.D. cal. 722–887). Some 58.8 g of burned bone was found in the hearth. Hut B is rectangular and measures 4 × 5.5 m. The floor area measures ca. 3 × 3.5 m. A 75 cm wide entrance opens

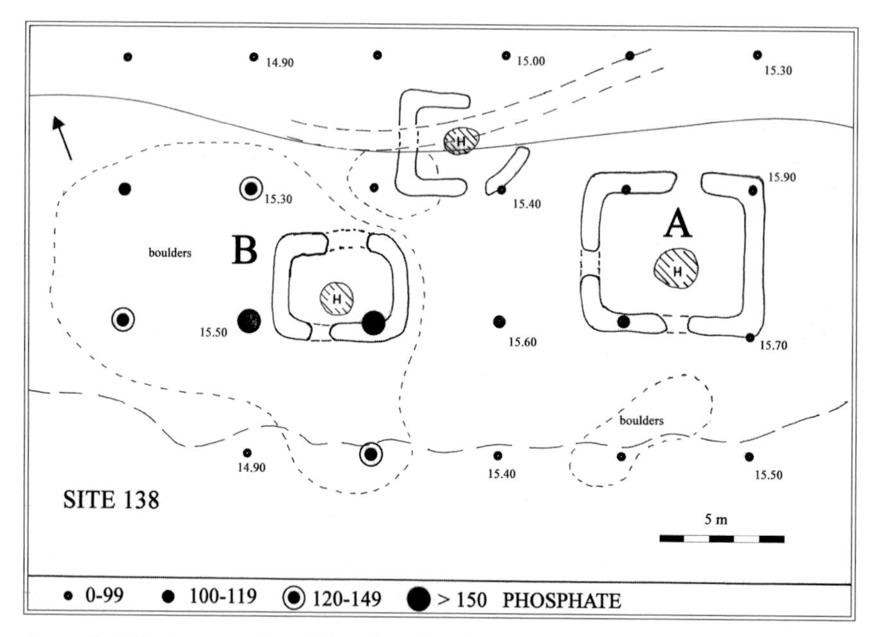


*Figure 60. Phosphate sampling of Site 138 conducted by Johan Linderholm. Values above 120 P° were obtained around Hut B.*

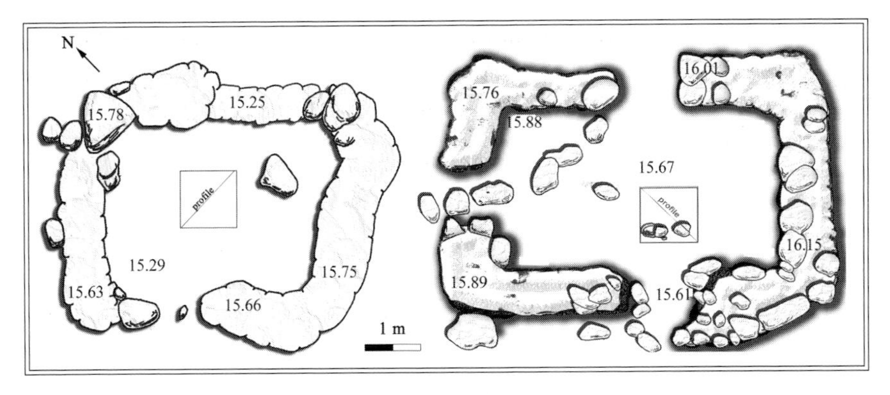


*Figure 61. Detailed maps of Huts A (right) and B (left).*

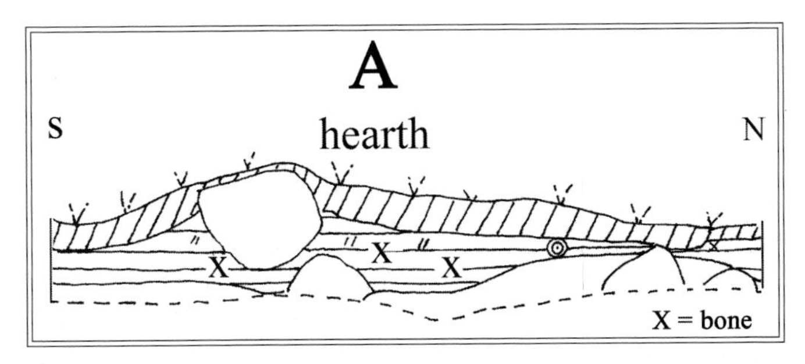


*Figure 62. Profile drawn diagonally through Hut A hearth.*

toward the south/southwest and faces the inlet. A 1 m² pit was excavated to sample the hearth and one radiocarbon date was obtained: (St. 11177) 1300±130 B.P. (A.D. cal. 636–886).

*Finds*

White (burned) flint chip (15mm)
Gray flint chip (10 mm)
Red brown flint chip (10 mm)
2 soapstone/asbestos (?) slivers (45 mm)

*Osteological Material*

The bone material from the two hearths weighs 195.59 g. All the bones were burned and were identified as ringed seal, undifferentiated seal, sheep/goat, a large ungulate, and a bird of unidentified species. Most of the material was found in Hut B, which was also more varied compared to Hut A.

Table 5. Site 138: Species by weight (g).

| SPECIES | HUT A | HUT B | TOTAL |
|---|---|---|---|
| Ringed seal | | 0.18 | 0.18 |
| Seal | 4.43 | 0.12 | 4.55 |
| Sheep/goat | 0.53 | | 0.53 |
| Large ungulate | | 2.31 | 2.31 |
| Bird | | 0.52 | 0.52 |
| Indeterminate | 53.92 | 133.58 | 187.5 |
| Total | 58.88 | 136.71 | 195.59 |

Table 6. Site 138: Species by fragment.

| SPECIES | HUT A | HUT B | TOTAL |
|---|---|---|---|
| Ringed seal | | 1 | 1 |
| Seal | 3 | 1 | 4 |
| Sheep/goat | 1 | | 1 |
| Large ungulate | | 2 | 2 |
| Bird | | 9 | 9 |
| Indeterminate | 436 | 903 | 1339 |
| Total | 440 | 916 | 1356 |

The anatomical breakdown of this material is difficult because of fragmentation and low number of species. It should be noted, however, that there were bones of the cranium, tibia and radius in Hut A, bones that are uncommon at, for example, Grundskatan. The radius is from a large adult seal. In addition, there is also a fragment of a tibia from a goat/sheep one to two years of age. Among the indeterminate bones, there is a dominance of long bones and vertebral fragments, probably from seals. In Hut B, a femoral fragment from a ringed seal and a seal phalanx were identified, as well as a fragment of a large ungulate shoulder blade and humerus. These appear to have been from the same animal (or cuts of meat), either an adult cow/moose or reindeer. The indeterminate bones appear to have mostly derived from seals, although some of the heavier long bones probably emanated from a large ungulate. There are also numerous small bones from birds.

Table 7. Site 138, Hut A: Anatomical distribution of burned bone fragments from seals.

| ANATOMY | SEAL |
|---|---|
| Cranium | 1 |
| Radius | 1 |
| Tibia | 1 |
| Total | 3 |

Table 8. Site 138, Hut B: Anatomical distribution of burned bone fragments.

| ANATOMY | RINGED SEAL | SEAL | LARGE UNGULATE | BIRD | TOTAL |
|---|---|---|---|---|---|
| Scapula | | | 1 | | 1 |
| Humerus | | | 1 | | 1 |
| Femur | | 1 | | | 1 |
| Ph3 post | 1 | | | | 1 |
| Ossa longa | | | | 9 | 9 |
| Total | 1 | 1 | 2 | 9 | 13 |

**Lappsandberget, Site 144**

The goal of the investigation of Site 144 was to document a circular stone feature on Lappsandberget found during survey in the late 1980s and later registered by the county. This rocky hill rises up to ca. 25 m above sea level. Excavation involved removal of vegetation and exposure of the circle and a 13 m² area outside of the circle (Figures 63, 64). The soil was sandy and barely covered the bedrock. Darker brown soil was observed in four patches within this circle. Twenty soil samples were taken,

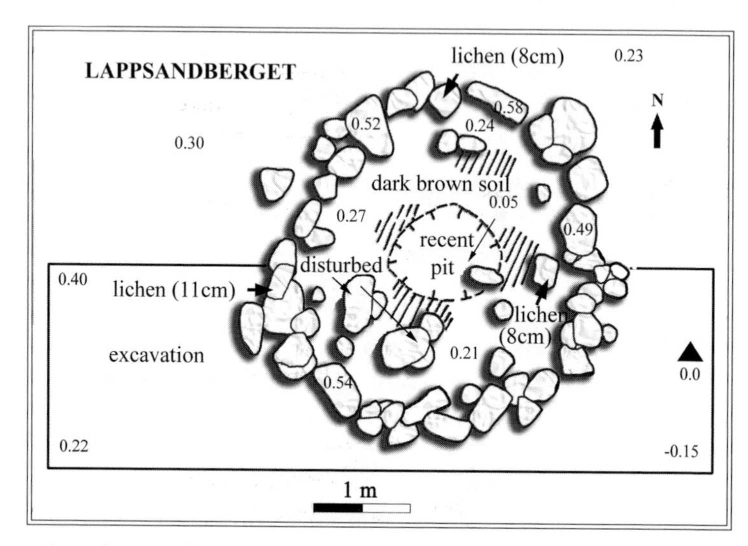


*Figure 63. Map of Site 144 and excavated areas.*

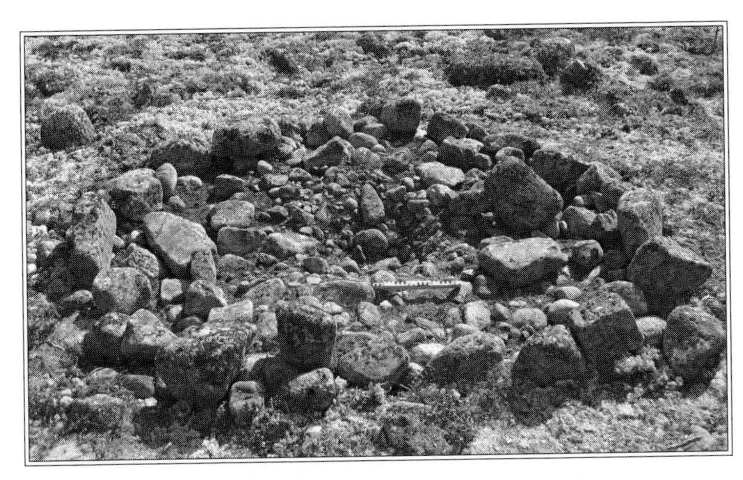

*Figure 64. Exposed surface within the stone circle. (Note depression due to a plundering attempt.)*

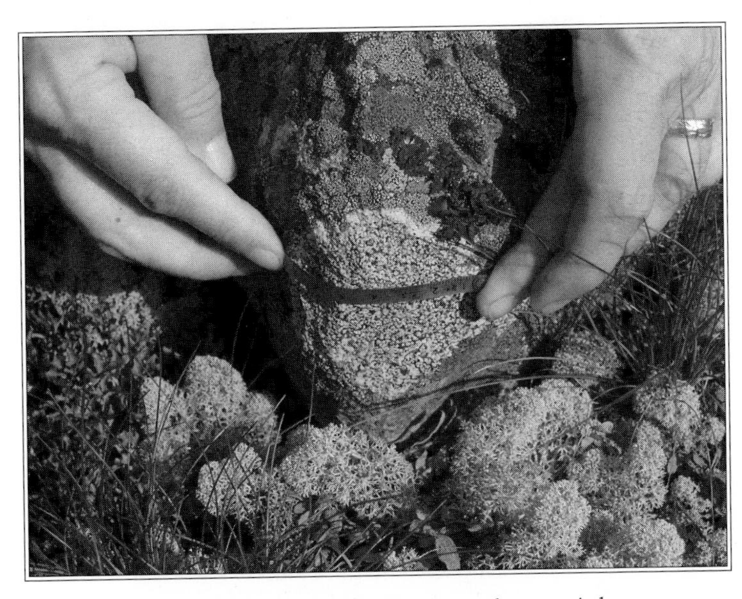

*Figure 65. Close-up of one of three lichens growing on the stone circle.*

13 from inside the circle and 6 from outside the circle. Three additional samples were taken from the dark soil deposits. A metal detector was also used but revealed no metal debris. The stone circle measures ca. 2.70 × 2.70 m and consists of some 50 stones 20–45 cm in size. Fourteen stones of comparable sizes were found within the circle. A 70–80 cm wide and ca. 10 cm deep depression was observed in the center of the circle and was likely to have been the result of a plundering attempt that pushed these stones aside. Three lichens of *Rhizocarpon geographicum* measuring 80–110 mm in diameter were observed on two *in situ* stones in the circle, and on a disturbed stone within the circle (Figure 65). These lichens date to A.D. 1480–1583 and provide a minimum date for the feature. The elevation above sea level (~25 m) is equivalent to ca. 300 B.C., but this locale was undoubtedly chosen because it overlooked the settlements and the sea. This feature does not appear to have been a grave and no traces of charcoal or bones were found in it. The brown soil deposits represent some kind of organic enrichment, and the phosphorus samples support this conclusion. The surrounding soil is very low in phosphorus by comparison. Nitrogen levels were high from within the circle, and this enrichment can potentially derive from organic sources such as blood, flesh and bone (Figure 66) The place-name itself suggests a Saami context, as do oral-historical accounts of Saami living on Bjurön (Wennstedt 1988), as well as the oval hearth of Saami type near Site 67 on Bjuröklubb. The age of the feature is most probably within the range of A.D. 1000–1600.

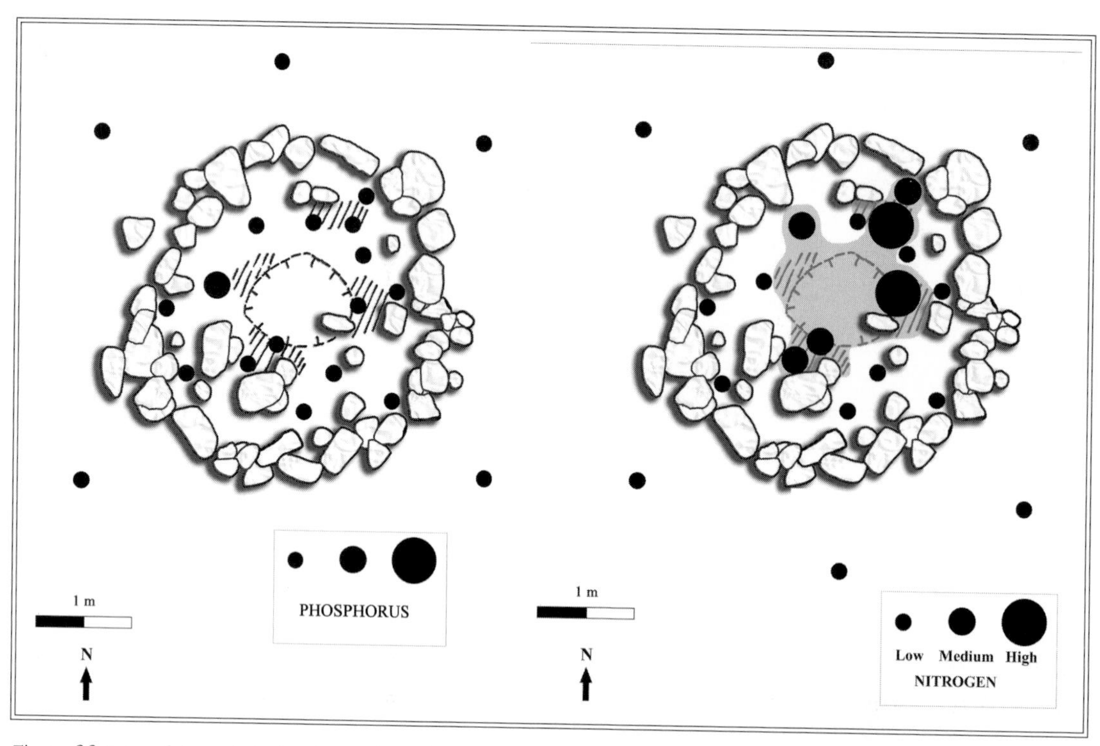


*Figure 66. Map of stone circle showing darker soil deposits within the circle and relative amounts of phosphorus and nitrogen enrichment.*

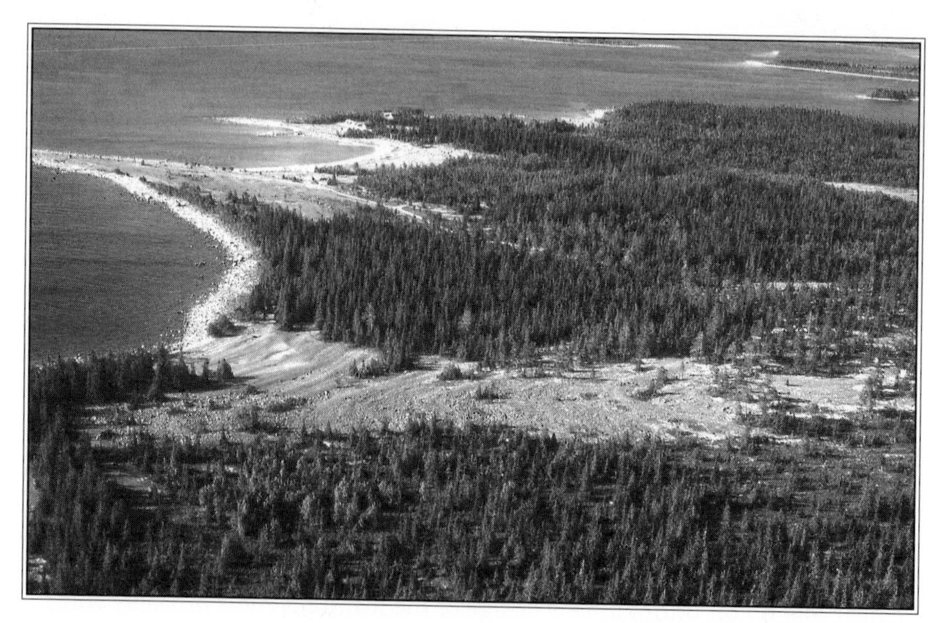

*Figure 67. Aerial view of wave-washed moraine beaches at the Grundskatan site, looking south.*

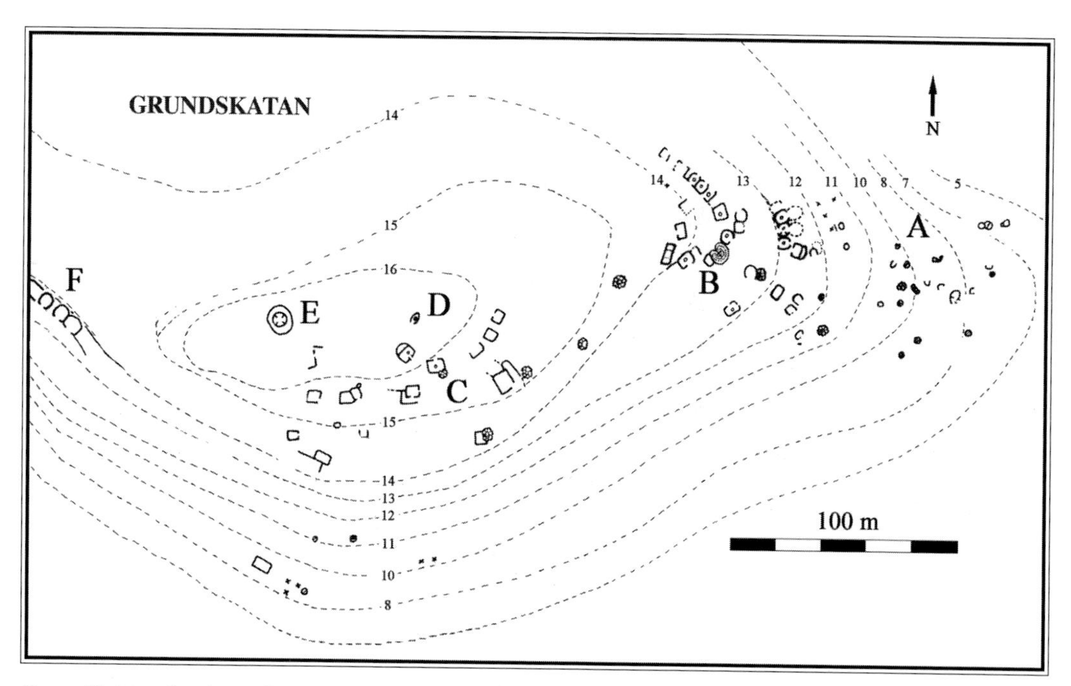


*Figure 68. Map showing archaeological features at the Grundskatan site. A, area with numerous hunting blinds and the Russian Oven (#10). B, location of the labyrinth (#14). C, location of the bear burial (#4). D, location of the circular feature (#17). E, location of the large pit (#15). F, location of Hut 2.*

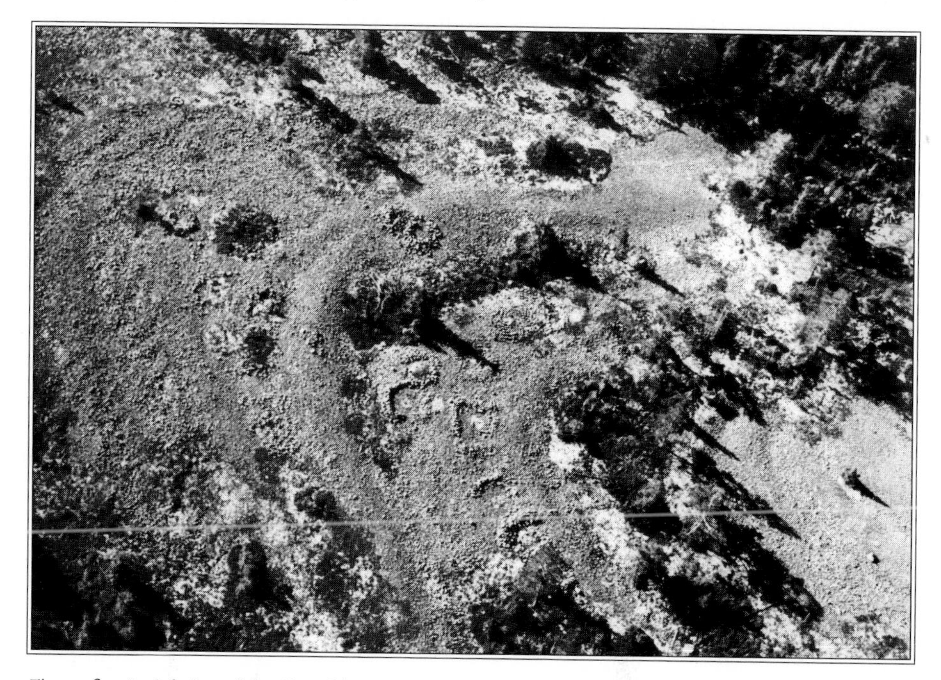

*Figure 69. Aerial view of the Grundskatan site with huts and hearths clearly visible at elevations between 12 m to 14 m above present sea level. A labyrinth can be seen near the center of the photo.*

## Grundskatan, Site 78

Grundskatan (Grundskataräften) lies on Bjurön at 64° 28′ N, 21° 35′ E. The site was described as early as 1882 but was first mapped in the 1940s by Carl Holm and Gustaf Hallström (Hallström 1942:250–257). There are more than 40 hut foundations, (Swedish *tomtningar*), cairns and other features, as well as a stone labyrinth and a Russian Oven (Figures 67, 68, 69). The site is situated on the northern half of a NNW–SSE oriented drumlin. The moraine has been wave-washed and consists of gravel and boulders mostly less than 1.0 m in diameter. The exposed beach toward the east has nine terrace formations up to 16.5 m above sea level. There is boggy and water-logged land north of the site. Grundskatan once formed a small peninsula when the sea level 10 m higher and was an ideal base for sealing.

### *Feature 1, Hut*

This hut is one of nine partly overgrown dwellings aligned in a single row between 13 m and 14 m above sea level (Figure 70). Ten cobble walls, 0.5–1.0 m in width, separate the floors. The huts were built so that a beach ridge forms the major portion of the back wall. Three huts have northeast-facing walls with door openings that measure 0.5–1.0 m in width. Five of the floors have central hearths. Hut 1 was in the middle of the row, was the most intact of these huts, and was therefore chosen for excavation. The floor area was completely overgrown by mosses, lichens, grass and brush. The floor measures 4.0 × 3.0 m and the hearth measures 1.0 m in diameter. The hearth was a round ashy deposit with a lens-shaped cross section up to 10 cm thick. There were no larger stones around it or beneath it, but there were a number of fire-cracked stones in it. A small ca. 20 cm wide and 15 cm deep cylindrical pit was found in the southwestern corner of the floor near the back wall. This straight-sided pit was tightly packed with smaller pebbles. An identical pit was observed in a

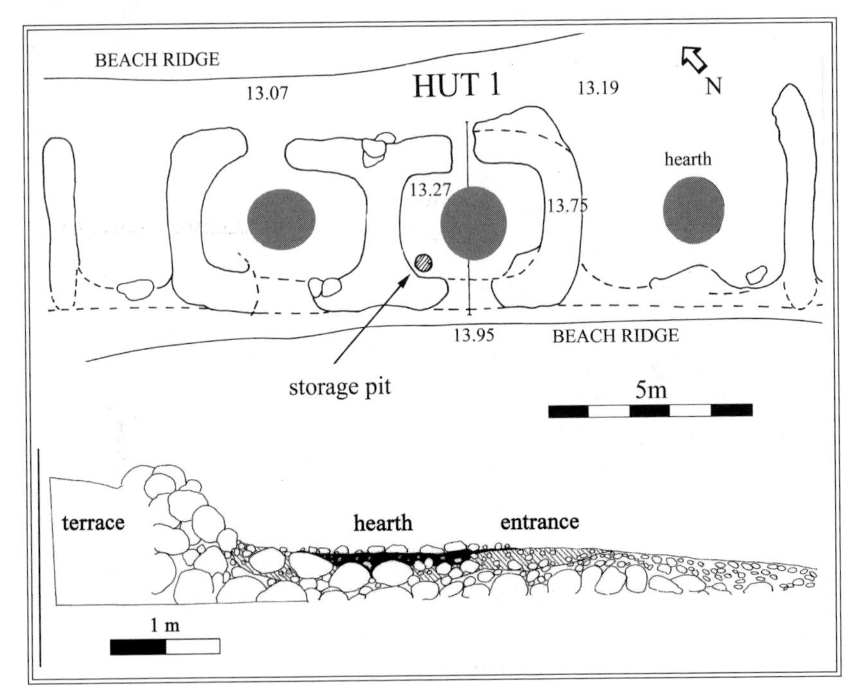


*Figure 70. (top) Map showing Hut 1 and profile excavated through the floor. This hut is one of approximately 9 built up against the same beach ridge. (bottom) Cross section of the hut and beach ridge.*

row of disturbed huts at Bjuröklubb Site 68 at about the same elevation. It had probably been for storage of some kind, but was completely sterile.

*Finds*
1 gray flint chip

*Chronology*
One charcoal sample from the hearth was radiocarbon dated to: 1160±70 B.P. (St. 10787). Calibrated date: A.D. cal. 779–968.

Table 9. Grundskatan, Hut 1: Anatomical distribution of bones.

| ANATOMY | SEAL | LARGE UNGULATE | BIRD | TOTAL |
|---|---|---|---|---|
| Cranium | | | | 2 |
| V caud | 2 | | | 2 |
| McV | 1 | | | 1 |
| Coxae | 3 | | | 3 |
| Talus? | | 2 | | 2 |
| Mt | 1 | | | 1 |
| Ph1 post | 1 | | | 1 |
| Ossa I | | | 2 | 2 |
| Total | 8 | 2 | 2 | 12 |

*Osteological Material*
Seal bone (*Phoca* sp.) dominated and included parts of the vertebrae, backbone, front and rear flippers and fragments that probably derived from the skull. One foot bone (a talus) from the rear flipper of an adult seal, two large ungulate heel bones (cow, moose, or reindeer), and two bird bones (*Aves* sp.) were also found. 336 bone fragments could not be identified.

*Macrofossil Analysis*
Seven seeds were identified, four of which were berries, and one of *chenopodium*, an edible plant. Their presence in the hearth suggest summer or fall. Crowberry and blueberry seeds were also found in the Hut 2 hearth (below).

Table 10. Grundskatan, Hut 1: Macrofossils.

| | CARBONIZED | NON-CARBONIZED |
|---|---|---|
| *Chenopodium* (goosefoot) | 1 | |
| *Stellearia graminea* (lesser stitchwort) | | 2 |
| *Rubus idaeus* (raspberry) | 1 | |
| *Arctostaphylos iva-ursi* (bearberry) | 1 | 4 |
| *Empetrum* (crowberry) | | 2 |
| *Picea* (spruce) | | 1 |
| *Vaccinium* (blueberry) | | 3 |

***Feature 2, Hut***
Feature 2 consists of a totally overgrown hut with a floor area measuring 4.0 × 4.0 m. Its elevation is 16 m above sea level (Figure 71). This hut is one in a row of three huts on the opposite end of the point and facing west. Two inwardly curving cobble walls 0.5 to 1.0 m in width give the hut a horseshoe shape with a southwesterly facing entrance. These structures had also been built up against a beach ridge. The floor is a natural pebble surface that had been cleared of larger stones. An area of ashy

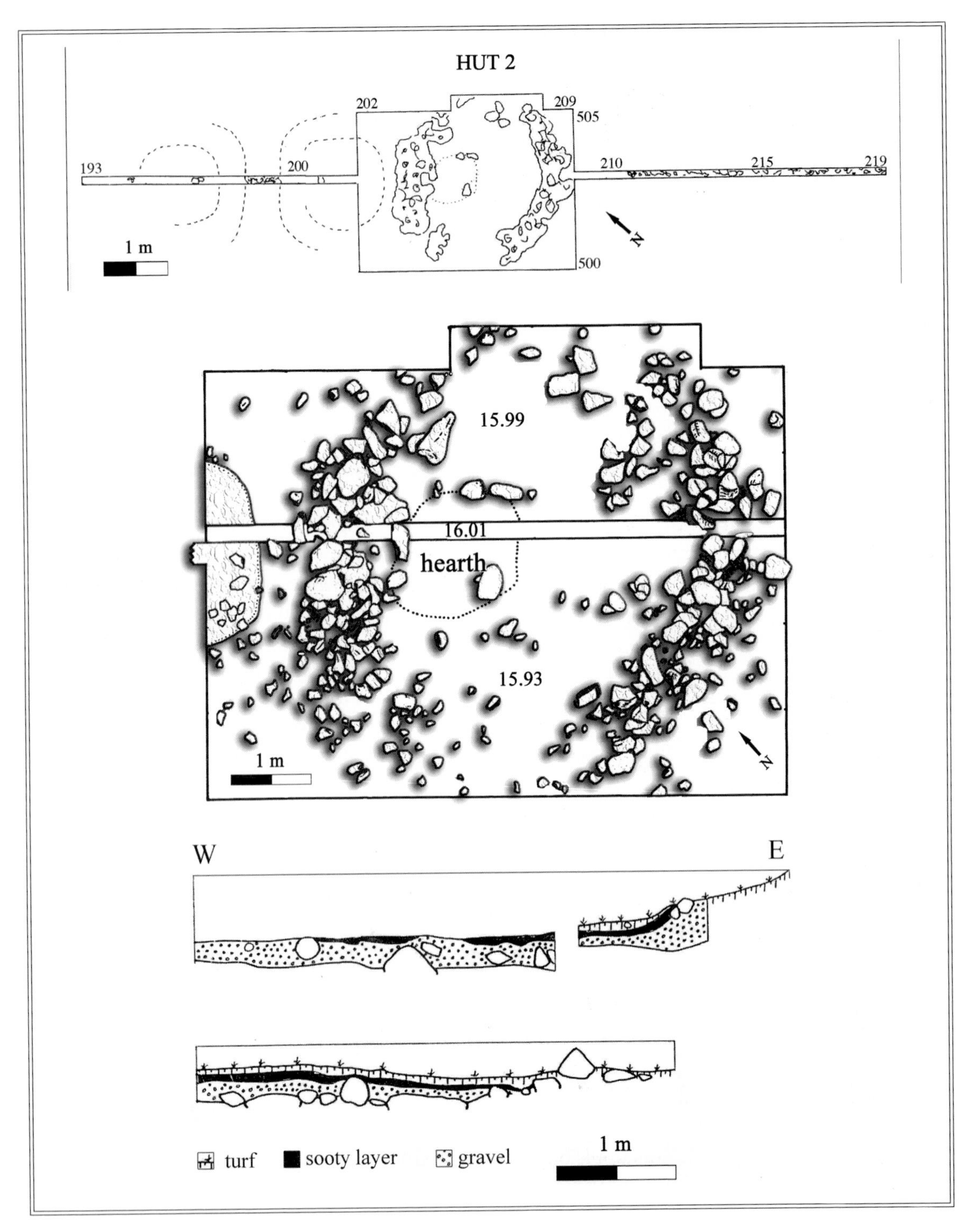


*Figure 71. Maps and profiles of Hut 2.*

soil measuring 1.7 m in diameter lay midway between the rear of the hut and its entranceway. Two additional floor depressions of approximately the same size lie parallel to the hut. Not enough un-

Table 11. Grundskatan, Hut 2: Macrofossils.

| | CARBONIZED | NON-CARBONIZED |
|---|---|---|
| *Arctostaphylos iva-ursi* (bearberry) | 1 | 3 |
| *Vaccinium* (blueberry) | | 3 |

contaminated charcoal was obtained for a date, but the form suggests these huts were contemporary with Hut 1.

*Macrofossil Analysis.*
Two types of berries were flotated from the hearth: bearberry and blueberry.

***Feature 3, Hut***
Feature 3 lies on level ground at ca. 16 m above sea level. It is a rounded rectangular cobble foundation with an outer measurement of 7 × 7 m and a floor area of 4 × 4 m (Figure 72). The foundation is 1.0 to 2.0 meters wide and up to 30 cm in height. The hut has a clearly marked entranceway in

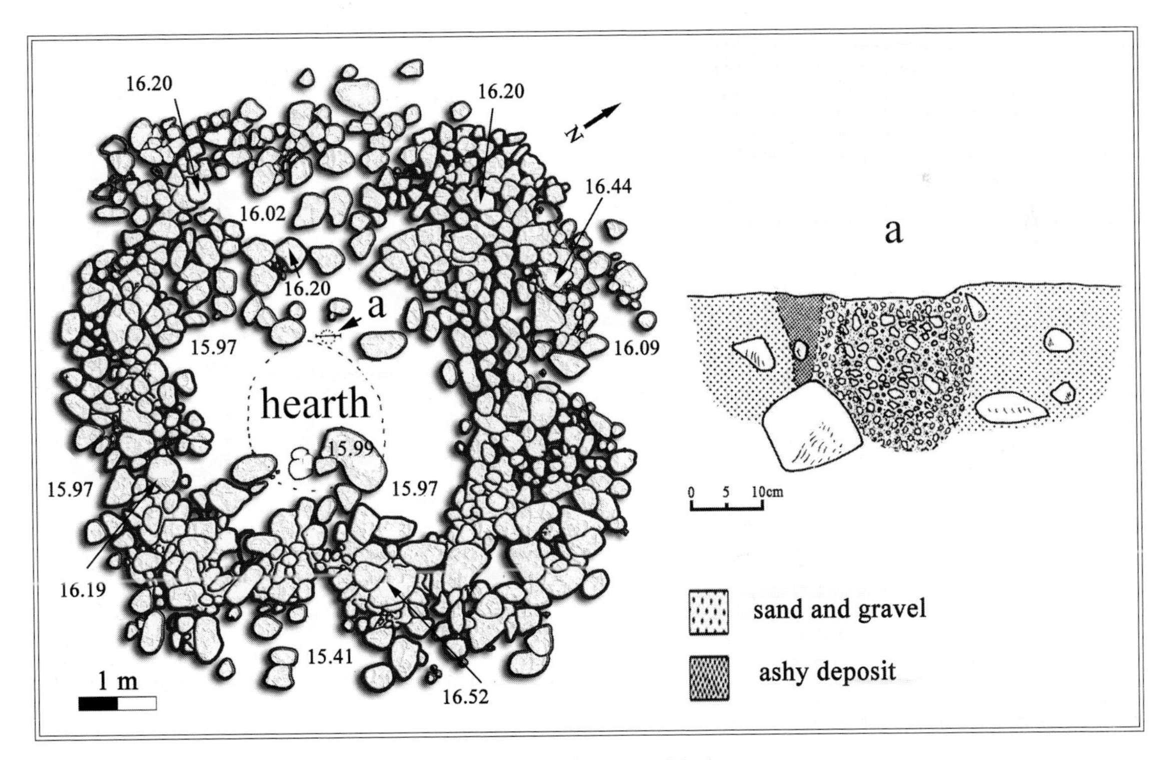


*Figure 72. Map of Hut 3 with section of a small posthole near the center of the hut.*

the southeast wall. At the rear of the hut is a 2.0 to 3.0 meter wide and relatively level layer of stones that may have supported a platform. The hearth lies in the center of the main floor in front of this platform as an irregular burned surface measuring 1.4 × 1.6 m. These deposits were 1 to 6 cm in thickness. There were no stones around the hearth, but several large stones look like they might have served as seats or served as "tables." One possible posthole was found between the hearth and the platform foundation, but was not large enough to have been a roof support.

*Finds*

Two white calcified flint chips (less than 5 mm)
One pebble (whetstone?)
23 pieces of iron slag (1-30 mm), 80 g.

Table 12. Grundskatan, Hut 3: Bones (fragments).

| SPECIES | HEARTH | FLOOR | TOTAL |
|---|---|---|---|
| Ringed seal | 1 | 4 | 5 |
| Seal | 65 | 64 | 129 |
| Hare | | 1 | 1 |
| Bird | | 1 | 1 |
| Indeterminate | 327 | 65 | 392 |
| Total | 393 | 135 | 528 |

*Osteological Material*

More than 500 fragments of burned bone were found in the hearth and on the floor that derived from ringed seal (*Phoca hispida*), seal (*Phoca* sp.) and hare (*Lepus* sp.). All of the skull bones were found on the floor together with most of the bones from the front flippers. Other bones from the front flippers and rear flippers, wrist, etc. were from the hearth.

*Chronology*

Two radiocarbon dates were obtained from the hearth: 1500±100 B.P. (St. 11907) and 1205±70 B.P. (St. 11906). The calibrated dates are: A.D. cal. 435–643, 695–894.

*Charcoal*

*Pinus* sp. (pine)

Table 13. Grundskatan, Hut 3: Anatomical representation for ringed- and indeterminate seals on the floor and in the hearth, burned bones (fragments).

| ELEMENT | HEARTH | FLOOR | TOTAL |
|---|---|---|---|
| Cranium | 1 | 28 | 29 |
| Dentes | | 1 | 1 |
| V caud | 1 | 1 | 2 |
| Costae | | 3 | 3 |
| Radius | 1 | | 1 |
| Cr+i | 1 | 3 | 4 |
| C2 | 1 | | 1 |
| C3 | | 1 | 1 |
| McI | 2 | | 2 |
| McII | 1 | | 1 |
| McIV | 1 | | 1 |
| Mc | 6 | | 6 |
| Ph1 ant | 7 | 2 | 9 |
| Ph2 ant | | 11 | 11 |
| Ph3 ant | | 8 | 8 |
| Fibula | 1 | | 1 |
| Calcaneus | | 1 | 1 |
| MtI | 1 | | 1 |
| MtII | | 1 | 1 |
| Mt | 2 | 1 | 3 |
| Mp | | 2 | 2 |
| Ph1 post | 20 | 3 | 23 |
| Ph2 post | 5 | | 5 |
| Ph3 post | 5 | 2 | 7 |
| Ph post | 9 | | 9 |
| Sesamoidea | 1 | | 1 |
| Total | 66 | 68 | 134 |

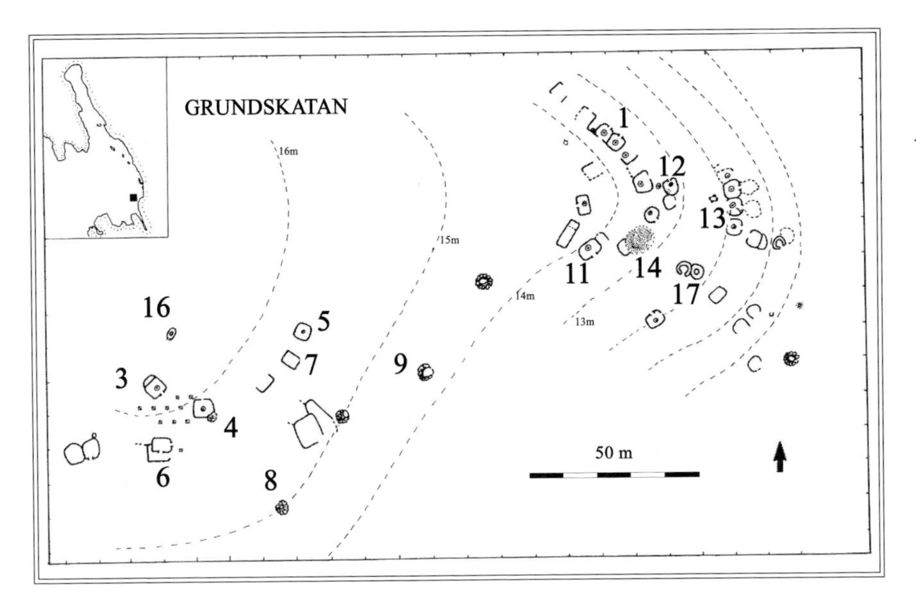


*Figure 73. Map of the central area of the Grundskatan site with feature numbers.*

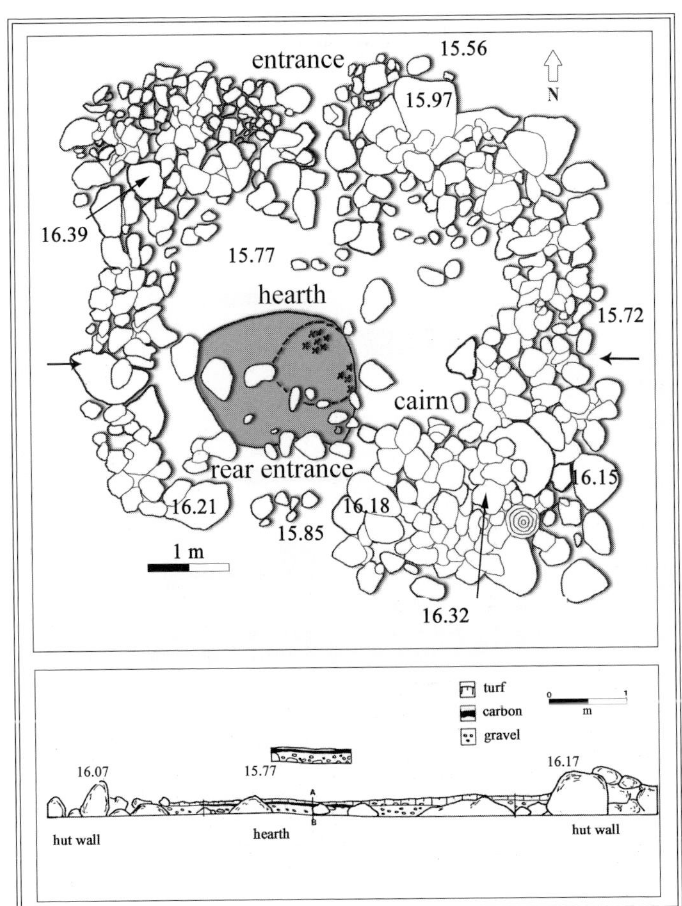


*Figure 74. Map and profile of Hut 4.*

### *Feature 4, Hut (Bear Burial)*

Hut 4 is situated at ca. 16 m above sea level and clusters together with three nearby dwellings and other foundations at the same elevation (Figures 73, 74). The outside measurements are 7.7 × 7.0 m and the floor area measures 4.0 × 3.0 m. The cobble walls average 1.0 m in width and 0.30–0.50 m in height. A ca. 1 m wide entranceway is observable in the north wall of the structure. A second opening is on the opposite (south) wall, but is more irregular and was probably disturbed when a cairn was constructed in the southeast corner of the dwelling. A 1.0 m diameter central hearth and an irregular area of sooty soil that could have been the result of secondary use were exposed on the floor. This hearth was not delimited by stones, although several large stones were found beside it. As will be described in more detail regarding the bear burial, the cairn that had been built directly on the floor had probably made the hut uninhabitable.

*Chronology*

Charcoal was obtained from the hearth and rendered a radiocarbon date: 1110±110 B.P. (A.D. cal. 780–1020) (St. 10785). A small indeterminate bone fragment found in a charcoal sample from the floor was AMS-dated. It proved to be older than the hearth, 1500±40 B.P. (A.D. 536–621) (Beta-210236), and was contemporary with Hut 3. Soils from under the walls of Hut 4 showed phosphorus enrichment in conjunction with several fire-cracked rocks, indicating the existence of cultural deposits that predated this hut foundation. Test pits between Huts 3, 6 and 4 also produced fire-cracked rocks. Hut 3 was thus both partly older than and contemporary with Hut 4. Two charcoal samples that had been collected in 1987 were dated in 2006: (Beta-196486) 190±40 B.P. and (Beta 196487) 420±B.P, but were almost certainly contaminated.

Table 14. Grundskatan, Hut 4: Identified species based on numbers of fragments (NISP) and weights (g) for burned bones in hearth.

| SPECIES | NISP | WEIGHT (G) |
|---|---|---|
| Ringed seal | 3 | 1.52 |
| Seal | 42 | 20.37 |
| Bird | 2 | 0.05 |
| Indeterminate | 338 | 38.8 |
| Total | 385 | 60.74 |

*Osteological Material*

Burned bones from the hearth (385 fragments) weighing 60.74 g were identified as ringed seal (*Phoca hispida*), seal (*Phoca* sp.) and bird (*Aves* sp.).

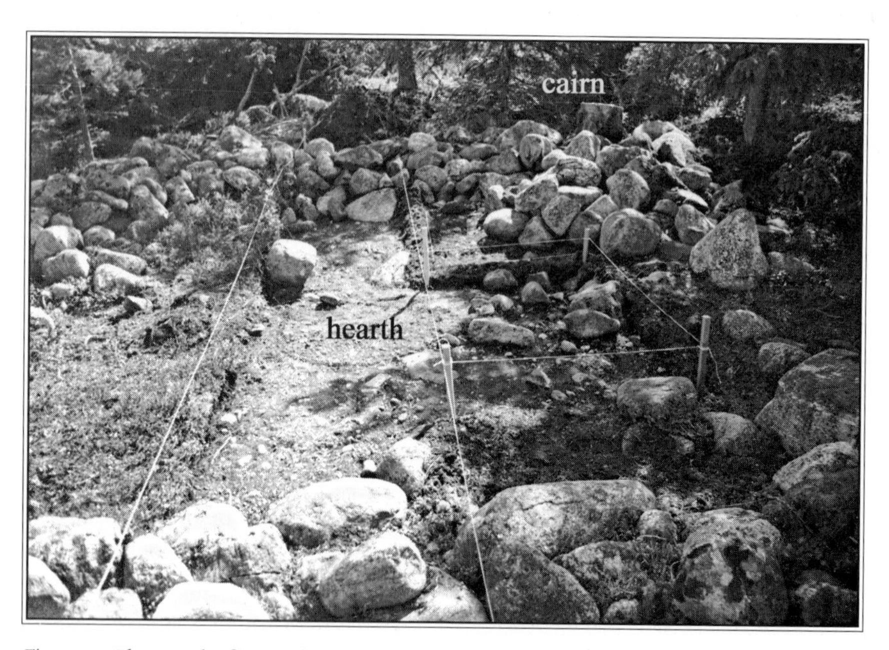


*Figure 75. Photograph of Hut 4 during excavation. View from west.*

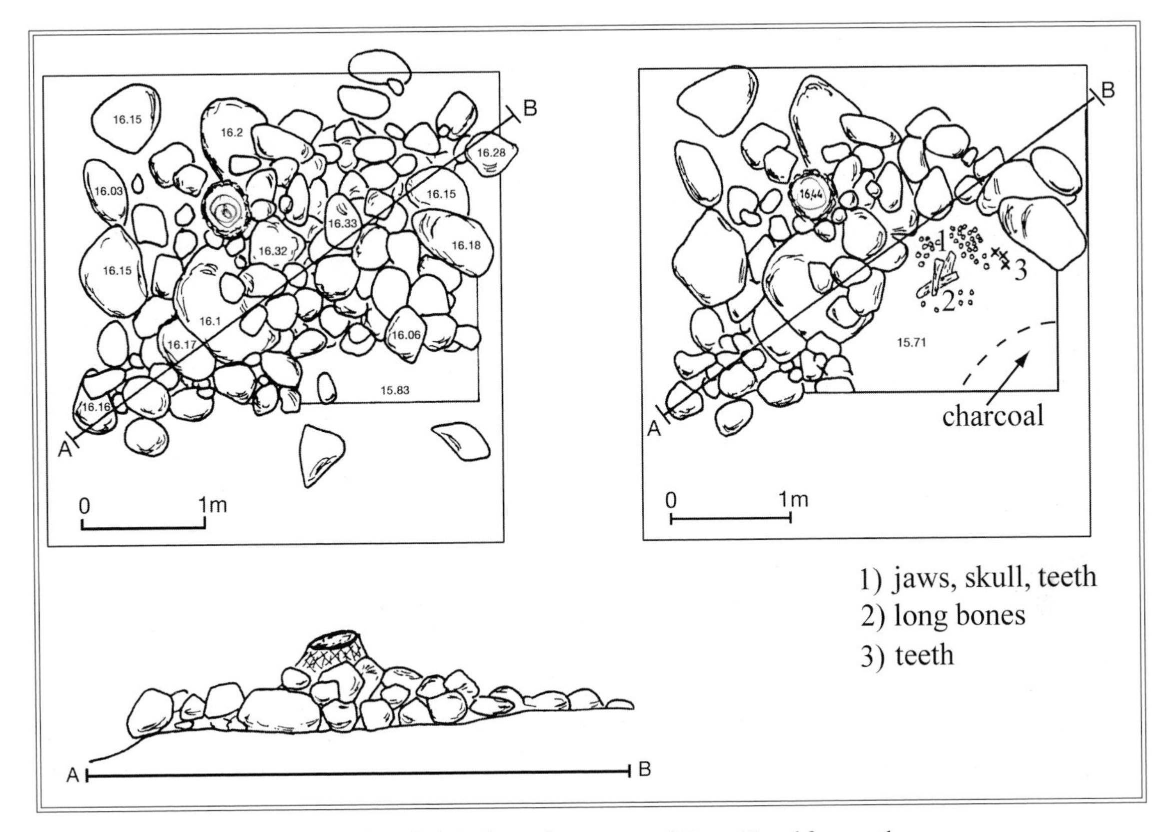


*Figure 76. Map of the cairn and bear bone finds in the southeast corner of Hut 4. Viewed from north.*

*A Cairn*

A trench was opened across the floor across the hearth and expanded to encompass the cairn (Figures 75, 76). The cairn measured ca. 3×3 m and was ca. 15 cm higher than the foundation. It was sectioned and excavated down to sterile gravel. A concentration of bones within an area of ca. 1.0×0.5 m was exposed directly beneath the cairn stones in the southeast corner of the hut. The

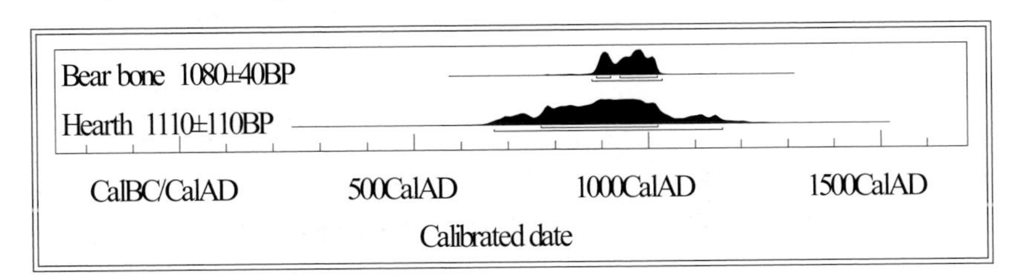


*Figure 77. Calibrated dates of the hearth and bear bones in Hut 4.*

bones were concentrated in a 10 cm thick layer between 15.71 and 15.74 m above sea level. This was approximately 10 cm below the former ground surface. At that time of discovery, the appearance of these bones was so dissimilar to the bones in the hearth, they were judged as being unrelated. They

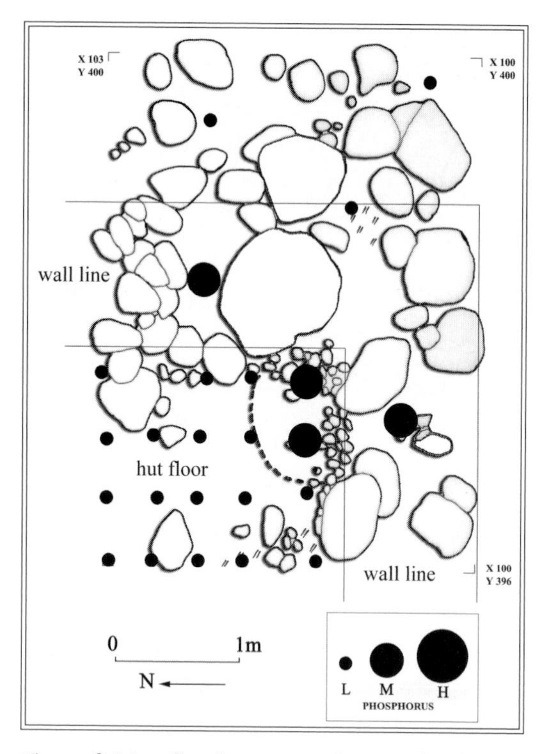


*Figure 78. Map of southeast corner of Hut 4. Phosphorus enrichment in the area of the bear bone deposition and under the hut walls. Fire-cracked stones were also found under the walls indicating an older settlement surface.*

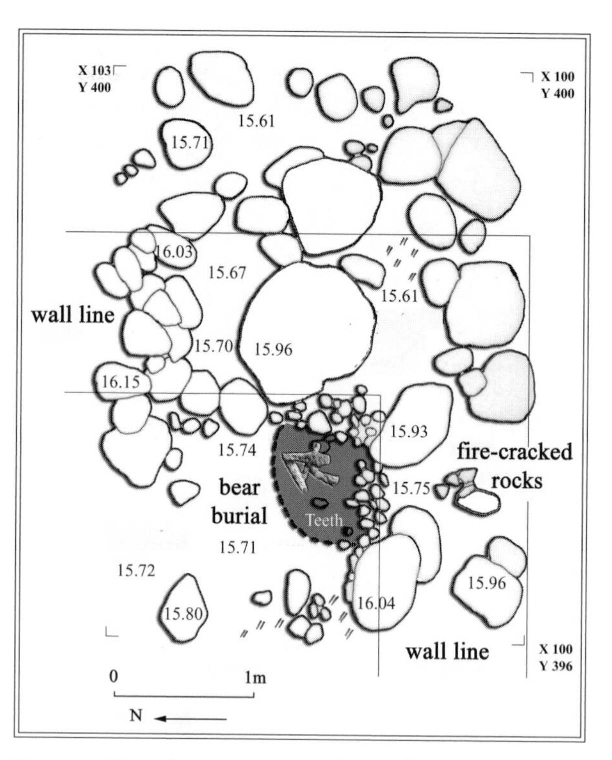


*Figure 79. Map of southeast corner of Hut 4 showing location of bear bone deposition.*

were subsequently AMS-dated to: 1080±45 B.P. (Ua-18930), indicating that the bear bones were contemporary with the hearth. This date calibrates to A.D. cal. 898–1014. Their median values are: A.D. cal. 912 and A.D. cal. 958.

Phosphorus sampling was undertaken in 2005 to additionally delineate the bone deposition. The La Motte system is based on a colorimetric scale indicating "Low," "Medium" or "High" levels of soil enrichment. Based on comparisons with previously analyzed phosphate samples on the site by Johan Linderholm (Broadbent 1987b:57), "Low" phosphorus levels correspond to 0–90 P°, "Medium" to 100–150 P° and "High" to >150 P°. The off-site values for the site were low using both methods. The highest measured phosphate enrichment on the site was 209 P° and the average for the huts was 108 P°. A sample from the southwest corner of Hut 4 measured 119 P°. The La Motte readings from Hut 4 are uniformly low except for two samples from the exact area where the bear bones had been lying when excavated in 1987 and in two samples from adjacent areas under the walls of the hut (Figures 78, 79, 80). This simple field test has thus rendered consistent information regarding the location of the bone deposition in the hut and has also confirmed that there had been an earlier occupation surface. The whole cairn was subsequently excavated and a tree stump in the foundation was removed. Although the tree had disturbed the outer part of the

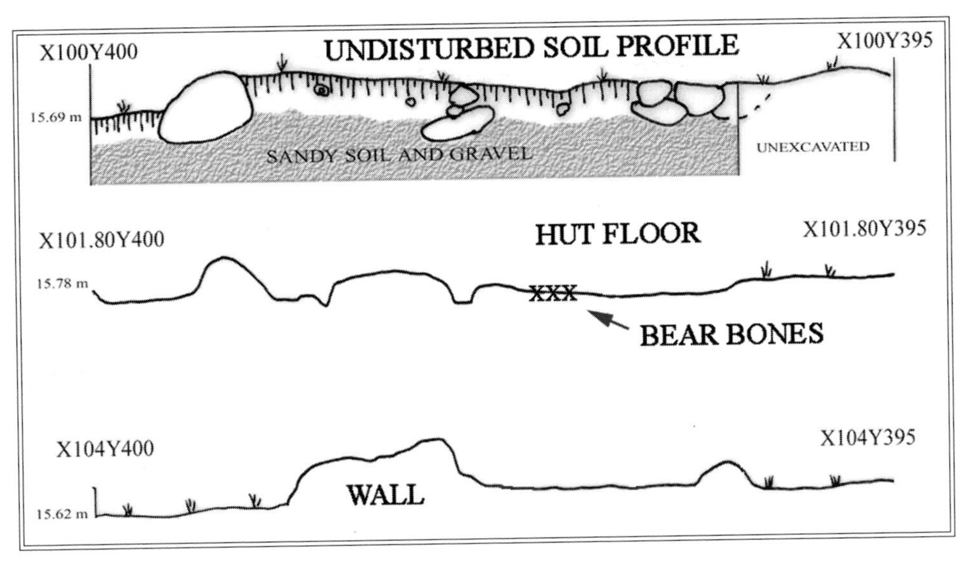


*Figure 80. Three profiles through Hut 4.*

cairn and foundation, the boulders that had been incorporated into the construction prevented any disturbance inside of the dwelling. The cairn was therefore mostly intact, as was the integrity of the bone find.

*Bear Bones*

A total of 66 bones weighing 949 g were found, of which 275 g could be identified as to skeletal element. The morphology and structure of the bone fragments indicate that they originated from the same individual. Judging from the sizes of the largest bones and the thickness of the cortex of the long bone fragments, they derived from an adult bear. Phosphorus enrichment was noted in this corner, as compared with the rest of the hut floor, and this localized buffering of soil acidity probably helped preserve the bones. The soils are otherwise quite acidic with pH values of 4.9 to 5.2. The bones lay in three separate piles surrounded by scattered fragments. In one pile lay parts of the cranium, both halves of the lower jaw, a few fragments of teeth and numerous small fragments of long bones. The second pile consisted of three larger long bones, and a third pile consisted of tooth fragments. There were no phalanges. Some of the bones were partly charred, dark colored and heavily fragmented. The tooth fragments also exhibit traces of heating (charring and discoloring) and the crowns had been broken due to heat. It is clear from the excavation that the bones had not been burned at the place of deposition.

Table 15. Bear (*Ursus arctos*) bones by weight (g).

| SPECIES | TOTAL |
|---|---|
| Bear | 275.4 |
| Indeterminate | 673.68 |
| Total | 949.08 |

*Bones and Teeth*

Although no skeletal elements lay in correct anatomical position, the deposition was not without structured elements. Most bone fragments had been placed without any specific order in the largest heap, but some larger leg bones, 2 tibia

Table 16. Bear bones by fragment.

| SPECIES | NO. FRAGMENTS | WEIGHT (G) |
|---|---|---|
| Bear | 66 | 275.40 |
| Indeterminate | 6* | 673.68 |
| Total | 72 | 949.08 |

*all indeterminate fragments not counted

Table 17. Bear bones by anatomy.

| ANATOMY | TOTAL |
|---|---|
| Mandibula | 5 |
| Dentes | 50 |
| Humerus | 1 |
| Radius | 1 |
| Ulna | 1 |
| Tibia | 2 |
| Long bone fragments | 6 |
| Total | 66 |

fragments, a radius, an ulna and a larger indeterminate fragment of a long bone, had been placed next to each other in a separate pile. A number of tooth fragments had been placed in a third concentration. There had been a conscious sorting of the bones. Marks on the bones provide some insights into how the bear carcass had been handled prior to burial. The radius and the ulna exhibit fresh fracture patterns, indicating that they had been broken or cracked shortly after the death of the bear when the carcass was in a fresh state. One of the charred fragments exhibits cut marks that show that the carcass had been slaughtered and severed prior to burning.

*Charcoal*
(From sooty deposits by the bear bones)
Yew (*Taxus* sp.)
Heather (*Erica* sp.)
Birch/Alder (*Betulaceae*)
Angiosperms (>13 small twigs)
Conifers (5 small twigs and wood remains).

The charcoal analysis from the area of the bear grave has produced some unexpected results. While most of the identified plants are typical of the area, the find of yew is totally out of its normal range. Yew grows in southern Sweden and this find could suggest that it had been part of a bow or had ritual meaning (refer to Chapter 8).

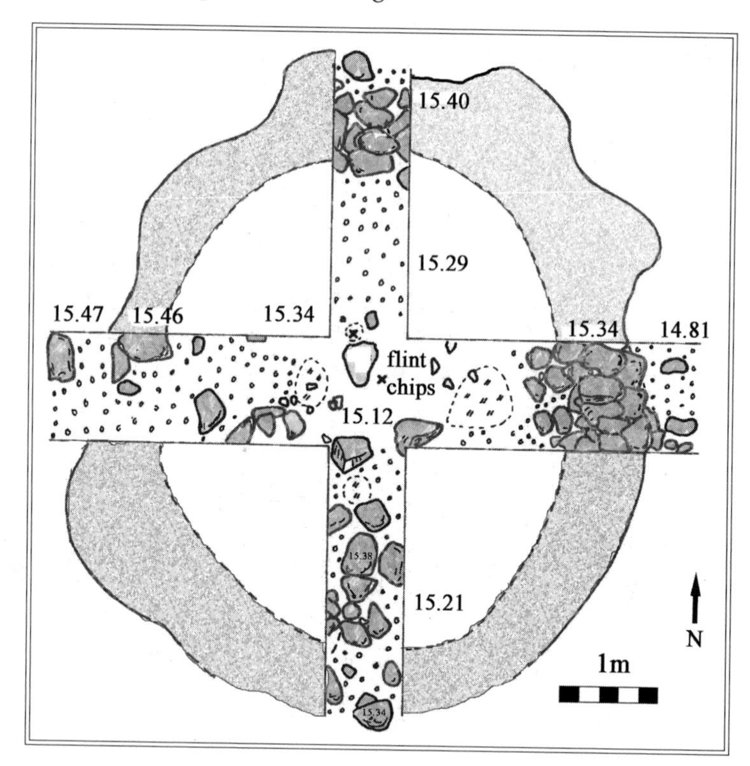


*Figure 81. Map of Hut 5.*

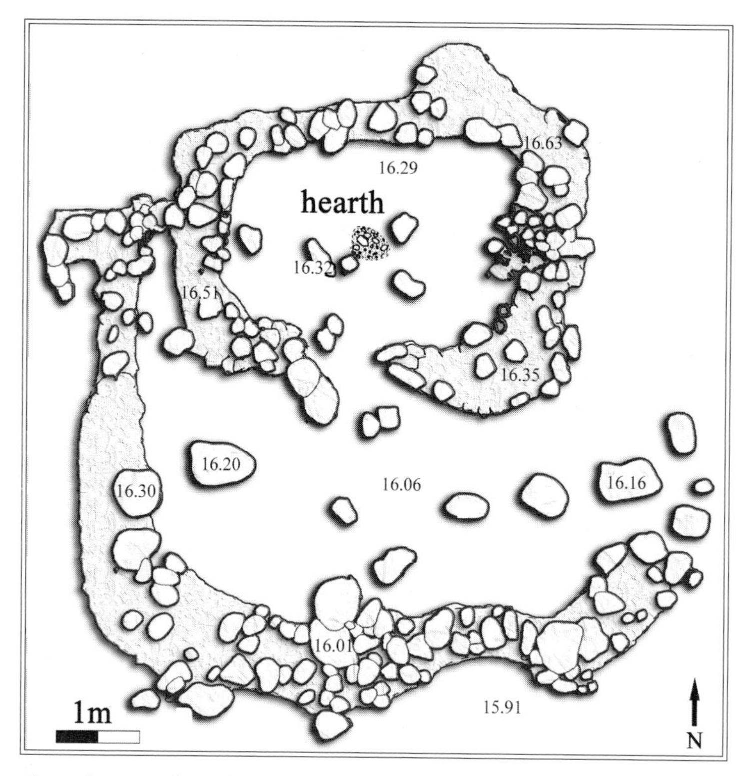


Figure 82. Map of Hut 6.

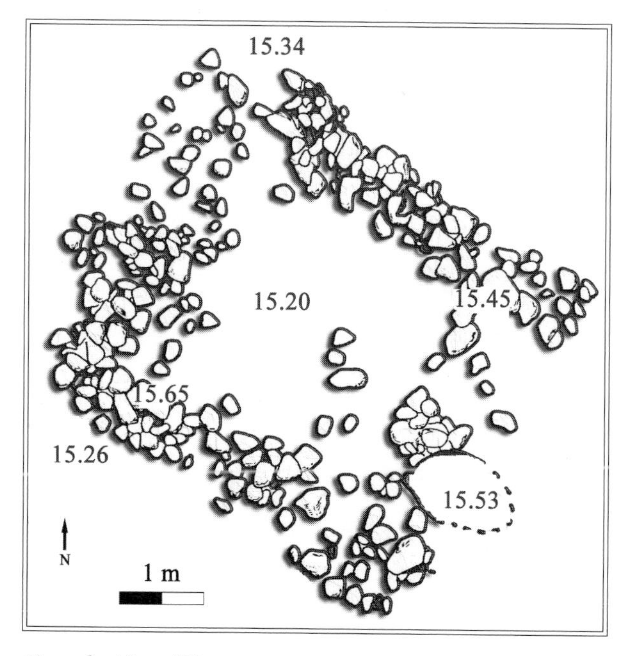


Figure 83. Map of Hut 7.

***Feature 5, Hut***

This oval hut was previously unregistered. It lies between 15–16 m above sea level and was built up against a beach ridge (Figure 81). It is one of three structures along the same beach ridge and probably belongs to the same complex of dwellings. It measures 5 × 6 m with a floor area of 4 × 4 m. Ashy deposits indicate a hearth area, but no bones or charcoal samples were obtained.

*Finds*

2 gray flint chips

***Feature 6, Hut***

This dwelling lies 10 m south of Huts 3 and 4. It consists of a rectangular foundation measuring 6 × 5 m with a floor area of 4.5 × 3 m (Figure 82). There is an opening toward the south, that was probably an entranceway, but there was possibly a second entranceway on the eastern short end of the dwelling. There was a small central hearth but there were no intact deposits. A large wall extension runs out of and parallel to the west wall of the dwelling, extending 4 m, and then running parallel with the southern wall for 8 m. This construction is interpreted as an addition to the dwelling, possibly a covered shed or porch. The wall also extends toward the west and could also be part of a stone alignment.

***Feature 7, Hut***

This foundation is located 5 m SSW of Hut 5 and on the same beach ridge. It measures 4.5 × 5 m with a floor area of 4 × 4 m

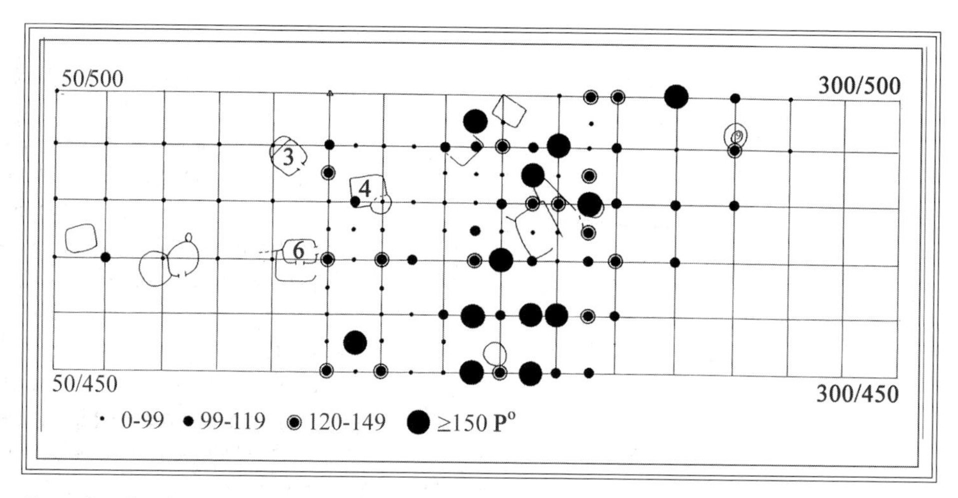


*Figure 84. Phosphate map showing enrichment to the southeast of the huts and near stone alignments.*

(Figure 83). There was no hearth but an entranceway toward the SE. It is probably the foundation of a storage shed.

***Phosphate Mapping***

Fifty-three phosphate samples were taken at 10 m intervals in an area of 50 × 150 m (7500 m²) (Figure 84). These were analyzed using standard laboratory methods. The samples showed some enrichment in the area between Huts 3, 4 and 6 but displayed the greatest concentrations to the east and south of the dwellings in a 25 m wide band that runs from the area of Feature 8 (a cairn), and around several stone alignments 20 m to the east of Hut 3. This pattern indicates organic enrichment near the cairns and what may possibly have been a livestock enclosure area. Finds of sheep/goat and other ungulate bones at five hut sites show that animal husbandry was indeed practiced by these seal hunters. Manure would create phosphate concentrations such as those seen at this site (greater than 150 P°) (cf. Aronsson 1991). What is curious about this enrichment is that it is not *inside* a potential enclosure, but around it. This could mean that if a fence had

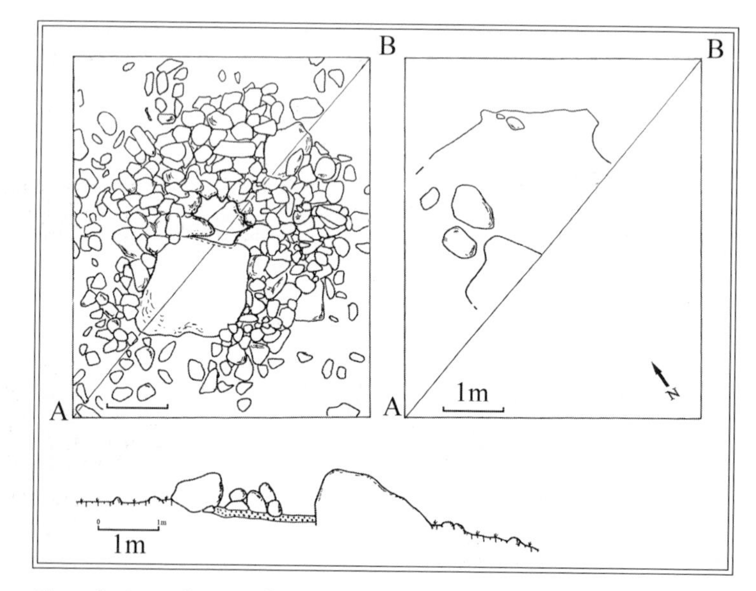


*Figure 85. Map of Feature 8.*

been supported by these stones it was intended to keep animals out, not in. This could thus have been a temporary holding pen used for marking or milking, or was perhaps a small garden plot.

### *Feature 8, Cairn*

This cairn is one of three that extend in a line to the north of Huts 3–7. The cairn measures ca. 3.5 × 3 m, is ca. 50 cm in height, and has a central chamber measuring 1 × 0.5 m (Figure 85). The opening is well constructed rather than the result of plundering. There were no finds of burned bones or charcoal. The feature is interpreted as a cache.

### *Feature 9, Cairn*

This cairn is almost identical to Feature 8. It measures 4 by 4 m and was built of cobbles and larger stones around a boulder (Figure 86). The height of the cairn is 50 cm and its central pit measures 60 by 85 cm. There were no traces of carbon, bone, or other organic residues. It is interpreted as a cache.

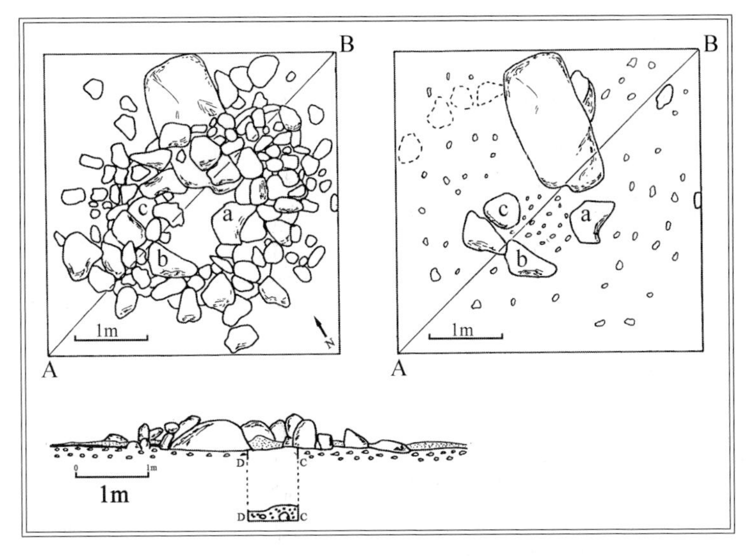


*Figure 86. Map of Feature 9.*

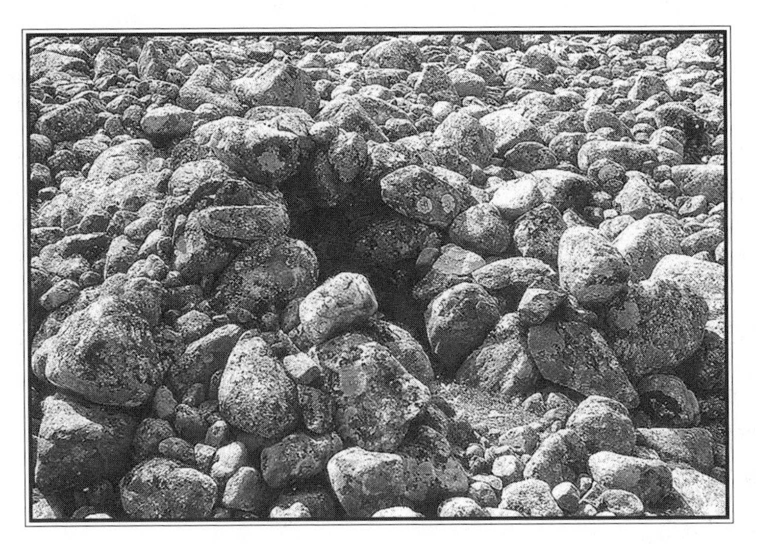

*Figure 87. Photo of Russian Oven (Feature 10) at Grundskatan.*

### *Feature 10, Baking Oven ("Russian" Oven)*

A distinctive oven with thick charcoal deposits lies at ca. 10 m above sea level and off to the side of the main site area (Figure 87). The soil was flotated, but revealed little except charcoal. The radiocarbon date (St. 10785) indicates an age of less than 250 years, which would be the 1700s, a period of Russian invasions in Västerbotten. There are two similar ovens near Site 67, but these were not dated. Two radiocarbon dates were obtained from an oven on Snöan Island, however, both indicating the fifteenth century, Site 92. This means that although these features were probably used for baking, they were not all associated with the Russian period.

***Feature 11, Hut***

Feature 11 is a rectangular hut foundation measuring ca. 7 × 5 m (Figure 88). The elevation above sea level is 14.0 m. The walls of the hut measure 1.0 m in width and 0.3 m in height. The floor measures 5.0 × 3.5 m. A 2 m wide entrance opens toward the southeast. A third parallel cobble wall forms a small additional room. This wall is 4.5 m long and 1.0 m wide. Another narrow rectangular foundation, possibly a storage shed, lies several meters behind Hut 11. Hearth deposits were found just beneath the humus and extended 10–20 cm below the surface, and somewhat off-center toward the back wall. Unfortunately, a tree had grown in the hearth area and several large roots had penetrated the deposits.

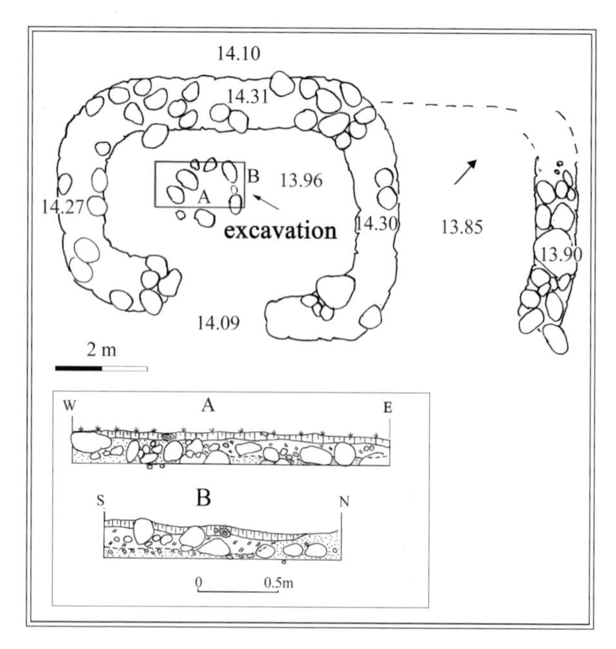


*Figure 88. Map of Hut 11 and profiles through the hearth area.*

*Finds*
300 g of iron slag

The find material consists of both homogeneous slag and slag with melted stones, red-burned clay and rusted iron. A technical analysis was performed by Grandin et al. (2005). The slag includes varying proportions of *wüstite*, olivine and glass flux. Fine-grained magnetite was also observed. Drops of metallic iron indicate that the iron content had been high. There had also been a good supply of oxygen. The slag derived from forging, and iron scales, the result of hammering, were picked up in the hearth using a magnet. A single radiocarbon date of charcoal (St. 11170) gave an age determination of: 1175± 100 B.P. (A.D cal. 723–972). No animal bones were found.

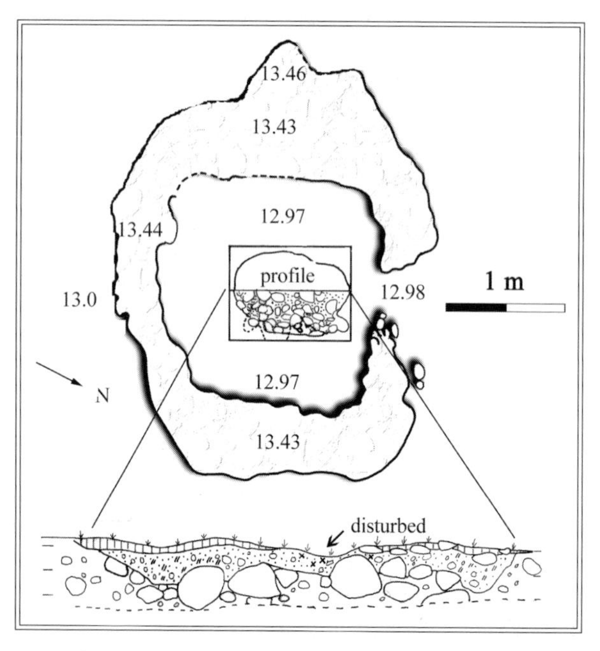


*Figure 89. Map of Hut 12 and profile of the hearth.*

*Charcoal*
*Betula* sp. (birch)
*Pinus* sp. (pine)
Angiosperm
Conifer

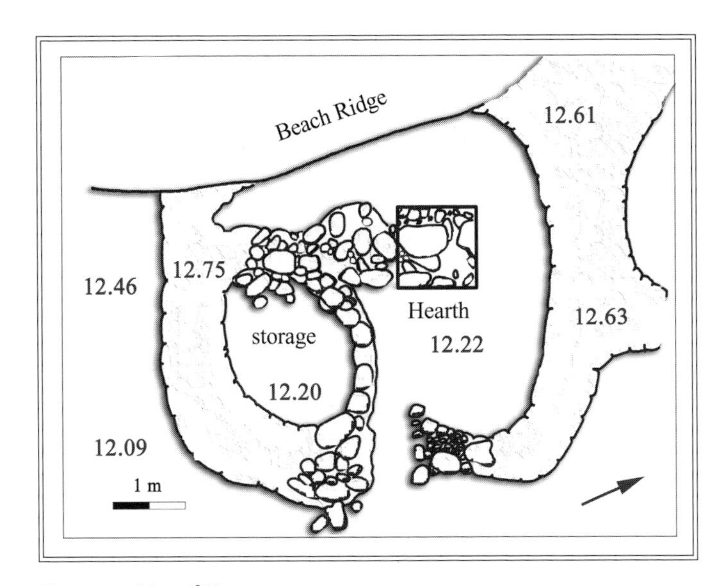


*Figure 90. Map of Hut 13.*

***Feature 12, Hut***
Feature 12 is a horseshoe-shaped hut foundation measuring ca. 8 × 6.5 m. The elevation is 13 m (Figure 89). The floor area measures 3.5 × 3.5 m. A single 1.0 m wide entrance faces north. An oval hearth measuring ca. 1 × 2 m had been partially disturbed. One half of the hearth was excavated and rendered animal bone (17.06 g, 391 fragments) and charcoal.

*Chronology*
One radiocarbon date was obtained: (St. 11171) 1430± 110 B.P. (A.D. cal. 437–760).

*Finds*
None

*Osteological Material*
None of the bones were identifiable.

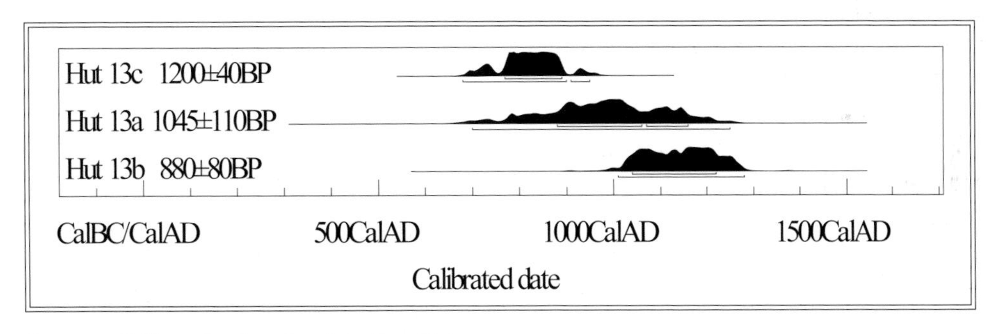


*Figure 91. Calibrated radiocarbon dates from Hut 13.*

***Feature 13, Hut***
Hut 13 lies at ca. 12 m above sea level and had been built up against a beach ridge. It measures 6.5 × 5 m (Figure 90). A well-marked entrance faces east toward the beach. A well-constructed oval chamber occupies almost one half of the floor space, presumably for storage. Hearth deposits were found in the rear of the structure and three carbon samples were collected: (Beta-198488), 1200±40 B.P., (St. 11908), 1045±110 B.P. and (St. 11172) 880±80 B.P. These calibrate respectively to: A.D. cal. 777–884, 880–1155, 1044–1220.

*Artifacts*
None

***Feature 14, Hut and Labyrinth***
Feature 14 is a labyrinth measuring 8 × 9 m. The labyrinth has 10 rows of stones and is situated at approximately 13 m above sea level. The entrance to the labyrinth faces north/northwest. The labyrinth overlies a hut wall measuring 6 m across (Figure 92). The exposed interior of the floor area is 4 m across. A 2 × 1 m trench and a 50 × 50 cm square were excavated across the labyrinth stones in order to expose the hearth beneath it. The hearth deposits extended to 20 cm below surface (Figure 93).

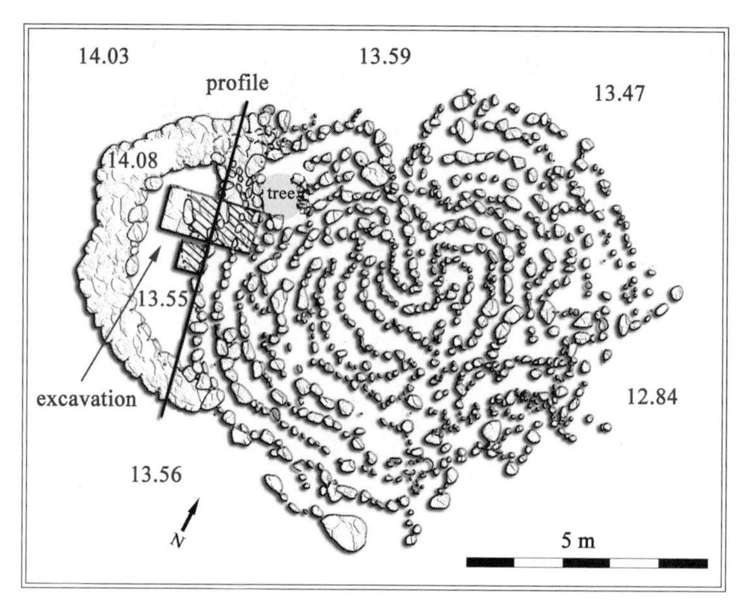


*Figure 92. Map of labyrinth and hut wall at Grundskatan, Feature 14. The labyrinth had been deliberately built on top of the hut and wall stones had been used for its construction.*

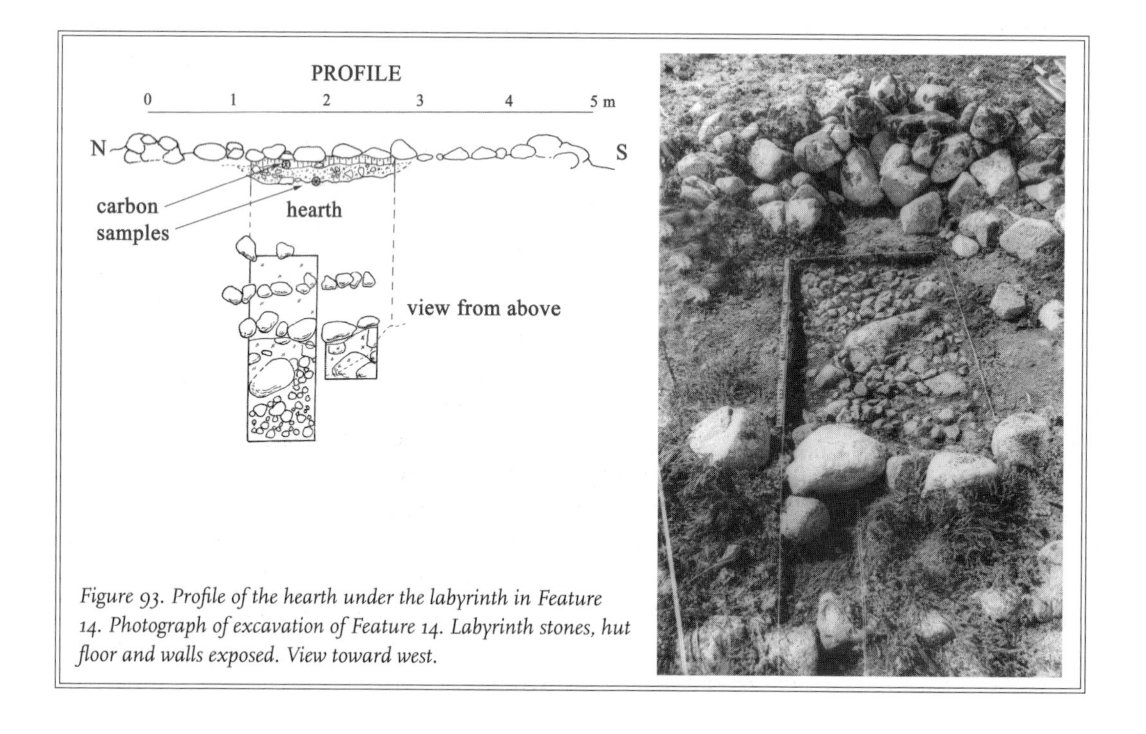


*Figure 93. Profile of the hearth under the labyrinth in Feature 14. Photograph of excavation of Feature 14. Labyrinth stones, hut floor and walls exposed. View toward west.*

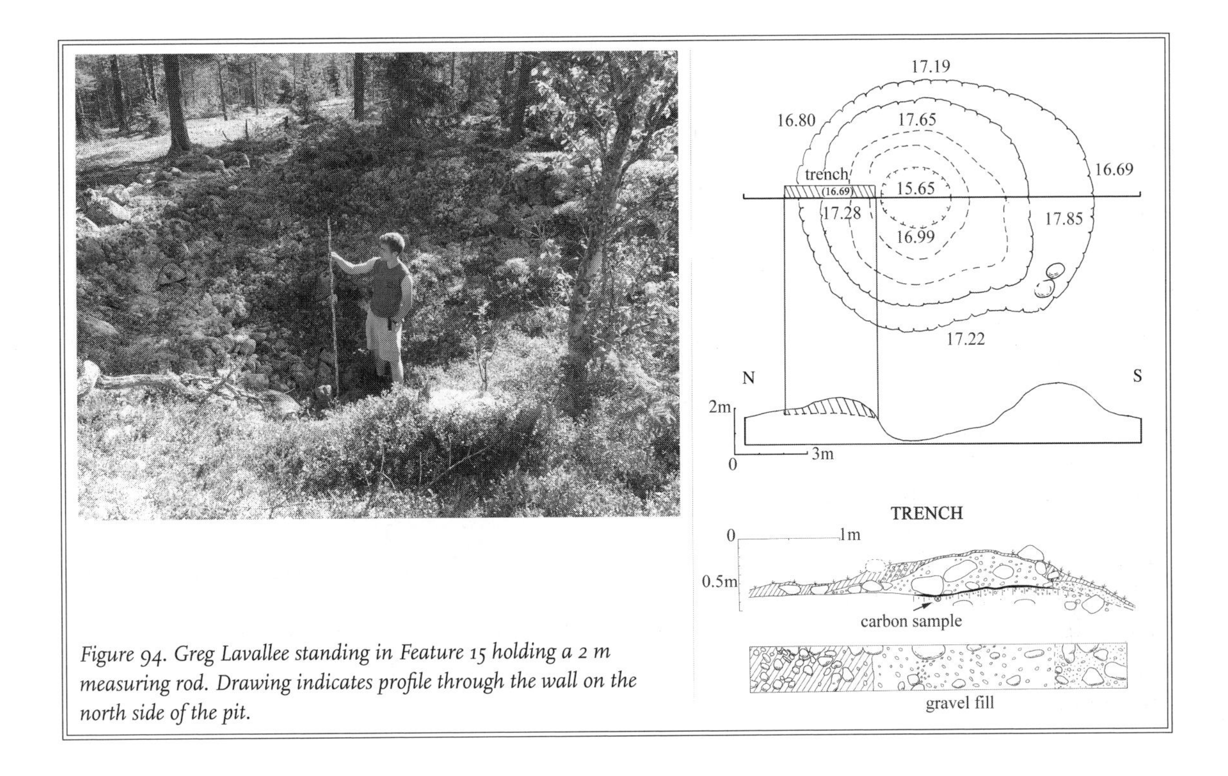


*Figure 94. Greg Lavallee standing in Feature 15 holding a 2 m measuring rod. Drawing indicates profile through the wall on the north side of the pit.*

*Chronology*

This excavation rendered two radiocarbon dates: (St.11173) 1145±100 B.P. (A.D. cal. 776–990) and (St. 11174) 1000±185 B.P. (A.D. cal. 870–1231). This complex feature established the chronological relationship between Iron Age huts and labyrinths in the region. It appears that the stones from the walls were, in fact, used to construct the labyrinth. The hut dates to the same period as the majority of huts at Grundskatan, the Late Iron Age. The labyrinth had a maximum lichen growth of 90–95 mm, giving the feature a minimum age of A.D. 1505 to 1523 ±31, using the formula in Chapter 4.

*Osteological Material*

Some 16.04 g of burned bone (205 fragments) were found in the hearth but were unidentifiable.

***Feature 15, Pit***

Feature 15 is a very large pit measuring 10 by 12 m across and 2.0 m in depth (Figure 94). The pit was dug at the highest level of the drumlin at 17 m above sea level. A surrounding earth wall averages 50 cm in height. A 4 m long and 50 cm wide trench was excavated through the north side of the wall to investigate its construction. The trench extended down to the former ground level where a thin charcoal layer was found. The radiocarbon date for the charcoal layer is: (St. 11175) 670± 245 B.P. (A.D. cal. 1033–1467). The median date is A.D. 1295. An older sample was analyzed in 2006 (Beta-196498), 320±40 B.P. (A.D. cal. 1515–1641), but is probably contaminated as were other improperly stored samples. Although the oldest date has an exceptionally wide range, it does show that the pit can be contemporary with the huts. Approximately half way down the inside of the pit there is a narrow ledge or offset. This suggests there could have been a construction, possibly a floor, at that level. There is no side access to this pit which shows it was not a tar-rendering pit. It is an unlikely place to dig a large solitary hunting pit, and is interpreted as most probably associated with seal oil production during the period A.D. 1033–1500 (1641?).

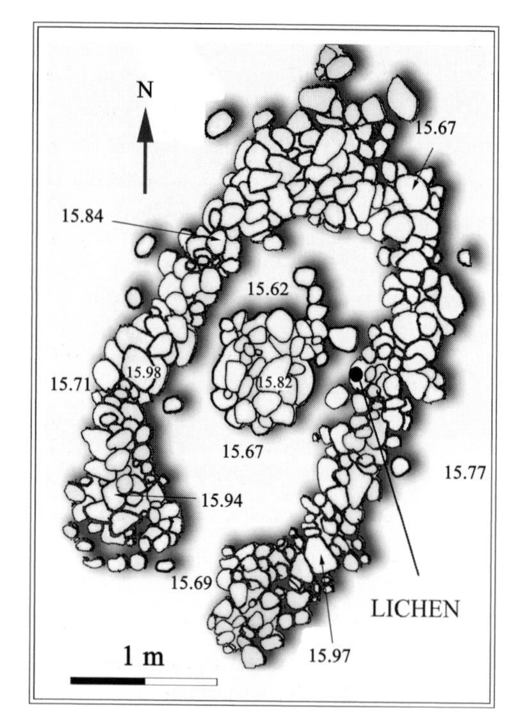


Figure 95. Map of Feature 16.

***Feature 16, Stone Circle***

Feature 16 is a 30 cm high cobble oval located ca. 10 m northwest of Hut 3 (Figure 95). It has a single opening facing south and a small central cairn. It measures 6 m in length and 3 m in width. The central cairn is approximately 80 cm in diameter. This enigmatic construction bears some resemblance to the so-called Jungfrugraven, located less than 2 km away. Its size and proximity to Huts 3–6 suggests it had a ritual function. The elevation above sea level, 16 m, gives it a maximum age of ca. A.D. 400. In 2006, a previously missed 220 mm diameter specimen of *Rhizocarpon geographicum* was discovered by Tim Bayliss-Smith on the inner wall of the construction. The stone with the lichen sat securely wedged in the wall and showed no evidence of having been moved since construction. On the basis of lichen growth curves specifically developed for Bjuröklubb and Grundskatan, this lichen is calculated as being 916 years old and dates to A.D. 1034±31 (with B.P. = 1950), which is almost identical to the radiocarbon- and AMS-datings of the adjacent bear burial and hearth in Hut 4.

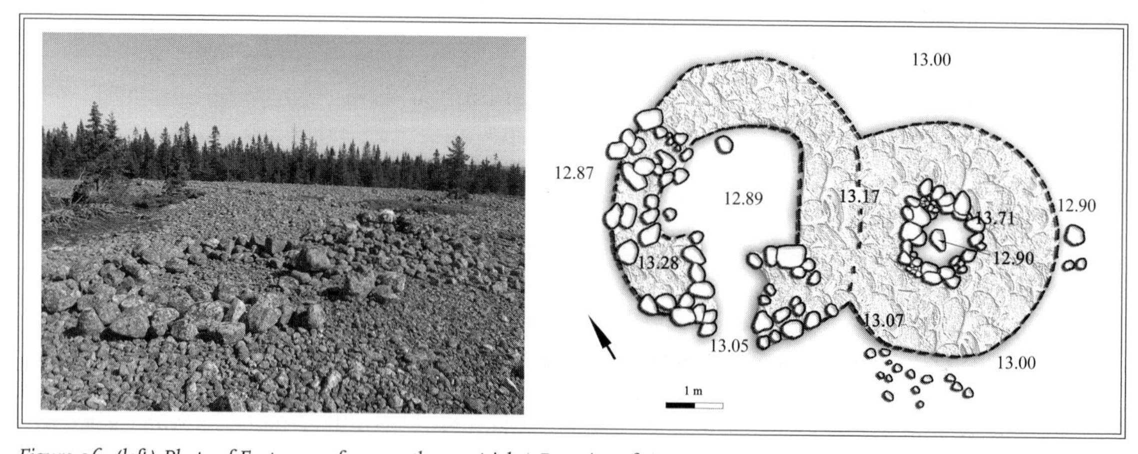


*Figure 96. (left) Photo of Feature 17, from southwest. (right) Drawing of Feature 17.*

*Feature 17, Cache and Hut*

This double feature consists of a 4 m wide cairn with a well-made central chamber about 1.5 m wide and 1 m deep (Figure 96). It lies at the 13 m level and is adjacent to Huts 13 and 14. It is tightly packed with smaller stones. The cairn was built together with a round wall foundation measuring 4.5 by 5 m, with a 2.4 by 2 m floor area, and a 1 m wide entranceway. The floor is level and has no traces of a hearth. A similarly built small hut stands near a cluster of 4 dwellings about 40 m to the east. Feature 17 is interpreted as a livestock (goat or reindeer) hut and a cache.

*Summary*

- Nineteen archaeological features were investigated at Grundskatan: eleven huts, six miscellaneous features (four cairns, a labyrinth and several stone alignments), a large pit and a Russian Oven. There is an assortment of hut forms, including round, rectangular and square shapes, structures with internal storage rooms, platforms and porch-like extensions. These occur in groups and in rows.
- Nine radiocarbon and two AMS dates were obtained from hearths, of which three calibrated with 95% probability to ca. A. D. 330–700. Seven of the dates fall within the eleventh century.
- The three oldest dates were obtained from Huts 3, 4 and 12, and the youngest dates were from Huts 13 and 14. There is a spread within individual hearths indicating multiple occupations. The medians of the 11 dates range between A.D. cal. 542–1019. Three samples had

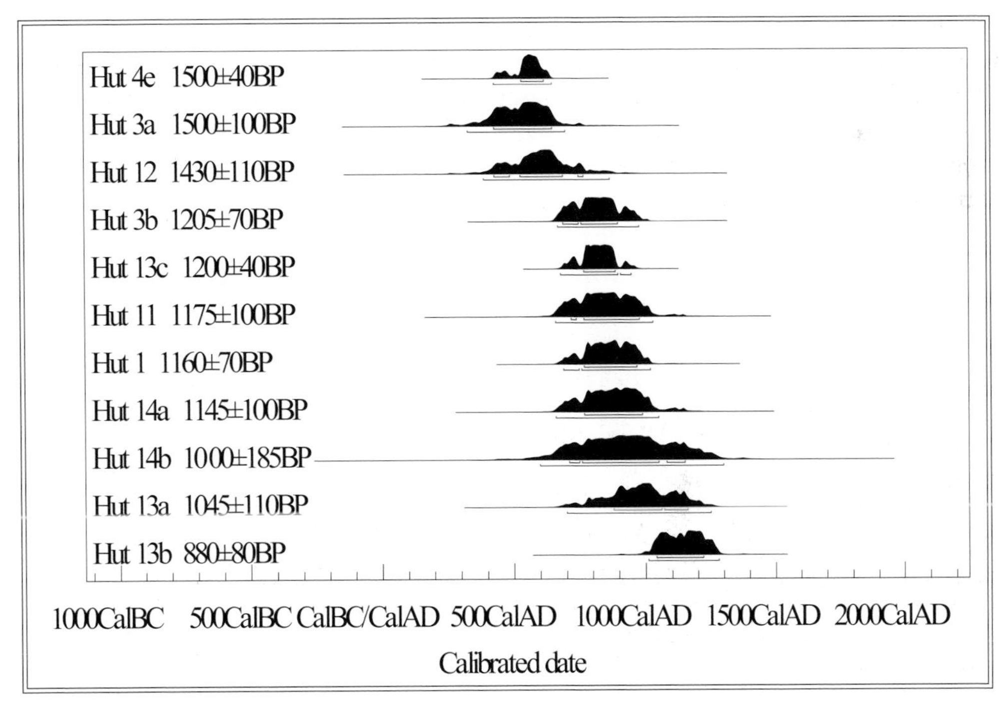


*Figure 97. Radiocarbon dates from the Grundskatan site.*

probably been contaminated by improper storage over fifteen years at room temperatures (Beta-196486, Beta-196487, Beta-196489).

- The date of the large pit (Feature 15) indicates that it was potentially contemporary with the huts.
- The Russian Oven radiocarbon dated to the eighteenth century and there are a number of hunting blinds etc. at lower levels on the beach that are not described here, but are also judged as being of relatively recent date.
- The labyrinth at Grundskatan (Feature 14) lichen dates to the early sixteenth century. This Late Medieval date is most plausible and borne out by other dated labyrinths in the project (Broadbent and Sjöberg 1990), as well as the historic context of Bjuröklubb. Most significant in this particular instance, however, is the fact that there is a stratigraphic association between a sealing hut and a labyrinth. The symbolic meaning of this super-positioning of stone constructions is discussed in Chapter 10.
- A stone circle (Feature 16) was dated using lichenometry to A.D. 1034±31, which is consistent with the dates of the hearth and bear bones in Hut 4. A full discussion of the stone circles is given in Chapter 8 and also in Wennstedt Edvinger and Broadbent (2006).
- Iron working is evidenced by slag in Huts 3 and 11. Hut 11 contained an iron furnace, which is discussed in Chapter 7.
- The most unusual find at Grundskatan is the bear burial in Hut 4, which dates to the eleventh century and the main period of site occupation. A detailed discussion of this find is presented in Chapter 8.
- The bone material from the hearths derives from five huts. There was approximately 700 g of bone, and the identified species or classes of animals were: bear, ringed seal, indeterminate seals, hare, large ungulates (moose/cattle or reindeer), as well as an indeterminate bird.
- The anatomical representation of bones from Hut 3 indicates that a selection of seal parts had been taken to the hut. Of the seal bones from the extremities, both front and rear flippers dominate. Bones from the cranium and backbone are few. Age determination, on the basis of closure of the epiphyses, shows the bones from adult seals dominate. Two phalanges have changes indicative of a high age. The same selection of bones was present in Huts 3 and 4. One long bone fragment of seal has cut marks.
- Macrofossils from Huts 1, 2 and 3 indicate berry harvesting, presumably in the fall, as well as an assortment of other plants.
- Charcoal analysis indicated that pine, birch, alder and rowan were burned. A find of yew from the Hut 4 is very unusual and can be the remains of a bow or relate to Eurasian shamanism (refer to Chapter 8).

## Stora Fjäderägg Island

Stora Fjäderägg Island is located ca. 14 km from the mainland and 3 km northeast of Holmön Island (63° 48′ N, 21° 00′ E). The island is roughly triangular in shape and measures 1.4 km in length and 1.2 km in width. It is the highest and oldest island in the Holmön Island group with an elevation of ca. 22 m (Figure 98). Its vegetation resembles the sub-alpine region with heaths, stunted stands of pine and spruce and exposed moraine and bedrock. Several larger ponds, and its location in the Bay of Bothnia, have made it a stopover for some 83 species of

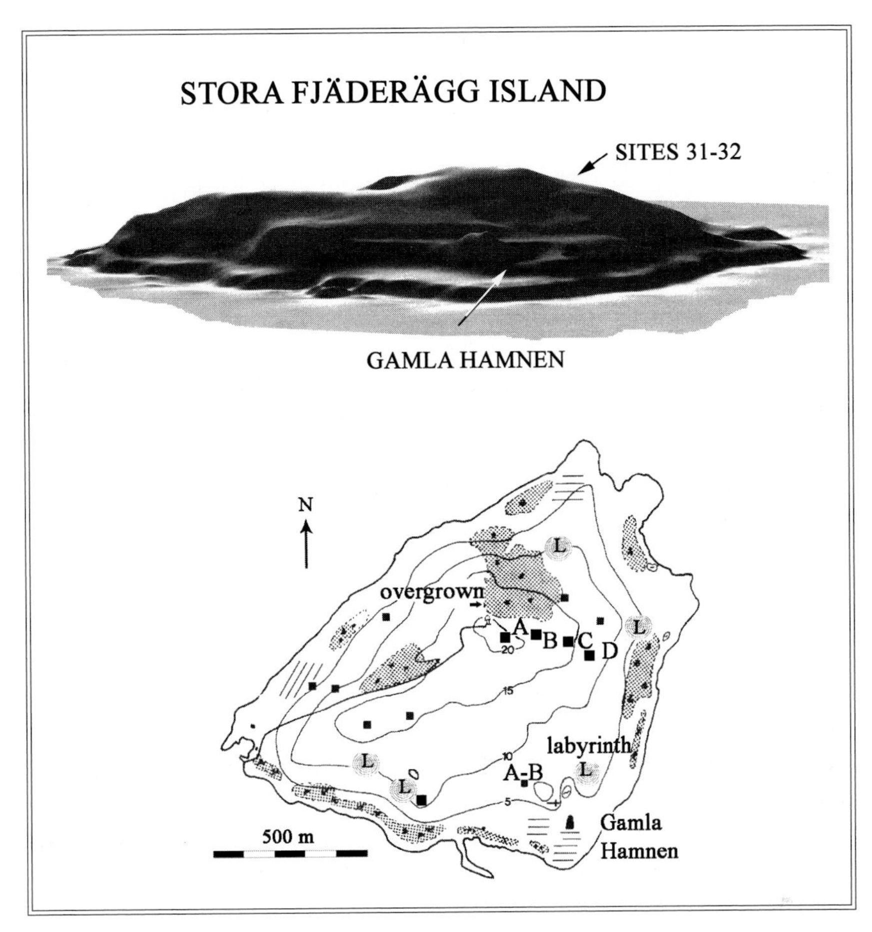


*Figure 98. (top) Three-dimensional rendition of topography of Stora Fjäderägg Island. Vertical scale exaggerated. Seen from the southeast. GIS by Katherine Rusk. (bottom) Map of island with locations of investigated huts and labyrinths.*

birds. The odd name probably derives from *fara*, which means "to travel," or might refer to danger or the appearance of the island.

Historical sources from the sixteenth and seventeenth centuries describe the island as the village territory of Holmön islanders, but it was also used by seasonal herring and salmon fishermen, and sealers from the mainland and Finland. During the most intensive fishing seasons more than 100 people are recorded as living there. It was even possible to grow potatoes. A small chapel had been built in 1729 by fisherman from Nykarleby in Finland (Jirlow 1930).

According to local oral history, the first settlers of Holmön were the "Fisher-Lapps" Håkan, Kerstop and Klemmet. These names (Håkansson, Christiern and Clemmeth) were still common in the sixteenth century (Sandström 1988:138). Other place-names on the island derive from these personal names, such as "Klemmetsgrundet" (Klemmet's Reef) and "Clemmets Myra" (Klemmet's Bog). Their original farmstead sites are still known.

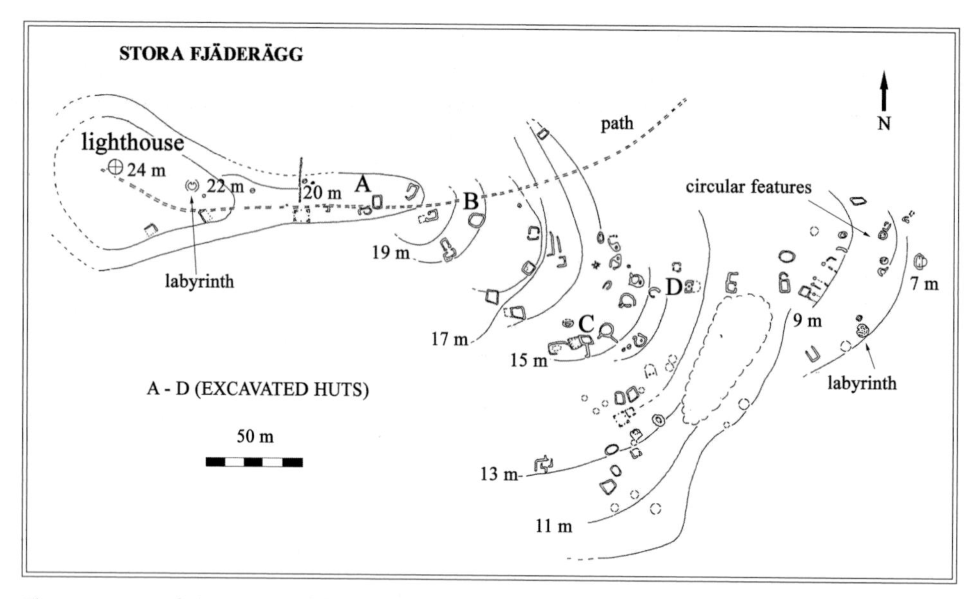


*Figure 99. Map of Sites 31–33 with hut locations and forms, pits, stone circles and excavations.*

Sandström judged the references to Fisher-Lapps to be credible. In fact, residents of Holmön were called Lapps by other villagers in the region, as were the people of Stöcke and Rånea on the mainland (Sandström 1988:138). This reference is reinforced by a unique Saami practice on Holmön of making ropes using roots, a technique also known in Råneå (Sandström 1988:139). Finally, it can be mentioned that the Örrskär cemetery on Holmön (with a squarish stone enclosure) was referred to as a "Viking nest" because of the heathen practices, including sacrifices, that were said to have occurred there (Sandström 1988:138). This was a chapel site but, like Jungfrugraven, could have an older pre-Christian ritual association.

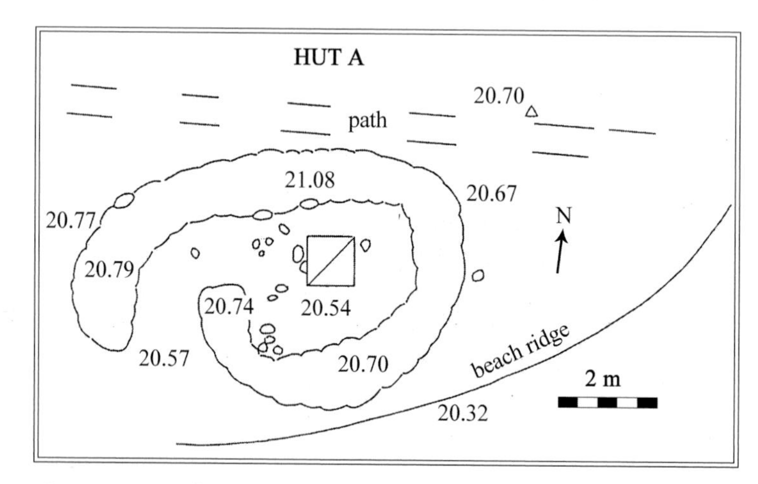


*Figure 100. Map of Hut A.*

## Archaeology of Stora Fjäderägg Island

A concentration of 35 huts lies on the eastern side of the island (Sites 31–32). This array of huts and features faces southeast and all have excellent views of the surrounding seas; they are situated without reference to any harbor basins (Figures 98, 99). Excavations were carried out at 20.5 m, 19 m, 15 m and

13 m above sea level. An area of 11 stone circles between 7 m and 9 m above sea level was also documented (Site 33). In addition, two small dwellings near the Old Harbor (Gamla Hamnen) were excavated (Site 34). They lie at ca. 8 m above sea level and overlook the harbor basin (Figures 110, 111, 112). Five labyrinths were lichen dated by Rabbe Sjöberg and range in age from A.D. 1525–1664 (Broadbent and Sjöberg 1990:295).

### *Hut A*

Hut A is located at 20.5 m above sea level. It has an inverted "G" form with an extended entranceway facing south (Figure 100). The feature measures ca. 8 × 5 m and has a floor area measuring 3 × 4 m. The walls are ca. 1 m wide and 0.30–0.50 m high. The entranceway is 1.5 m wide and the most distinctive aspect of the hut is its unusual form. A 1 m² pit was excavated in the hearth area.

Table 18. Sites 31–32, Hut A: Faunal remains by weight (g).

| BONES | BURNED (G) | BURNED, NISP |
|---|---|---|
| Indeterminate seal | 0.18 | 2 |
| Indeterminate seal | 10.91 | Not counted |
| Total | 11.09 | |

*Finds*

None

*Osteological Material*

Bone was recovered (11.09 g) and two specimens could be identified, both fragments of metatarsal bones from the rear flippers of an adult seal.

*Chronology*

13.8 g of charcoal was obtained. This sample (St. 11181) produced one radiocarbon date: 1015±100 B.P. (A.D. cal. 898–1155).

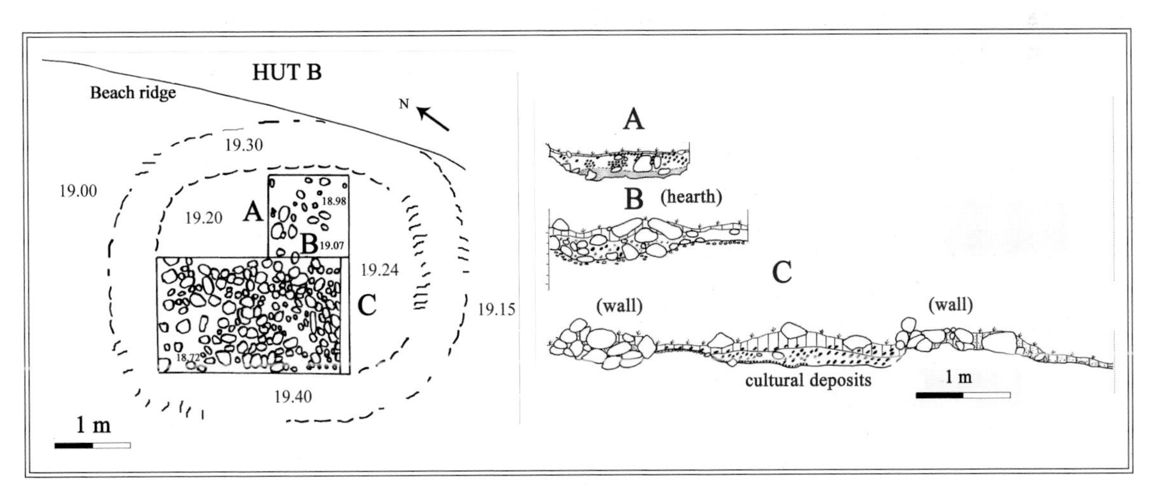


*Figure 101. Map of Hut B excavation and locations of profiles. (A) Section through the hearth in the center of the dwelling. (B) Shows the hearth depression. (C) Cross section of the dwelling.*

### *Hut B*

Hut B is situated at 19 m above sea level. The heavily overgrown hut is approximately 11 m in diameter with a floor area of 7 × 6 m (Figure 101). The walls are thick, up to 2.0 m wide, and there is no obvious entrance. The hearth was excavated as a unit (a 1 m² pit) and this sampling area was then expanded to cover 19 m².

*Finds*

Red clay/slag (iron furnace wall)
Gray flint chip (11 mm)
Gray flint chip (less than 10 mm)
Gray flint chip (less than 10 mm)
Slag (21x23 mm)
Slag (34x23 mm)
Fragment of whetstone (36 × 13 × 15 mm)

*Chronology*

Charcoal was recovered (18.7 g), and two radiocarbon dates were obtained: (St. 11900), 1660±70 B.P. (A.D. cal. 259–529), and (St. 11182), 1235±315 (A.D. cal. 465–1154). The medians are: A.D. cal. 386 and 779.

*Osteological Material (by Jan Storå)*

A total of 7.9 kg of bones were recovered from the hut. Approximately 0.6 kg was either unburned or charred. 5.2 kg of bones were recovered from the floor area and 3.2 kg from the hearth. The floor area contained a slightly smaller proportion of charred fragments than the hearth and the pit (according to weight). The bones came from the original 1 m² excavation pit, the hearth, the floor area and the profile wall.

Most of the bones from Hut B could only be identified as unspecified seal. The most common species was harp seal, followed by ringed seal, cattle, sheep/goat and duck. The representation of species is similar on the floor area and in the hearth, while the pit contained only bones of seals. There are also some differences in species representation between the burned and unburned bones. The minimum numbers of individuals for the identified species are: 4 harp seals, 2 ringed seals,

Table 19. Sites 31–32, Hut B: Bones recovered in different areas, by weight (g).

| BONES | PIT | HEARTH | SECTION* | FLOOR | TOTAL |
|---|---|---|---|---|---|
| Burned | 29.29 | 2181.84 | 752.7 | 4946.93 | 7910.76 |
| Unburned | 0.99 | 11.55 | 8.57 | 15.81 | 36.92 |
| Charred | 2.86 | 248.47 | 40.7 | 276.77 | 568.8 |
| Soil sample (Indeterminate fragments) | | | | | 1029.65 |
| Total | 33.14 | 2441.86 | 801.97 | 5239.51 | 9546.13 |

* from hearth.

Table 20. Sites 31-32, Hut B: Species by weight (g).

| SPECIES | BURNED | UNBURNED | CHARRED | SOIL SAMPLE | TOTAL |
|---|---|---|---|---|---|
| Harp seal | 22.31 | 0.44 | 54.74 | | 77.49 |
| Ringed seal | 10.41 | 8.82 | | | 19.23 |
| Indet. seal | 1986.1 | 24.96 | 510.06 | | 2521.12 |
| Cattle | | 2.7 | | | 2.7 |
| Sheep/goat | 0.42 | | | | 0.42 |
| Large ungulate | 1.82 | | | | 1.82 |
| Indet. duck | 0.15 | | | | 0.15 |
| Bird | 0.2 | | | | 0.2 |
| Bird? | 0.27 | | | | 0.27 |
| Indeterminate | 5889.08 | | 4 | | 5893.08 |
| Not analyzed (indeterminate) | | | | 1029.65 | 1029.65 |
| Total | 7910.76 | 36.92 | 568.8 | 1029.65 | 9546.13 |

* from hearth.

Table 21. Sites 31–32, Hut B: Species, NISP.

| SPECIES | BURNED | UNBURNED | CHARRED | TOTAL |
|---|---|---|---|---|
| Harp seal | 9 | 1 | 7 | 17 |
| Ringed seal | 4 | 3 | | 7 |
| Indeterminate seal | 3474 | 15 | 623 | 4112 |
| Cattle | | 1 | | 1 |
| Sheep/goat | 1 | | | 1 |
| Large ungulate | 1 | | | 1 |
| Indeterminate duck | 1 | | | 1 |
| Bird | 1 | | | 1 |
| Bird? | 2 | | | 2 |
| Total | 3493 | 20 | 630 | 4143 |

Table 22. Sites 31–32, Hut B: Species in the floor area, NISP.

| SPECIES | BURNED | UNBURNED | CHARRED | TOTAL |
|---|---|---|---|---|
| Harp seal | 5 | | 4 | 9 |
| Ringed seal | 3 | | | 3 |
| Indet. seal | 2580 | 6 | 255 | 2841 |
| Cattle | | 1 | | 1 |
| Bird? | 2 | | | 2 |
| Indeterminate | 162 | | 5 | 167 |
| Total | 2752 | 7 | 264 | 3023 |

Table 23. Sites 31–32, Hut B: Species in the hearth (including the finds from the profile), NISP.

| SPECIES | BURNED | UNBURNED | CHARRED | TOTAL |
|---|---|---|---|---|
| Harp seal | 4 | 1 | 3 | 8 |
| Ringed seal | 1 | 2 | | 3 |
| Indet. seal | 884 | 9 | 364 | 1257 |
| Sheep/goat | 1 | | | 1 |
| Large ungulate | 1 | | | 1 |
| Indet. duck | 1 | | | 1 |
| Bird | 1 | | | 1 |
| Indeterminate | 109 | | | 109 |
| Total | 1002 | 12 | 367 | 1381 |

Table 24. Sites 31–32, Hut B: Species in the 1 m² pit, NISP.

| SPECIES | BURNED | UNBURNED | CHARRED | TOTAL |
|---|---|---|---|---|
| Ringed seal | | 1 | | 1 |
| Indet. seal | 10 | | 4 | 14 |

Table 25. Sites 31–32, Hut B: Species and skeletal elements, unburned bones.

| ELEMENT | HARP SEAL | INDET. SEAL | RINGED SEAL | CATTLE | TOTAL |
|---|---|---|---|---|---|
| Cranium | | 2 | | | 2 |
| Mandibula | 1 | 1 | 3 | | 5 |
| Hyoideum | | 1 | | | 1 |
| Atlas | | 1 | | | 1 |
| Vertebrae | | 1 | | | 1 |
| Costae | | 1 | | | 1 |
| Cr+i | | 1 | | | 1 |
| Coxae | | 1 | | | 1 |
| Femur | | 1 | | 1 | 2 |
| Talus | | 1 | | | 1 |
| Calcaneus | | 1 | | | 1 |
| T4 | | 1 | | | 1 |
| Mtv | | 1 | | | 1 |
| Ph3 post | | 1 | | | 1 |
| Total | 1 | 15 | 3 | 1 | 20 |

Table 26. Sites 31–32, Hut B: Species and skeletal elements, charred bones.

| ELEMENT | HARP SEAL | INDET. SEAL | TOTAL |
|---|---|---|---|
| Cranium | 5 | 19 | 24 |
| Mandibula | 1 | 4 | 5 |
| Atlas | | 3 | 3 |
| Axis | | 1 | 1 |
| V caud | | 8 | 8 |
| Vertebrae | | 510 | 510 |
| Costae | | 3 | 3 |
| Humerus | | 1 | 1 |
| Cr+i | | 2 | 2 |
| Cu | | 1 | 1 |
| C1 | | 1 | 1 |
| C2 | | 1 | 1 |
| C3 | | 1 | 1 |
| Mc II | | 1 | 1 |
| Mc V | | 2 | 2 |
| Ph1 ant | | 2 | 2 |
| Ph2 ant | | 4 | 4 |
| Ph3 ant | | 1 | 1 |
| Coxae | | 4 | 4 |
| Sacrum | | 2 | 2 |
| Femur | 1 | 7 | 8 |
| Patella | | 1 | 1 |
| Fibula | | 2 | 2 |
| Talus | | 7 | 7 |
| Calcaneus | | 2 | 2 |
| Tc | | 2 | 2 |
| T1 | | 1 | 1 |
| T2 | | 3 | 3 |
| T3 | | 4 | 4 |
| T4 | | 2 | 2 |
| Mt I | | 2 | 2 |
| Mt II | | 4 | 4 |
| Mt V | | 3 | 3 |
| Mt | | 1 | 1 |
| Ph1 post | | 6 | 6 |
| Ph2 post | | 1 | 1 |
| Ph3 post | | 4 | 4 |
| Total | 7 | 623 | 630 |

Table 27. Sites 31–32, Hut B: Species and skeletal elements, burned bones.

| ELEMENT | HARP SEAL | RINGED SEAL | INDET. SEAL | SHEEP/ GOAT | LARGE UNGULATE | INDET. DUCK | BIRD | BIRD? | TOTAL |
|---|---|---|---|---|---|---|---|---|---|
| Cranium | 5 | 2 | 92 | | | | | | 99 |
| Mandibula | 1 | | 23 | | | | | | 24 |
| Dentes | 1 | | 8 | | | | | | 9 |
| Hyoideum | | | 9 | | | | | | 9 |
| Atlas | | | 2 | | | | | | 2 |
| Axis | | | 14 | | | | | | 14 |
| V cerv | | | 4 | | | | | | 4 |
| V caud | | | 196 | | | | | | 196 |
| V thor | | | 1 | | | | | | 1 |
| Vertebrae | | | 506 | | | | | | 506 |
| Costae | | | 5 | | | | | 1 | 6 |
| Cartil. Costae | | | 1 | | | | | | 1 |
| Scapula | | | 1 | | | | | | 1 |
| Humerus | | | 2 | | 2 | | | | 3 |
| Ulna | 1 | | | | | | | | 1 |
| Carpometacarpus | | | | | | 1 | 1 | | 2 |
| Cr+i | | | 4 | | | | | | 4 |
| C2 | | | 1 | | | | | | 1 |
| C4 | | | 1 | | | | | | 1 |
| Mc I | | | 6 | | | | | | 6 |
| Mc II | | | 2 | | | | | | 2 |
| Mc IV | | 1 | 1 | | | | | | 2 |
| Mc | | | 5 | | | | | | 5 |
| Ph1 ant | | | 14 | | | | | | 14 |
| Ph2 ant | | | 5 | | | | | | 5 |
| Ph3 ant | | | 6 | | | | | | 6 |
| Ph ant | | | 2 | | | | | | 2 |
| Coxae | | | 31 | | | | | | 31 |
| Sacrum | | | 2 | | | | | | 2 |
| Femur | | | 15 | | | | | | 15 |
| Patella | | | 4 | | | | | | 4 |
| Tibia | | 1 | 37 | | | | | | 38 |
| Fibula | 1 | | 19 | | | | | | 20 |
| Talus | | | 22 | | | | | | 22 |
| Calcaneus | | | 9 | | | | | | 9 |
| Tc | | | 30 | | | | | | 30 |
| T1 | | | 23 | | | | | | 23 |
| T2 | | | 54 | | | | | | 54 |
| T3 | | | 43 | | | | | | 43 |
| T4 | | | 27 | | | | | | 27 |
| Mt I | | | 33 | | | | | | 33 |
| Mt II | | | 42 | | | | | | 42 |
| Mt III | | | 30 | | | | | | 30 |
| Mt IV | | | 22 | | | | | | 22 |
| Mt V | | | 45 | | | | | | 45 |
| Mt | | | 193 | | | | | | 193 |
| Mp | | | | 1 | | | | | 1 |
| Ph1 post | | | 469 | | | | | | 469 |
| Ph2 post | | | 301 | | | | | | 301 |
| Ph3 post | | | 310 | | | | | | 310 |
| Ph post | | | 198 | | | | | | 198 |
| Tarsi/carpi | | | 127 | | | | | | 127 |
| Sesamoidea | | | 472 | | | | | | 472 |
| Baculum | | | 3 | | | | | | 3 |
| Ossa longa | | | 2 | | | | | 1 | 3 |
| Total | 9 | 4 | 3474 | 1 | 2 | 1 | 1 | 2 | 3494 |

1 cow, 1 sheep/goat and 1 duck. If the seal bones are treated as one unit regardless of species, the material contains bones from at least 21 different individuals. Epiphyseal fusion data of the first toe bone (Ph1 post) indicate that sixteen of them were adults while the other five were sub-adults. Some of the bones of both harp seals and ringed seals exhibit skeletal lesions characteristic of old age, indicating that there are at least a few very old adults among them. The other species identified in Hut B are represented by one individual each.

There are noteworthy differences in the anatomical representation of seals between the different find contexts and between the burned, charred and unburned bones. The differences are obvious, according to both the number of specimens and the weight distributions. The burned bones exhibit a higher representation from the rear flippers. The charred fragments are mostly from the vertebral column, while the unburned bones are from the cranium (and rear flippers). The bones identified as deriving from cattle or large ungulates come from the upper extremities, i.e. the meatiest parts of the animals, while the bones from sheep/goats are from the meat-poor lower extremities. One femoral fragment comes from a calf. These finds probably represent food resources brought to the island. Eight seal bones exhibited marks associated with butchery. One element is from a front flipper, two elements are from a rear extremity, and five are from rear flippers. Seven of the elements exhibit chop marks and two have superficial cut marks. One fragment exhibits both types of marks. The character of the marks indicates rather crude partitioning techniques using heavy tools, probably axes. Poor preservation of the bone surfaces may, however, mask the true frequencies of lighter cut marks.

The differences in anatomical representation are not related to the different numbers of bones in each anatomical region. A comparison of anatomical units of seals shows that there was

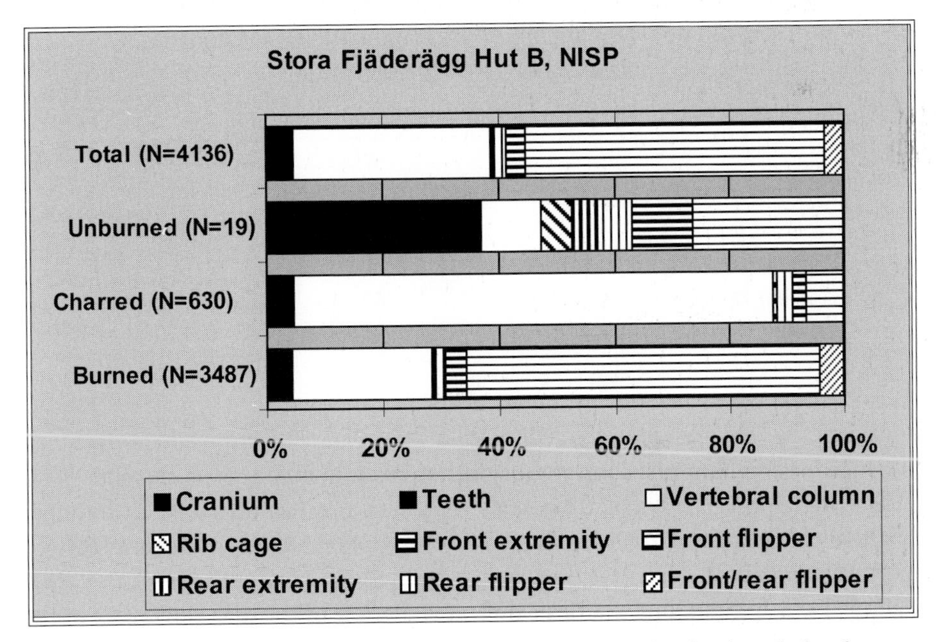


*Figure 102. Anatomical representation by NISP (excluding 472 sesamoids, 3 bacula and 2 long bone fragments).*

Table 28. Sites 31–32, Hut B: Species and skeletal elements, unburned bones.

| ANATOMY | ELEMENT | HARP SEAL | INDET. SEAL | RINGED SEAL | CATTLE | TOTAL |
|---|---|---|---|---|---|---|
| Cranium | Cranium | | 2 | | | 2 |
| | Mandibula | 1 | 1 | 3 | | 5 |
| | Hyoideum | | 1 | | | |
| Backbone | Atlas | | 1 | | | 1 |
| | Vertebrae | | 1 | | | 1 |
| Rib cage | Costae | | 1 | | | 1 |
| Front flipper | Cr+i | | 1 | | | 1 |
| Rear extremity | Coxae | | 1 | | | 1 |
| | Femur | | 1 | | 1 | 2 |
| Rear flipper | Talus | | 1 | | | 1 |
| | Calcaneus | | 1 | | | 1 |
| | T4 | | 1 | | | 1 |
| | MtV | | 1 | | | 1 |
| | Ph3 post | | 1 | | | 1 |
| Total | | 1 | 15 | 3 | 1 | 20 |

Table 29. Sites 31–32, Hut B: Anatomical representation for seals by MAU (minimum anatomical unit). Burned, charred and unburned bones not separated.

| ANATOMY | STORA FJÄDERÄGG B (N=60) |
|---|---|
| Cranium | 6 |
| Front extremity | 3 |
| Front flipper | 4 |
| Rear extremity | 5 |
| Rear flipper | 42 |
| Total | 60 |

a clear preference for rear flippers. This comparison takes into account the number of skeletal elements in each body region. The bones from seals represent a minimum of 60 different anatomical units; 42 of these are rear flippers. Note that this comparison excludes the vertebral column (see discussion, this chapter).

There are also differences in anatomical representation in the different areas of the hut. The burned fragments exhibit relatively great differences between the hearth and the floor area; the hearth contained a larger proportion of burned fragments from the vertebral column as compared

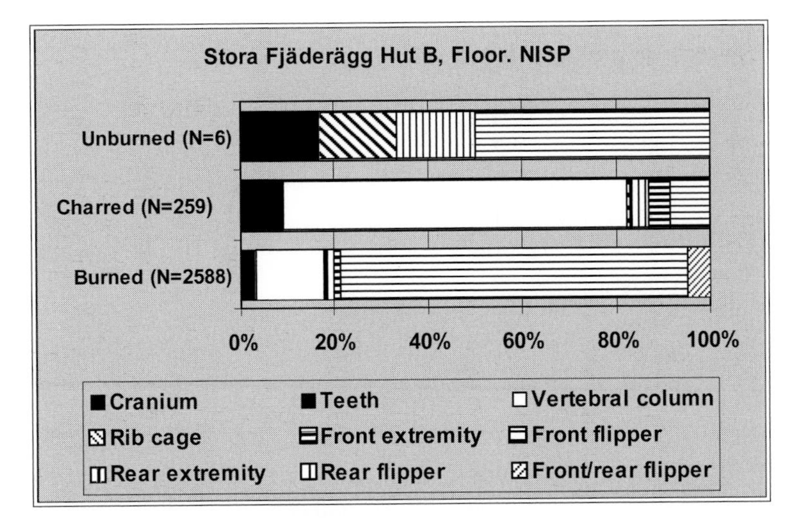


*Figure 103. Anatomical representation in the floor area according to NISP (excluding 472 sesamoids, 3 bacula and 2 long bone fragments).*

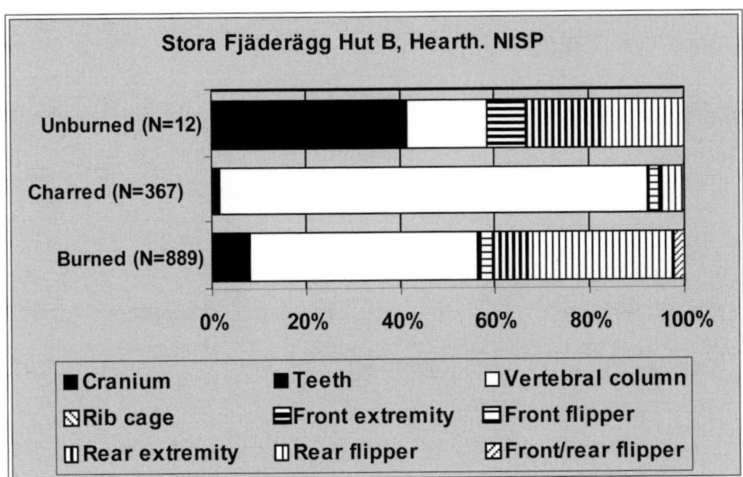


*Figure 104. Anatomical representation in the hearth by NISP (excluding 472 sesamoids, 3 bacula and 2 long bone fragments).*

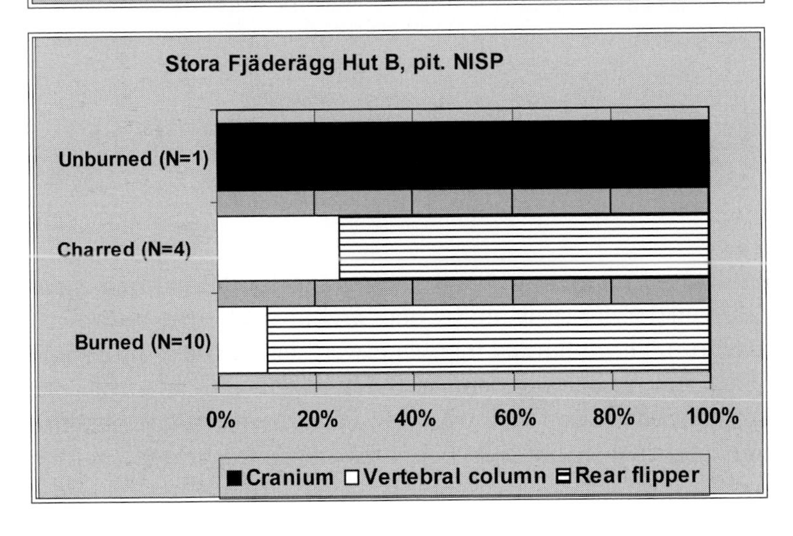


*Figure 105. Anatomical representation in the storage pit by NISP (excluding 472 sesamoids, 3 bacula and 2 long bone fragments).*

Table 30. Sites 31–32, Hut B: Anatomical representation for seals, NISP.

| ANATOMY | BURNED | UNBURNED | CHARRED | TOTAL |
|---|---|---|---|---|
| Cranium+teeth | 132 | 7 | 29 | 168 |
| Vert. Column | 725 | 2 | 524 | 1251 |
| Rib cage | 6 | 1 | 3 | 10 |
| Front extr. | 13 | 1 | 1 | 15 |
| Rear extr. | 108 | 2 | 15 | 125 |
| Front flipper | 48 | 1 | 16 | 65 |
| Rear flipper | 1851 | 5 | 42 | 1898 |
| Front or rear flipper | 127 | | | 127 |
| Sesamoidea, baculum | 475 | | | 475 |
| Long bone fragments | 2 | | | 2 |
| Total | 3487 | 19 | 630 | 4136 |

Table 31. Sites 31–32, Hut B: Anatomical representation for seals by weight (g).

| ANATOMY | BURNED | UNBURNED | CHARRED | TOTAL |
|---|---|---|---|---|
| Cranium+teeth | 132.22 | 12.80 | 79.34 | 224.36 |
| Vert. Column | 382.51 | 6.72 | 368.52 | 757.75 |
| Rib cage | 5.11 | 3.09 | 3.83 | 12.03 |
| Front extr. | 5.26 | 0.17 | 1.45 | 6.88 |
| Rear extr. | 172.03 | 1.77 | 33.15 | 206.95 |
| Front flipper | 36.98 | 0.62 | 24.40 | 62.00 |
| Rear flipper | 1145.54 | 9.05 | 54.11 | 1208.7 |
| Front/rear flipper | 60.13 | | | 60.13 |
| Sesamoidea, baculum | 80.60 | | | 80.60 |
| Long bone fragments | 1.71 | | | 1.71 |
| Total | 2018.82 | 34.22 | 564.80 | 2617.84 |

with the floor area, which mainly contained bones from the rear flippers. The charred fragments displayed a similar anatomical representation for seals on the floor and in the hearth, with most bone fragments from the vertebral column. The unburned fragments were dominated by fragments from the rear flippers in the floor area, and cranial fragments in the hearth. The small number of unburned fragments probably makes the comparison somewhat unreliable, however. The anatomical representation in the pit is more restricted than the on floor area and in the hearth, but this

Table 32. Sites 31–32, Hut B: Burned bones, anatomical representation for seals, NISP.

| ANATOMY | HEARTH | PIT | FLOOR | TOTAL |
|---|---|---|---|---|
| Cranium | 67 | | 56 | 123 |
| Teeth | 3 | | 6 | 9 |
| Vertebral column | 410 | 1 | 314 | 725 |
| Rib cage | 4 | | 2 | 6 |
| Front extremity | 2 | | 11 | 13 |
| Front flipper | 20 | | 28 | 48 |
| Rear extremity | 73 | | 35 | 108 |
| Rear flipper | 255 | 9 | 1587 | 1851 |
| Front/rear flipper | 18 | | 109 | 127 |
| Long bone fragments | | | 2 | 2 |
| Sesamoids, baculum | 37 | | 438 | 475 |
| Total | 889 | 10 | 2588 | 3487 |

Table 33. Sites 31–32, Hut B: Burned bones, anatomical representation for seals by weight (g).

| ANATOMY | HEARTH | PIT | FLOOR | TOTAL |
|---|---|---|---|---|
| Cranium | 72.72 | | 57.62 | 130.34 |
| Teeth | 1.04 | | 0.84 | 1.88 |
| Vertebral column | 247.30 | 0.09 | 135.12 | 382.51 |
| Rib cage | 4.00 | | 1.11 | 5.11 |
| Front extremity | 0.94 | | 4.32 | 5.26 |
| Front flipper | 15.33 | | 21.65 | 36.98 |
| Rear extremity | 121.99 | | 46.77 | 168.76 |
| Rear flipper | 190.68 | 3.99 | 950.87 | 1145.54 |
| Front/rear flipper | 7.92 | | 52.21 | 60.13 |
| Long bone fragments | | | 1.71 | 1.71 |
| Sesamoids, baculum | 7.26 | | 73.34 | 80.60 |
| Total | 669.18 | 4.08 | 1345.56 | 2018.82 |

comparison is also affected by the small numbers of fragments. It general, it appears from this material that there was some form of spatial organization and related activities in Hut B.

### *Hut C*

Hut C is located at 15.5 m above sea level. It measures ca. 5.5 × 5.5 m and the floor area is ca. 3 × 3 m (Figure 106). The walls are heavily overgrown and measure ca. 1.0 m in width. A single

Table 34. Sites 31–32, Hut B: Unburned bones, anatomical representation for seals, NISP.

| ANATOMY | HEARTH | PIT | FLOOR | TOTAL |
|---|---|---|---|---|
| Cranium | 5 | 1 | 1 | 7 |
| Vertebral column | 2 | | | 2 |
| Rib cage | | | 1 | 1 |
| Front extremity | 1 | | | 1 |
| Front flipper | | | 1 | 1 |
| Rear extremity | 2 | | | 2 |
| Rear flipper | 2 | | 3 | 5 |
| Total | 12 | 1 | 6 | 19 |

Table 35. Sites 31–32, Hut B: Unburned bones, anatomical representation for seals by weight (g).

| ANATOMY | HEARTH | PIT | FLOOR | TOTAL |
|---|---|---|---|---|
| Cranium | 10.93 | 0.99 | 0.88 | 12.80 |
| Vertebral column | 6.72 | | | 6.72 |
| Rib cage | | | 3.09 | 3.09 |
| Front extremity | 0.17 | | | 0.17 |
| Front flipper | | | 0.62 | 0.62 |
| Rear extremity | 1.77 | | | 1.77 |
| Rear flipper | 0.53 | | 8.52 | 9.05 |
| Total | 20.00 | 0.99 | 13.11 | 34.22 |

Table 36. Sites 31–32, Hut B: Charred bones, anatomical representation for seals, NISP.

| ANATOMY | HEARTH | PIT | FLOOR | TOTAL |
|---|---|---|---|---|
| Cranium | 6 | | 23 | 29 |
| Vertebral column | 333 | 1 | 190 | 524 |
| Rib cage | 1 | | 2 | 3 |
| Front extremity | | | 1 | 1 |
| Front flipper | 7 | | 9 | 16 |
| Rear extremity | 3 | | 12 | 15 |
| Rear flipper | 17 | 3 | 22 | 42 |
| Total | 367 | 4 | 259 | 630 |

Table 37. Sites 31–32, Hut B: Charred bones, anatomical representation for seals by weight (g).

| ANATOMY | HEARTH | PIT | FLOOR | TOTAL |
|---|---|---|---|---|
| Cranium | 35.26 | | 44.08 | 79.34 |
| Vertebral column | 200.62 | 0.48 | 167.42 | 368.52 |
| Rib cage | 0.61 | | 3.22 | 3.83 |
| Front extremity | | | 1.45 | 1.45 |
| Front flipper | 12.12 | | 12.28 | 24.40 |
| Rear extremity | 9.30 | | 23.85 | 33.15 |
| Rear flipper | 31.26 | 2.38 | 20.47 | 54.11 |
| Total | 289.17 | 2.86 | 272.77 | 564.80 |

Table 38. Sites 31–32, Hut B: Bones exhibiting marks of butchery. All fragments from the floor area.

| ANATOMY | ELEMENT | MARK |
|---|---|---|
| Front flipper | McI | Cut marks at distal epiphysis |
| Rear extremity | Tibia | Chop mark at distal end |
| | Tibia | Chop mark on diaphysis |
| Rear flipper | Tc | Chop mark and cut mark |
| | Tc | Chop mark |
| | T2 | Chop mark |
| | T2 | Chop mark |
| | MtIII | Chop mark |

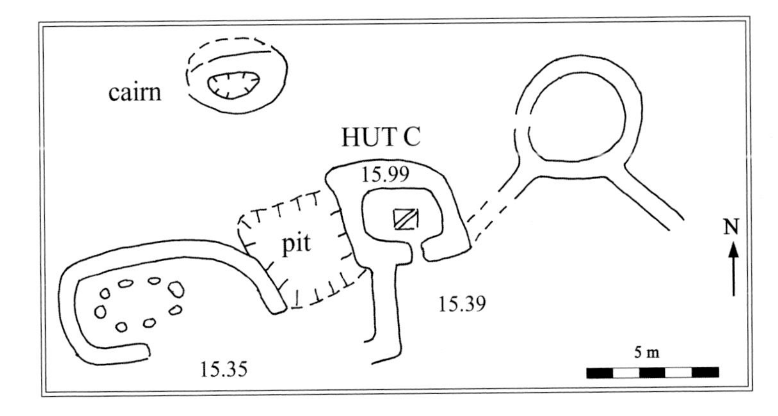


*Figure 106. Map of Hut C with alignments, huts and a storage cache.*

entrance, measuring 1.0 m in width, faces southeast. The excavated hut is one of three constructions with external wall alignments, a depression and a cairn. One of the huts resembles the inverted "G" shape of Hut A and is roughly contemporary with it. This appears to be a small cluster of contemporary structures.

*Finds*
One chip of gray flint was found and measures 15 mm in length.

*Chronology*
A 1 m² pit was excavated in the hearth and 15.7 g of charcoal was found. One radiocarbon date (St. 11183) was obtained: 955±75 B.P. (A.D. cal. 1018–1163).

*Osteological Material*
No bone was recovered.

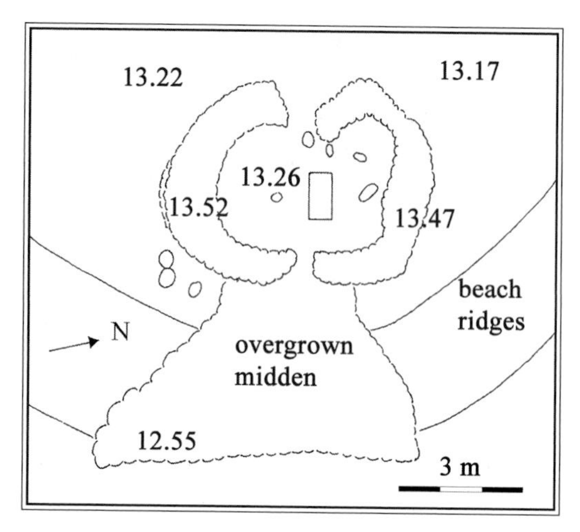

*Figure 107. Map of Hut D.*

### *Hut D*

Hut D is situated at the 13 m elevation. It is roughly oval in shape and has two opposite-lying entrances facing east and west. The features measures ca. 6 × 4.5 m (Figure 107). The floor area measures ca. 4 × 3 m. The doors are ca. 0.75 m wide. A 1 × 0.50 m pit was excavated in the hearth. This rendered 205.8 g of bone. Charcoal was found (10.6 g) and radiocarbon dated (St. 11184): 1110±145 B.P. (A.D. cal. 714–1036).

Table 39. Sites 31–32, Hut D: Identified species, NISP.

| SPECIES | HEARTH | SAMPLE 1 | SAMPLE 2 | SAMPLE3 | SAMPLE 4 | TOTAL |
|---|---|---|---|---|---|---|
| Indeterminate seal | 1.67 | 27.95 | 1.23 | 1.03 | 0.08 | 31.96 |
| Indeterminate | 93.43 | 12.2 | 6.81 | 6.25 | 2.06 | 120.75 |
| Total | 95.1 | 40.15 | 8.04 | 7.28 | 2.14 | 152.71 |

*Finds*
One gray flint chip
Red brown clay furnace fragment (1.5 cm)

*Osteological Material*
The hearth soils and 4 additional soil samples were collected from Hut D.

Table 40. Sites 31–32, Hut D: Anatomical representation for indeterminate seals, burned bones, NISP.

| ELEMENT | HEARTH | SAMPLE 1 | SAMPLE 2 | SAMPLE 3 | SAMPLE 4 | TOTAL |
|---|---|---|---|---|---|---|
| Cranium | 1 | 2 | | | | 3 |
| V caud | | 5 | | | | 5 |
| Vertebrae | | | 1 | | | 1 |
| C2 | | 1 | | | | 1 |
| Tc | | 1 | | | | 1 |
| T1 | | 1 | | | | 1 |
| T2 | 1 | 2 | 1 | | | 4 |
| Mt I | | 3 | | | | 3 |
| Mt II | | 1 | | | | 1 |
| Mt III | | | | | 1 | 1 |
| Mt V | 2 | 1 | | | | 3 |
| Mt | 1 | 7 | | | | 8 |
| Ph1 post | | 20 | 1 | 4 | | 25 |
| Ph2 post | | 8 | | | | 8 |
| Ph3 post | | 4 | | | | 4 |
| Tibia | | 1 | | | | 1 |
| Ph post | 1 | 3 | | | | 4 |
| Sesamoidea | | 21 | 2 | 1 | | 24 |
| Total | 6 | 81 | 5 | 5 | 1 | 98 |

Table 41. Sites 31–32, Hut D: Anatomical representation for seals by MAU (minimum anatomical unit).

| ANATOMY | STORA FJÄDERÄGG D (N=6) |
|---|---|
| Cranium | 1 |
| Front extremity | 0 |
| Front flipper | 1 |
| Rear extremity | 1 |
| Rear flipper | 3 |
| Total | 6 |

The bones derive from seals of indeterminate species, and the rear flippers were most common. The minimum number of individuals is two (based on three rear flippers). Epiphyseal fusion of the toe bones indicates that one of them was an adult and the other, a sub-adult. One element from the rear flipper (MtII) exhibits cut marks on the diaphysis.

**Circular Features**

A group of ten ring-shaped stone settings measuring 3 to 5 m in diameter is recorded in the archaeological surveys (Site 33). The rings are on two beach ridges within an area of ca. 50 × 112 m between 7 and 9 m above sea level (Figures 108). The largest feature is an oval wall measuring 0.75 m to 1 m in height, with a diameter of 4.9 × 3.7 m (Figure 109). The wall is ca. 50 cm in width and incorporates a large unusual looking boulder. Fifteen meters to the northwest of this feature are two simpler stone rings, one measuring 3.5 × 4.1 m in diameter, and a smaller ring measuring 2 × 3 m. Fifty meters to the northeast, and on a terrace at the 9 m elevation, is an additional cluster of stone constructions, including a small cairn of stones lying up against a boulder. Five meters to the northwest are three smaller rings. One of these consists of three small chambers. Five meters above them is a 5.8 m long cobble wall, an oval depression measuring 4 × 3.3 m,

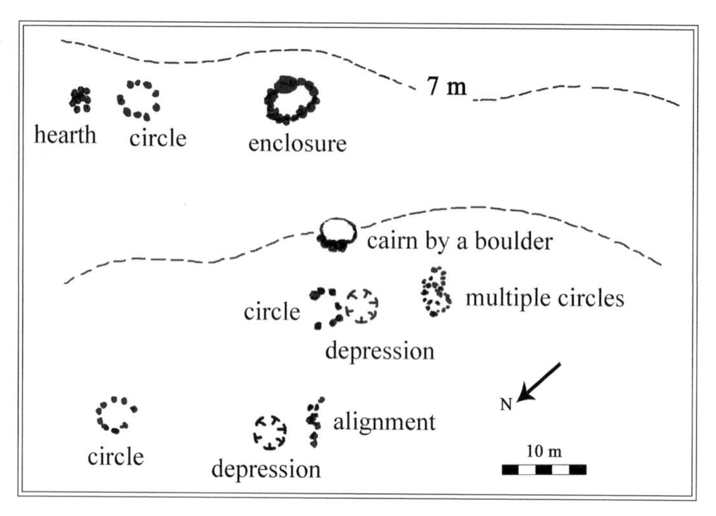


*Figure 108. Sketch map of Site 33 with stone circles and related constructions and depressions.*

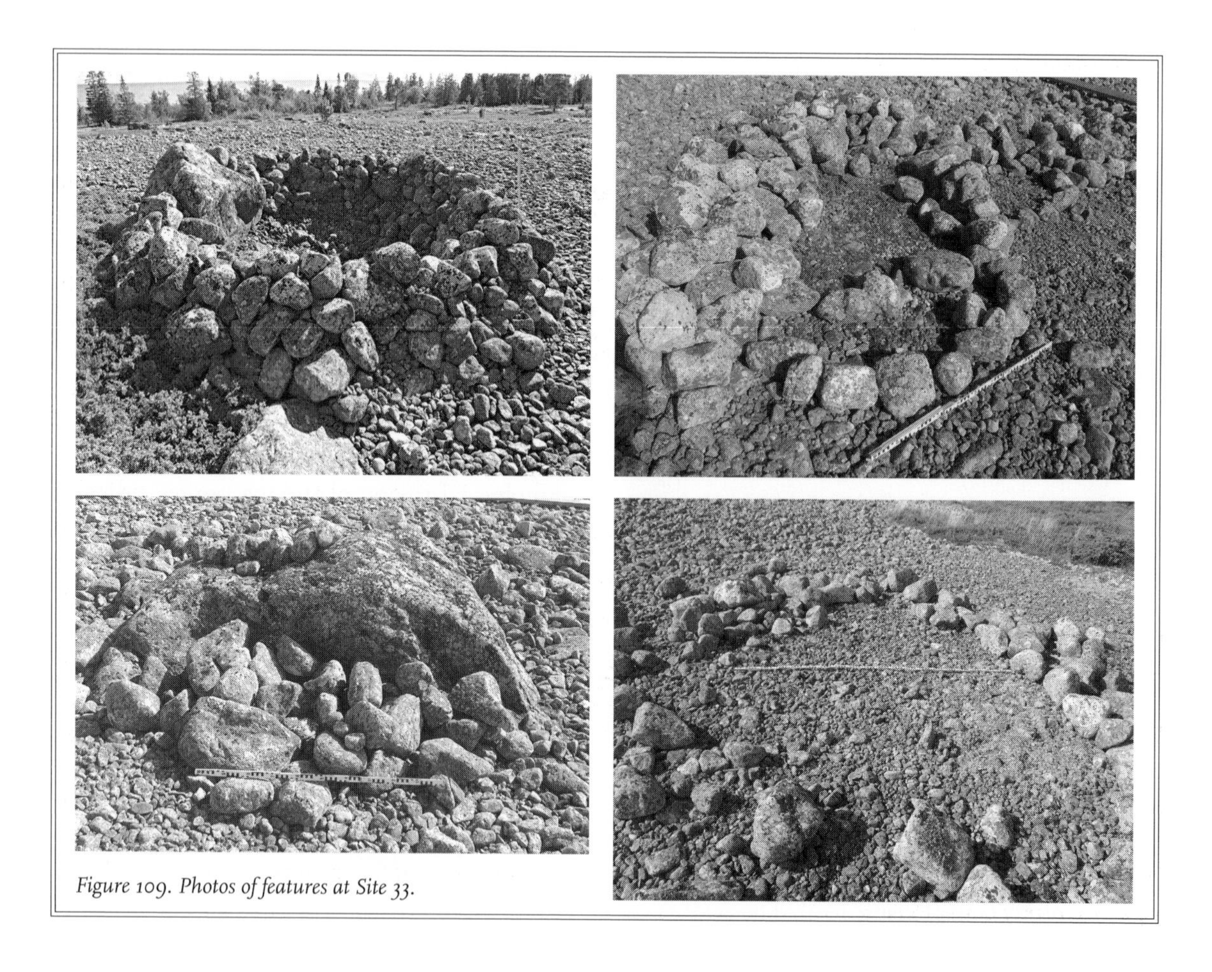

*Figure 109. Photos of features at Site 33.*

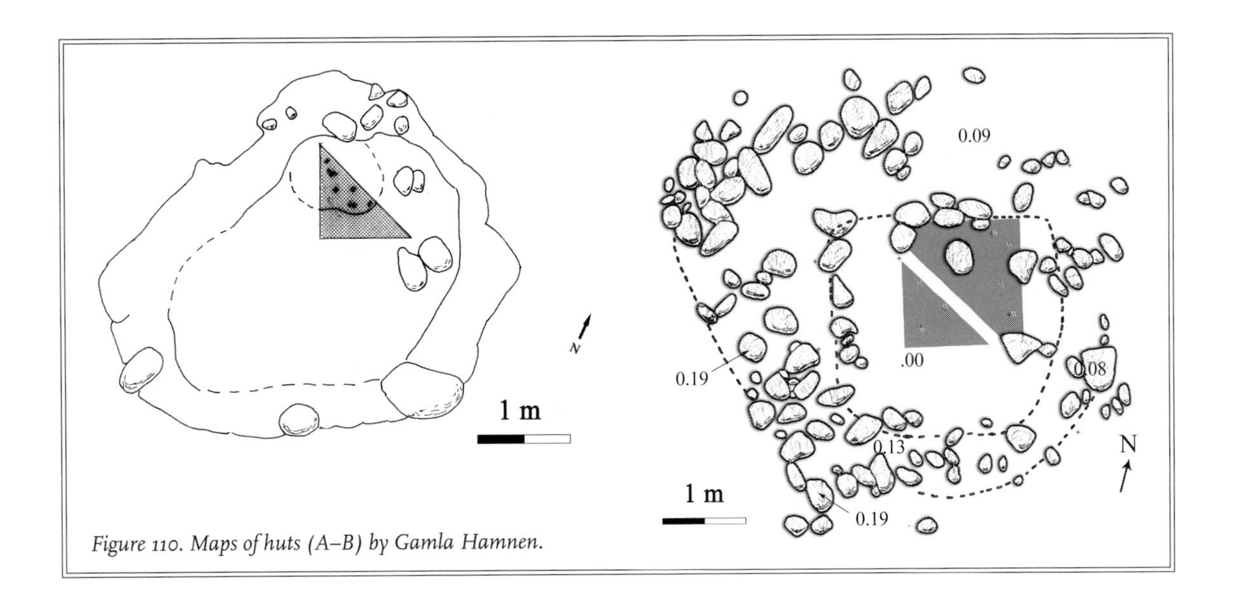

Figure 110. Maps of huts (A–B) by Gamla Hamnen.

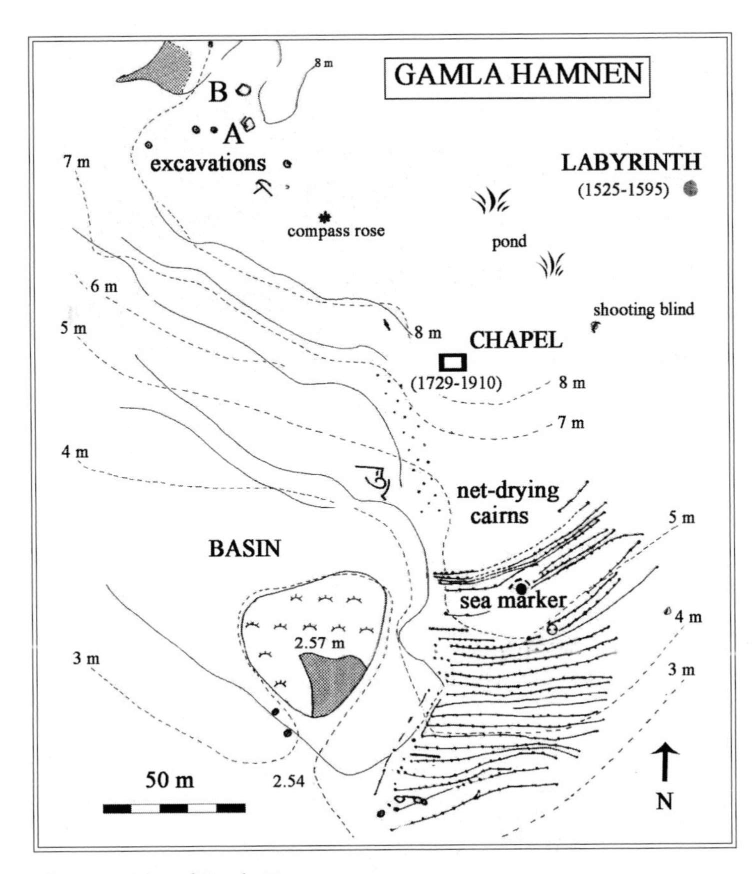

Figure 111. Map of Gamla Hamnen.

and a stone ring measuring 4 × 3.7 m. The complex faces in the same direction as the settlement as a whole, southeast. The shore level suggests a date analogous to the radiocarbon dates from Huts B–D., approximately A.D. 900–1200. Only two of the stone rings can be seen as dwellings (tent rings). The other circular features do not appear to have had any practical functions. These features parallel other finds documented within the project that are interpreted as Saami in origin (cf. Wennstedt Edvinger and Broadbent 2006). The most remarkable feature at the site is the cobble-built enclosure and a large boulder with odd eye-like holes (Figure 109). According to early written sources (Leem 1767), these circular constructions could be

Table 42. Stora Fjäderägg: Bones from Gamla Hamnen.

| SPECIES | WEIGHT (G) | NISP | ELEMENT |
|---|---|---|---|
| Large ungulate | 22.28 | 2 | 1 centrotarsale; 1 long bone fragment |
| Indeterminate seal | 1.66 | 1 | Part of the claw of the third toe bone, Ph3 posterior |
| Total | 23.94 | 3 | |

covered over to prevent dogs or predators from desecrating the offerings. These interpretations are discussed in Chapter 8.

**Gamla Hamnen**

Two small overgrown huts lying at the ca. 8 m level above the Gamla Hamnen area were investigated. Hut A is an irregular oval hut measuring ca. 4 × 3.5 m. The low walls measure ca. 0.50 m in width. A small hearth was found in the northwest corner of the hut. Hut B is also irregular feature and measuring ca. 4 × 4.5 m (Figures 110, 111).

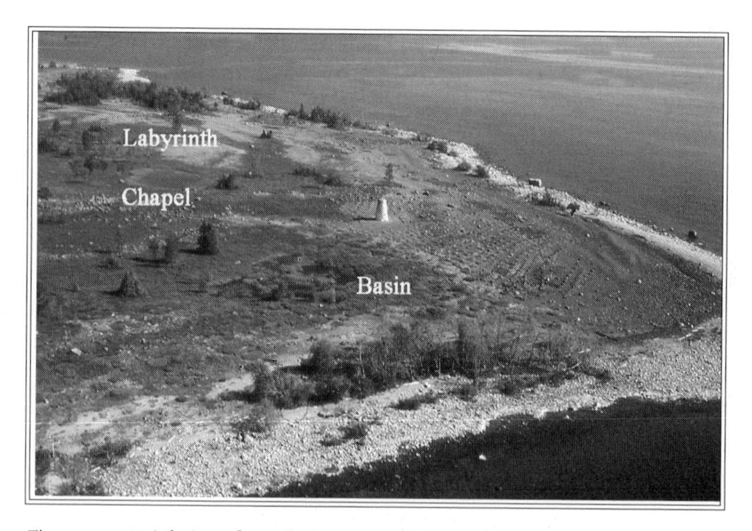


Figure 112. Aerial view of Gamla Hamnen, looking east.

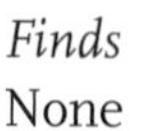

*Finds*
None

*Chronology*
One radiocarbon date was obtained from Hut B (St. 11901): 310±70 B.P. (A.D. cal. 1490–1650).

*Osteological Material*
All bones were unburned: one tarsal bone and a long bone fragment of a large ungulate (cattle or moose) and the claw (nail) of a third toe bone of an indeterminate seal were identified.

The harbor basin has a threshold elevation of 2.54 m above present sea level, which dates to ca. A.D. 1650. A beach ridge at its entrance is 50 cm higher than this level and is probably the result of storm surges. The chapel by the basin dates to 1729. As a whole, the radiocarbon date from the huts and the lichen dates of the labyrinths, suggest that the harbor could date as early as 1490 to 1650. As noted earlier, Sandström (1988:136–141) has undertaken an extensive analysis of the elevations of place-names on Holmön and found they start at the 6 m level, or ca. A.D. 1300.

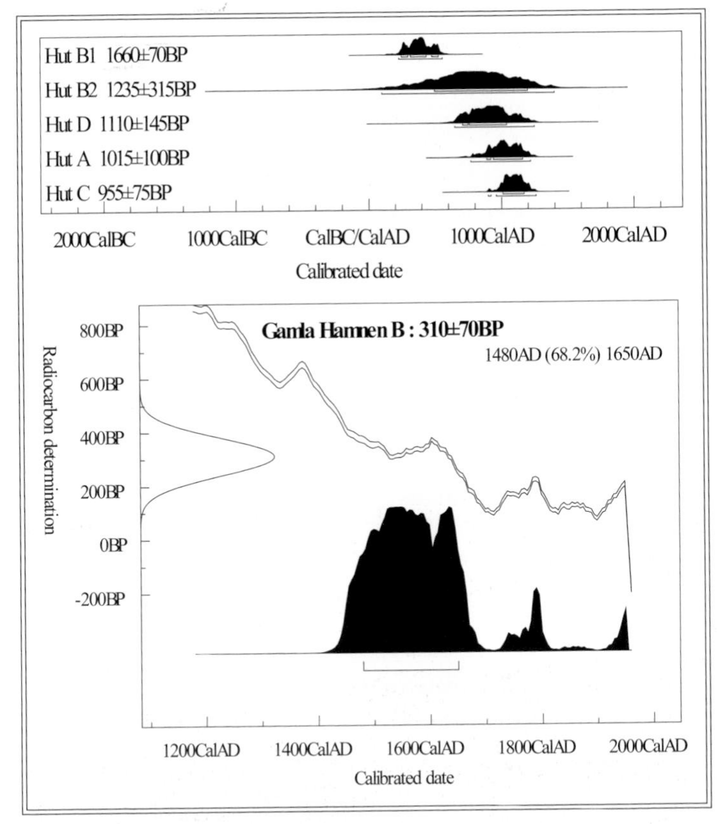


*Figure 113. Calibrated dates of huts at Sites 31–32. Below, calibrated date of hut by Gamla Hamnen.*

**Summary Discussion**

The highest-lying huts and the stone circles from Stora Fjäderägg Island date to the period ca. A.D. 200 to 1200. This range is fully consistent with the other investigated sites with similar elevations. The harbor and associated features date to the late sixteenth century, in line with the lichenometric dating of the labyrinths on the island.

The artifacts from the huts show evidence of iron working, both slag and furnace clay. This material was found in Huts B and C, ranging in age from 1660 to 1015 B.P. Flint chips from strike-a-lights were found in Huts B, C and D. The two stray finds from the island, a silver ring and bronze bells, date to the late Viking Period and are contemporary with the huts (cf. Serning 1960:150).

In addition to the seal bones discussed below, there were finds of cattle, sheep/goat and duck bones. This evidence of husbandry parallels the finds of sheep/goat bones from Jungfruhamn Site 138. Even stone alignments, as found at Bjurön Site 70 and Grundskatan Site 78, were in evidence at Hut C on Stora Fjäderägg, and are seen at other huts on the island as well. The circular features, combined with the oral history regarding Lapp settlers on Holmön and Saami traditions in rope- and net making, make the island a key locale in this analysis of coastal Saami culture in Västerbotten.

**Comparative Analysis of the Osteological Material (by Jan Storå)**

***Harp Seal Populations***

Earlier analyses have shown that prehistoric harp seals in the Baltic exhibited a smaller body size than extant ones from the Atlantic (Storå and Ericson 2004; Storå and Lõugas 2005). Due to the high level of fragmentation it has been difficult to document osteometric data from Stora Fjäderägg. The (greatest) diagonal breadth of *pars mastoideus* of two temporal bones (42.7 and 37.15 mm) are the only measurements providing information on the sizes of the harp seals. One of the elements comes from a rather large adult individual, in fact larger than most individuals from the

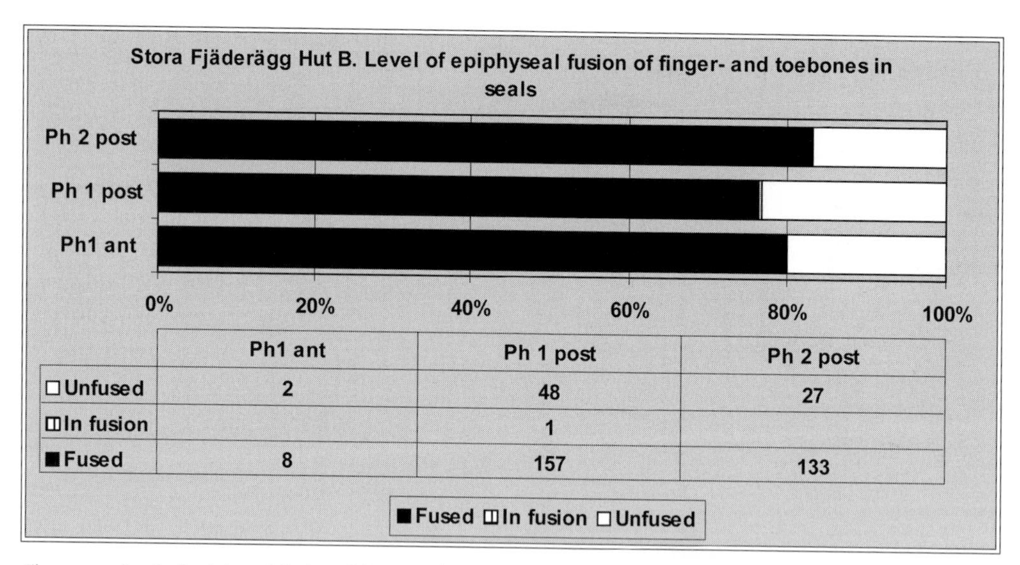


| | Ph1 ant | Ph 1 post | Ph 2 post |
|---|---|---|---|
| Unfused | 2 | 48 | 27 |
| In fusion | | 1 | |
| Fused | 8 | 157 | 133 |

*Figure 114. Level of epiphyseal fusion of finger and toe bones in seals. The unfused elements most probably derive from sub-adult seals while the fused bones come from adult seals (Aging according to Storå 2001a).*

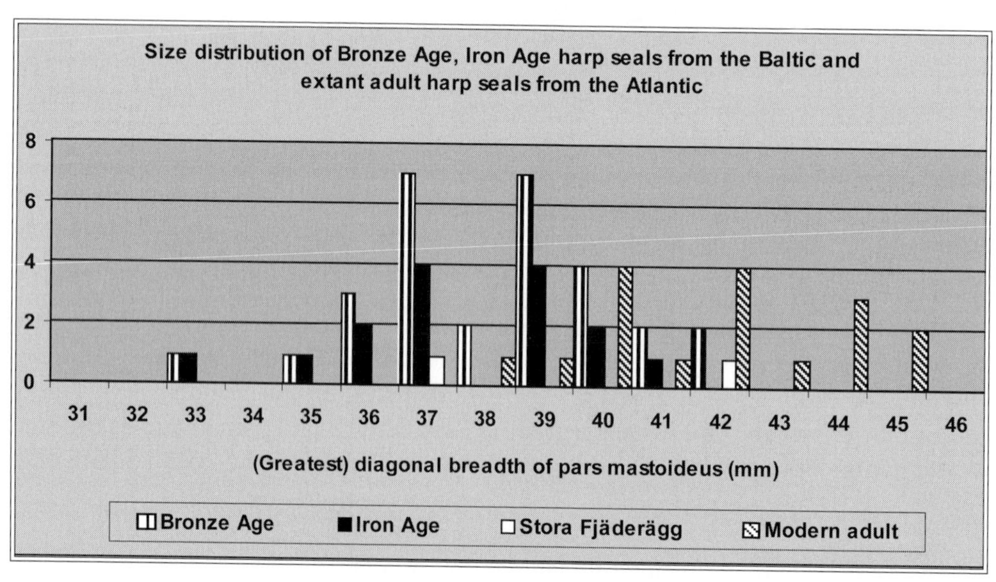


*Figure 115. Size comparison of two temporal bones (37.15 and 42.7 mm) from Stora Fjäderägg with bones from the Åland Islands and Estonia, and extant harp seals from the Atlantic (Modified from Storå and Lõugas 2005).*

Bronze Age and Iron Age. The size nevertheless corresponds to that of the smallest adults of extant harp seals from the Atlantic. A small temporal bone from Stora Fjäderägg probably derives from a sub-adult individual. Approximately 31% of the material by weight could be identified as to species or class of animals. Bones from ringed seals (*Phoca hispida*), harp seals (*Phoca*

Table 43. Stora Fjäderägg: Combined species by weight (g). Material in soil samples excluded.

| SPECIES | BURNED | UNBURNED | CHARRED | TOTAL |
|---|---|---|---|---|
| Ringed seal | 10.41 | 8.82 | | 19.23 |
| Harp seal | 22.31 | 0.44 | 54.74 | 77.49 |
| Indeterminate seal | 2018.24 | 26.62 | 510.06 | 2554.92 |
| Cattle | | 2.7 | | 2.7 |
| Large ungulate | 1.82 | 22.28 | | 24.1 |
| Sheep/goat | 0.42 | | | 0.42 |
| Indeterminate duck | 0.15 | | | 0.15 |
| Bird | 0.2 | | | 0.2 |
| Bird? | 0.27 | | | 0.27 |
| Indeterminate | 6020.74 | | 4 | 6024.74 |
| Total | 8074.56 | 60.86 | 568.8 | 8704.22 |

Table 44. Stora Fjäderägg: Combined species, NISP (indeterminate fragments not counted). Material in soil samples excluded.

| SPECIES | BURNED | UNBURNED | CHARRED | TOTAL |
|---|---|---|---|---|
| Ringed seal | 4 | 3 | | 7 |
| Harp seal | 9 | 1 | 7 | 17 |
| Indeterminate seal | 3574 | 16 | 623 | 4213 |
| Cattle | | 1 | | 1 |
| Large ungulate | 1 | 2 | | 3 |
| Sheep/goat | 1 | | | 1 |
| Indet. duck | 1 | | | 1 |
| Bird | 1 | | | 1 |
| Bird? | 2 | | | 2 |
| Total | 3593 | 23 | 630 | 4246 |

*groenlandica*) and indeterminate seals (*Phoca sp.*) by far dominate the material, together with solitary occurrences of cattle (*Bos taurus*), sheep/goat (*Ovis aries/Capra hircus*) and bird bones.

There are only minor differences in the species compositions among the burned, charred and unburned bones. Some bones could be identified as to class of animals or group of animals only. The bones identified as large ungulates may originate from moose (*Alces alces*), cattle or reindeer (*Bos taurus, Rangifer tarandus*). The possibility of horse (*Equus caballus*) can, with some certainty, be excluded.

The osteological analysis of the finds from Stora Fjäderägg has given new insights into the activities at these coastal sites. This is the first time that harp seal has been identified at such a location, and this is rather surprising. Previously, only ringed seals have been identified on sites this far north dating to Late Iron Age or Medieval period. Ethnographic records show that the ringed seal was also important in historic times, together with gray seal (*Halichoerus grypus*). The latter species is surprisingly rare in archaeological records from the Bothnian Sea and the Bay of Bothnia (see Ekman and Iregren 1984; Ukkonen 2002). At present, it seems that the hunting for gray seals has a rather recent history.

The discovery of harp seals from Stora Fjäderägg is chronologically one of the youngest in the Bothnian Sea. In the most comprehensive survey of faunal remains from archaeological sites in northern Sweden published in 1984, no finds of harp seal were reported (Ekman and Iregren 1984). However, harp seal bones were later identified at other sites. Some finds of harp seals have, for example, been reported from the Neolithic sites of Lillberget in Norrbotten (Halén 1994; Wallander 1992) and Bjurselet in Västerbotten (Lepiksaar 1975), and in recent years the species has been identified at several coastal sites in the southern (and middle) coastal areas of the Bothnian Sea, i.e. Bjästamon in Ångermanland (Olson *et al.* 2008) and Fräkenrönningen in Gästrikland (Holm 2006). The harp seal is very common in coastal site refuse faunas dating to the Neolithic period in the Baltic Sea (e.g. Storå and Ericson 2004).

Table 45. Stora Fjäderägg: Combined burned bones by species, NISP (indeterminate fragments not counted).

| SPECIES | HUT A | HUT B | HUT D | TOTAL |
|---|---|---|---|---|
| Harp seal | | 9 | | 9 |
| Ringed seal | | 4 | | 4 |
| Seal sp. | 2 | 3474 | 98 | 3574 |
| Sheep/goat | | 1 | | 1 |
| Large ungulate | | 1 | | 1 |
| Indeterminate duck | | 1 | | 1 |
| Bird | | 1 | | 1 |
| Bird? | | 2 | | 2 |
| Indeterminate | | 271+ | | 271+ |
| Total | 2 | 3764+ | 98 | 3864+ |

Table 46. Stora Fjäderägg: Combined unburned bones by species, NISP.

| SPECIES | HUT B | OLD HARBOR | TOTAL |
|---|---|---|---|
| Harp seal | 1 | | 1 |
| Ringed seal | 3 | | 3 |
| Seal sp. | 15 | 1 | 16 |
| Cattle | 1 | | 1 |
| Large ungulate | | 2 | 2 |
| Total | 20 | 3 | 23 |

Table 47. Stora Fjäderägg: Combined charred bones by species, NISP.

| SPECIES | HUT B |
|---|---|
| Harp seal | 7 |
| Seal sp. | 623 |
| Undetermined | 5 |
| Total | 635 |

The number of finds of harp seal in the Baltic decreases after the Neolithic Period. New studies suggest, however, that the species may have been present in the region more recently. Two sub-fossil harp seal skeletons on the Finnish West Coast of the Bothnian Bay have been radiocarbon dated to the Bronze Age (Ukkonen 2002). Another find of harp seal in Finland was recovered in a cairn dating to the Early Iron Age (Mäkivuoti 1986). More numerous finds in archaeological contexts have also been reported in the Baltic. Iron Age finds of the harp seal have been reported from the Åland Islands, the Estonian Islands, the Islands of Gotland, Öland and Bornholm (Storå and Lõugas 2005 and references therein). The finds from Stora Fjäderägg are contemporary with these finds. The size of one adult harp seal at Stora Fjäderägg is amongst the largest found compared with other Iron Age harp seals from the Baltic. The finds from Stora Fjäderägg provide some support that remnants of large Neolithic Period harp seal populations were still present in different areas of the Baltic Sea during the Late Iron Age.

The uniqueness of the harp seal finds at Stora Fjäderägg makes it difficult to generalize about hunting patterns. The harp seal is obviously the most common seal found in Hut B. The minimum number of individuals for ringed seals is two. However, the minimum number of seals of all species in Hut B is at least 21. In contrast to the most often solitary ringed seal, the harp seal is both migratory and gregarious. It breeds in late winter/early spring and is unable to keep breathing holes open in fast ice. This latter behavior is similar to that of the gray seal. The behavioral patterns of the harp seal are rather different from those of the ringed seal and in Neolithic times hunting patterns differed for the two species (Storå 2001b). The behavioral patterns almost certainly affected hunting strategies during the Iron Age, but unfortunately it has not been possible to pinpoint seasonality using only the seal bones from Stora Fjäderägg. If behavioral patterns of the harp seal are considered, the most suitable period for hunting would have been during periods with open water, the summer and fall. The harp seals in Hut B were found together with bones of a duck; the latter would have also been in the area during the warmer seasons of the year.

Whether the Stora Fjäderägg find is unique remains to be seen. Hut B is in several respects different from other studied hut structures of similar date and in corresponding locations. The presence of harp seal is certainly significant and the amount of faunal remains in Hut B exceeds that of all the other examined hut structures (e.g. Storå and Broadbent 2001). It appears that not all body parts of the seals were transported to Hut B. Bones from the rear flippers clearly dominate the assemblage. Interestingly enough, the meat of the flippers has often been considered the tastiest by hunters, and sometimes even the only edible parts of seals. At Stora Fjäderägg there was an obvious preference for rear flippers, while the front flippers were uncommon. Hut D on Stora Fjäderägg shows a similar (although not as obvious) preference for the same anatomical parts as that seen in Hut B.

The vertebral column is also fairly well represented, especially among the charred remains. Due to the level of fragmentation it has not been possible to estimate the minimum number of anatomical units for the different sections of the vertebral column (cervical, thoracic, lumbar and caudal). It is possible that the different regions of the vertebral column are not represented in similar proportions in Hut B. Due to the high level of fragmentation, most fragments have been identified as indeterminate vertebrae only. Considering a complete seal, it would be expected that thoracic vertebrae would be best represented. Also noteworthy is the fact that most vertebral fragments, identified to a specific region, are caudal vertebrae and cervical vertebrae also seem to be well represented. The second cervical vertebra, the axis, is represented by at least 10 individuals. Thoracic and lumbar vertebrae are not absent, but they appear to be underrepresented by comparison with the caudal and cervical regions. The few fragments of ribs at Stora Fjäderägg are an indication that this was the case, as the ribs are anatomically associated with thoracic vertebrae. It is also possible that rib fragments are rare because this part of the seal not was processed in Hut B. Indeed, the caudal vertebrae and rear flippers may have been be connected if the rear body parts of the seals were handled as a single unit.

It seems plausible that only parts of seals were brought to Hut B for preparation and consumption. The character of the cut marks from slaughter indicates rather crude methods for partitioning the body parts. The anatomical parts of seals that are missing in Hut B (as compared with the numbers of rear flippers), are the crania, front extremities and front flippers, thoracic vertebrae, ribs and rear extremities; these parts were taken somewhere else. The missing parts at Hut B roughly comprise the articulated trunk. One aspect that needs more attention is a possible bias in preservation. The burned fragments exhibit a clear dominance of bones from the rear flippers, while the charred fragments were dominated by vertebral fragments. This indicates that the vertebrae were subjected to a lower level of burning. Many vertebral fragments are burned, but the proportion of charred fragments is higher as compared to other anatomical units. The few unburned fragments came from several different anatomical regions, but they are too few to highlight further. The lower level of burning of vertebrae may also be because they were more deeply embedded in soft tissue than the more superficial bones, e.g. the toe bones of the rear flippers. If the vertebrae (and other more embedded bones) were not burned to the same extent as the rear flippers, this could mean these bones are underrepresented. This possibility has to be taken into account, but most probably

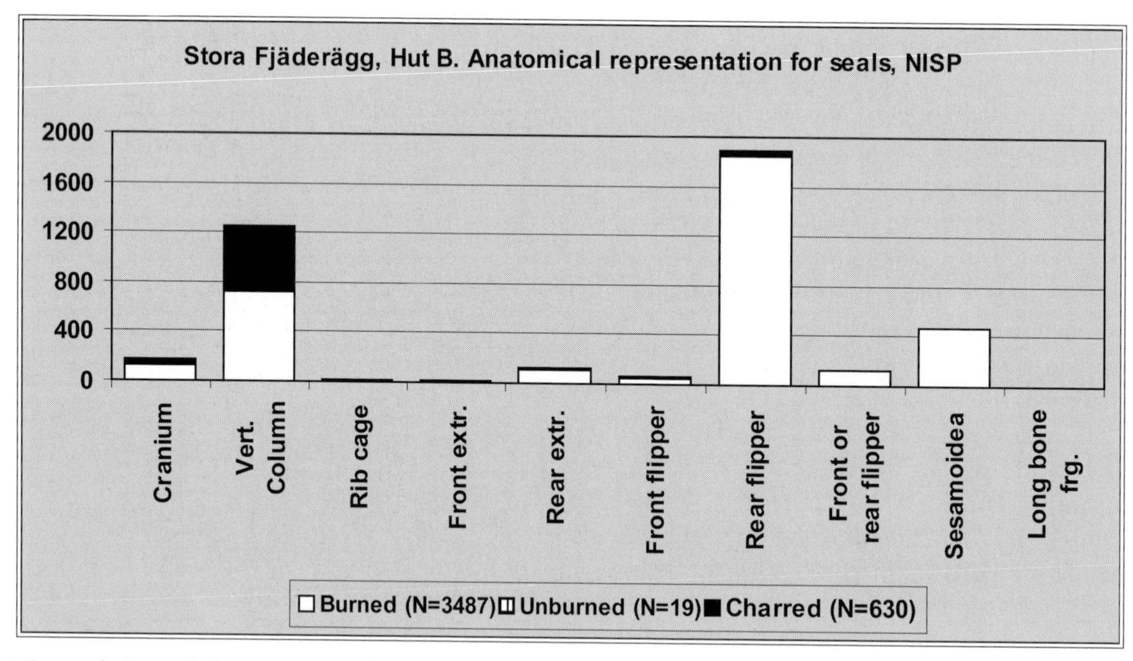


*Figure 116. Anatomical representation of seal bones in Hut B, NISP.*

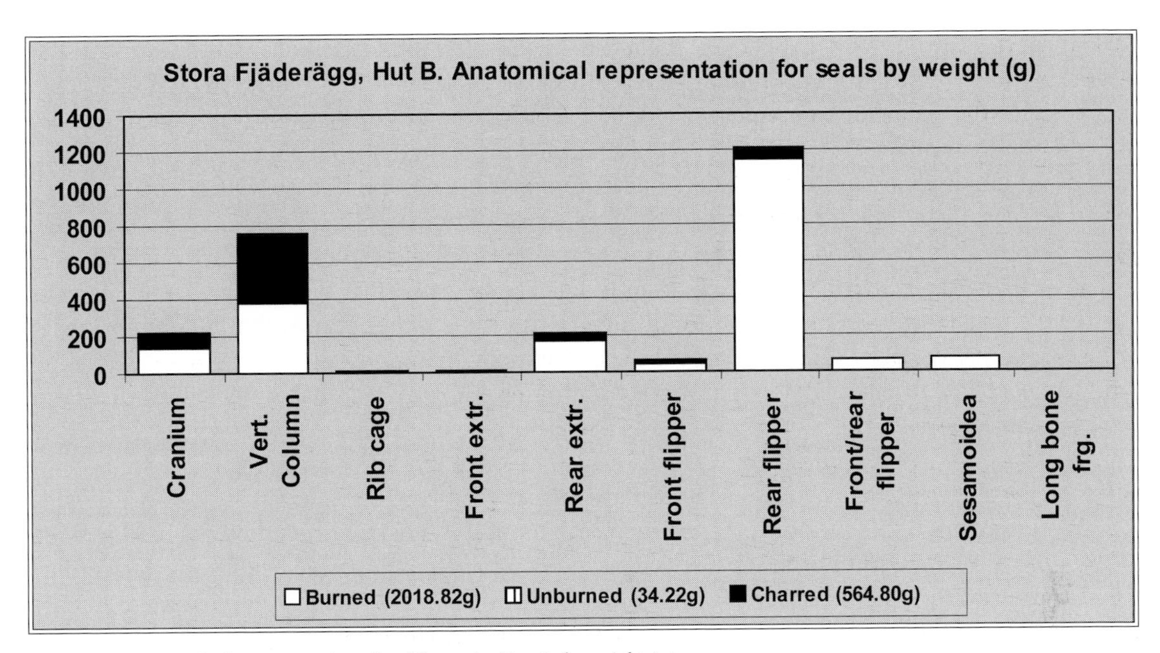


*Figure 117. Anatomical representation of seal bones in Hut B, by weight (g).*

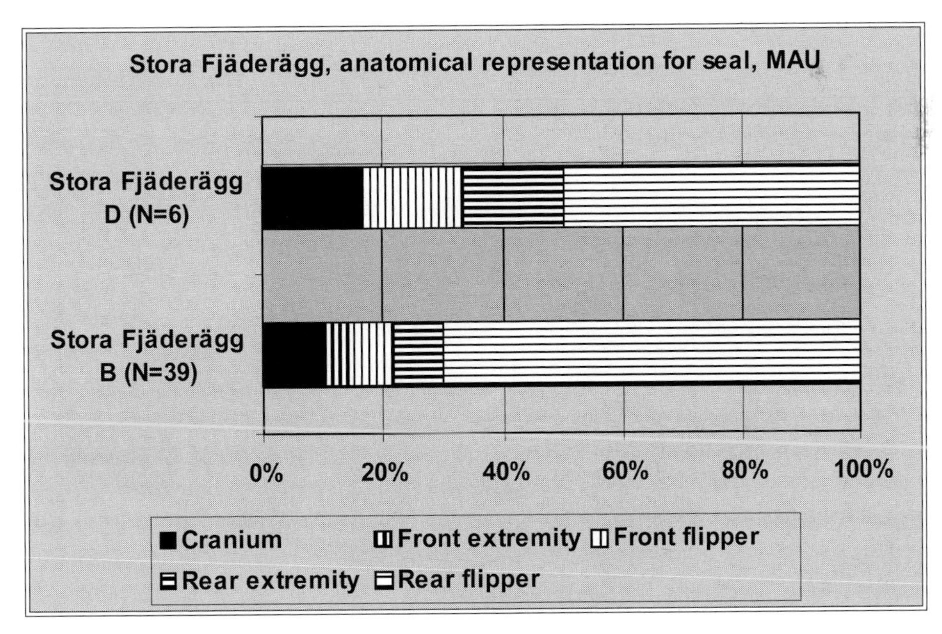


*Figure 118. Anatomical representation of seal bones in Hut B and Hut D according to minimum anatomical units.*

cannot explain the observed patterns of anatomical representation for seals at Stora Fjäderägg. The absence of finger bones from the fore flippers cannot be explained in this manner. The finger bones (and also the cranial bones) were not embedded in thick layers of soft tissue.

The faunal material from Hut B has highlighted the complicated taphonomic history of this kind of assemblage. It is obviously one of the more intriguing faunal assemblages from such a location and time period. It is of interest that there are differences in anatomical representation in Hut B between the hearth and the floor area. This has some implications regarding the character of carcass utilization. If the archaeological excavations had targeted either the floor area or the hearth, the results would have been different. Additionally, the analysis has shown that it is important to relate the faunal remains as closely as possible to the overall find context.

To conclude, the faunal assemblage from Stora Fjäderägg Island has provided new insights on a number of issues:

1) For the first time harp seal (*Phoca groenlandica*) has been identified in such a location and time period this far north. The ringed seal is not the most common species in Hut B, indicating that seal hunting patterns during the Iron Age may have been more varied than previously believed.
2) The amount of faunal remains in Hut B exceeds that of any other previously analyzed coastal hut structure. Hut B contains the body parts from at least 21 different seals indicating a planned utilization of the seals and use of the hut structure. The meat of the 60 anatomical regions identified in Hut B would have been a considerable food resource.
3) The anatomical representation of seals indicates that selected body parts were brought to Hut B for specific processing and probably consumption. The large parts of the seals that are missing in Hut B indicate strategies beyond immediate use. The missing parts of the 21

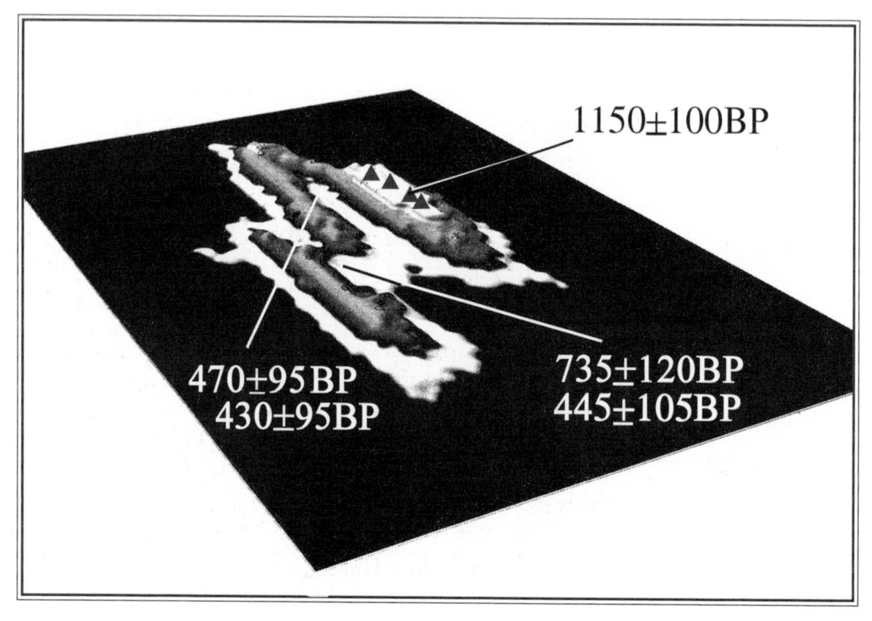


*Figure 119. Three-dimensional rendition of Snöan Island with radiocarbon dates.*

individuals represent a considerable amount of meat, blubber and skins.

4) Differences in anatomical representation in the find contexts of Hut B indicate spatial organization. The differences observed between the burned and charred bones, as well as the differences between the hearth and the floor, have been established for a rather large faunal material. This suggests a repeated behavioral pattern inside the hut.
5) All of the above indicates that Hut B must be regarded as a rather permanent structure in a well-organized hunting complex. The activities that produced this faunal assemblage were also well planned. Stora Fjäderägg contains many kinds of material remains indicative of the importance of the island over a long time period of time.

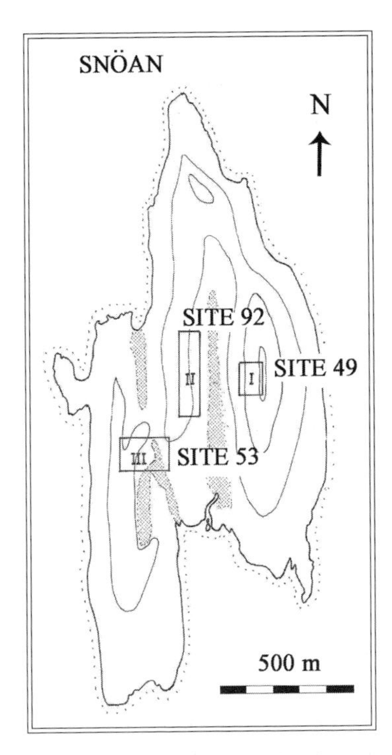


*Figure 120. Map of Snöan Island, Umeå Municipality, Västerbotten. Investigated areas indicated by rectangles.*

## Snöan Island

Snöan Island is outermost in the Snöan archipelago at 63° 29′ N, 20° 53′ E, and is ca. 7 km from the mainland. The island consists of two parallel glacial ridges and is arrowhead shaped (Figures 119, 120). It measures 2.8 km in length, 0.9 km in width, and rises up to 17 m above sea level. Snöan Island was surveyed by the National Heritage Board in 1981 and an excellent account of this work was published by Löfgren and Olsson (1983). Five locales with huts, eight labyrinths and an equal number of

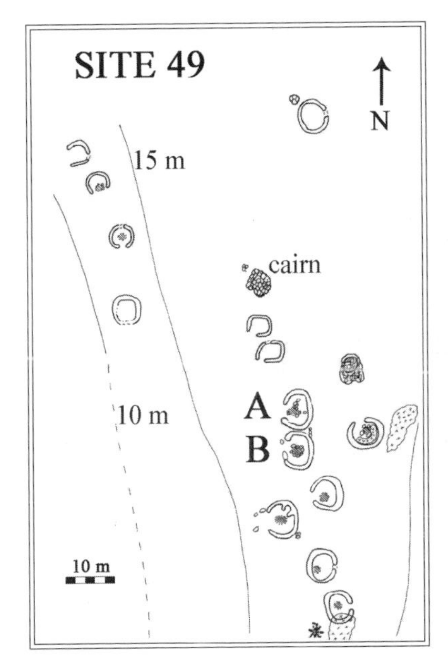


*Figure 121. Map of Site 49.*

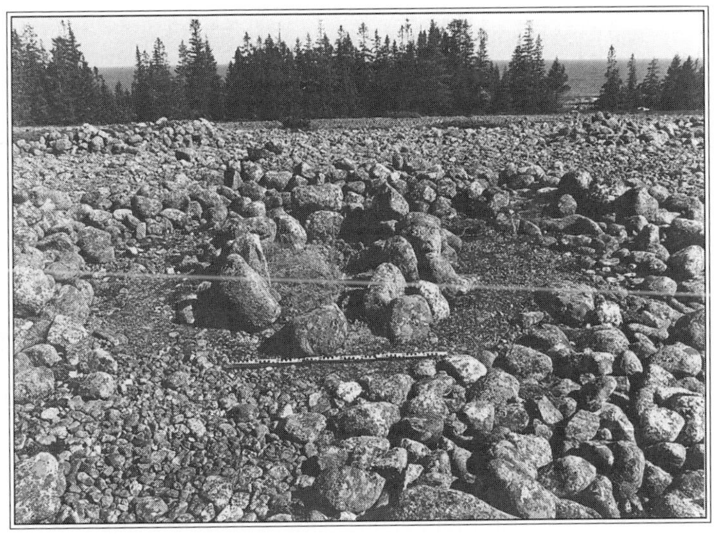

*Figure 122. Photo of Hut B with distinctive hearth, facing east.*

compass roses were recorded. The main hut concentration of some 50 structures lies above the 8 m curve within an area of 650 × 100 m (Site 49). The first historical account/map of the island dates to 1646. The name was written as *Snödan* and means "barren." Nine fishing sheds and a chapel were recorded in 1821 and there was cultivatable land in the central part of the island.

The goal of my investigation was to obtain charcoal for radiocarbon dates, animal bones and artifacts from different shoreline elevations. Two huts were investigated at the 10–15 m elevation, Site 49. Extensive mapping was undertaken at Sites 53 and 92, which are Late Medieval fishing harbors between 3–8 m above present sea level. Two dates were obtained from a Russian Oven at the 5 m level, and two dates were obtained from a hut by a harbor basin at the 3–5 m levels.

Table 48. Stor-Rebben: Bones in Huts A and B.

| SPECIES | HUT A | HUT B | TOTAL |
|---|---|---|---|
| Seal | | 2 | 2 |
| Large ungulate | 1 | | 1 |
| Hare | | 1 | 1 |
| Indeterminate. | 64+* | | 64* |
| Total | 65+* | 3 | 68* |

* not all small fragments counted

## Site 49

These oval huts form a cluster of features near the highest part of the island. Fourteen huts cluster above the 10 m level (Figure 121). Five of the huts face west, three east, one north and two south. Nine of the huts have hearths. Hut 49A measures 7 × 8 m and has an inner measurement of 5 × 6 m. The entrance is 2–3 m wide. Hut 49B has the same measurements. Hut 49B has a large built-up hearth measuring 2 × 3 m that nearly fills the floor (Figure 122). Charcoal was recovered from Hut 49B and dated: (Ua-1323), 255±100 B.P. This recent date suggests that the hearth was contaminated by later re-use. One artifact was found, a white-gray burned flint piece measuring 22 × 15 mm. Hut 49A (Ua-1322) rendered a date of: 1150±100 B.P. (A.D. cal. 775–988), which is consistent with its elevation. Burned bone was found in both huts. In Hut A, a large ungulate was identified. In Hut B seal and hare bones were identified. There was only 16 g of bone from the two huts, including those of a large ungulate (moose or reindeer), two rear flipper bones, including one

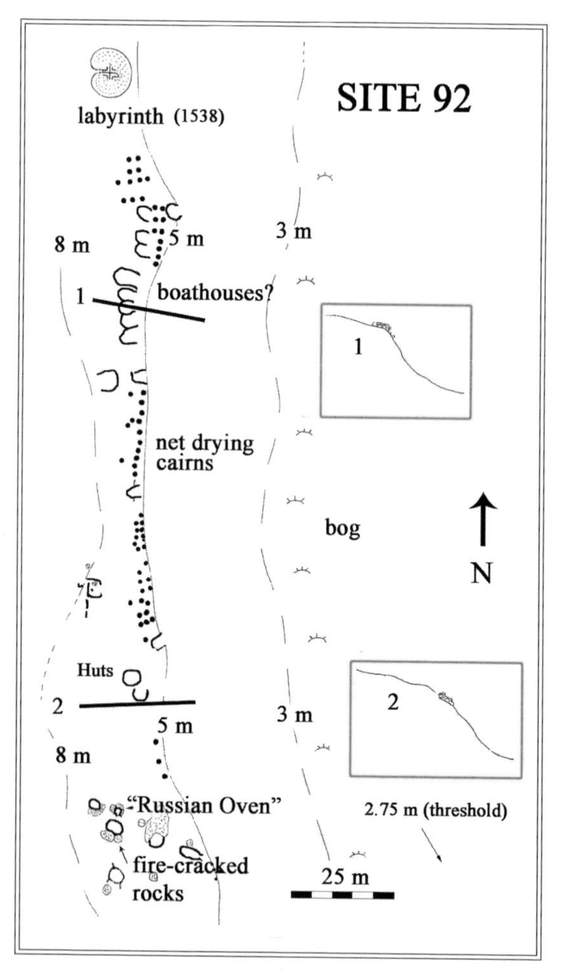


*Figure 123. Map of fishing harbor, Site 92.*

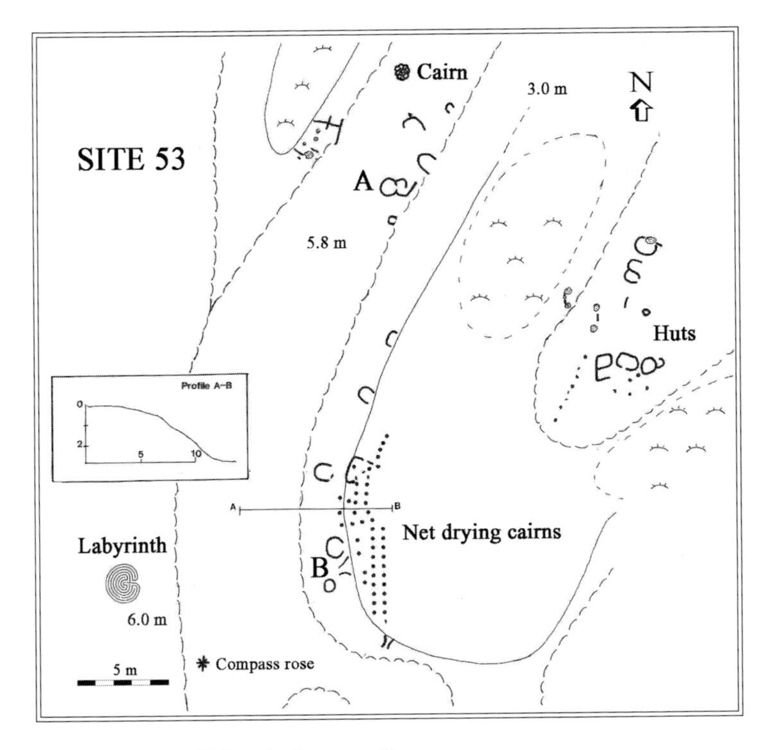


*Figure 124. Map of fishing harbor area, Site 53.*

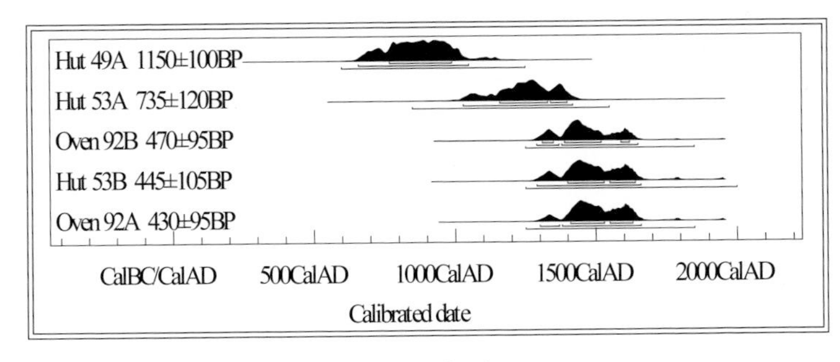


*Figure 125. Calibrated dates from Snöan Island.*

from an adult seal, and an adult hare. Although this is a small sample, this pattern is most similar to that of Grundskatan.

### Site 92

Site Area II is located in the center of the island and by a narrow former inlet. Numerous features lie on the west side of the inlet and follow the 5 m elevation (Figure 123). The entrance to the inlet has a threshold of 2.75 m above sea level, which means it could not have been used after ca. 1700. The stone features consist of U-shaped stone structures that open toward the former inlet. They were probably boat slips and it is possible they once had boat houses attached to them. There are also many small cairns that supported posts for drying nets. A number of small hut-like shelters, fire-cracked rocks and a Russian Oven were found as well. Two radiocarbon dates were obtained for the oven:. (St. 11902): 430±95 B.P. (A.D. cal. 1413–1630) and (St. 11903) 470±95 B.P. (A.D. cal. 1320–1618). These are among the few radiocarbon-dated Russian Ovens in the region and their association with a fishing harbor shows them to pre-date the Russian invasions. The 5 m level dates to ca. A.D. 1450 and the labyrinth dates to A.D. 1538±35. Sjöberg measured lichen growth on seven labyrinths on the island that dated them to A.D. 1388–1816 (Broadbent and Sjöberg 1990:295).

### Site 53

Site 53 is a complex of small net-drying post cairns, hut-like enclosures, boat slips, a labyrinth and a compass rose (Figure 124). This site (Area III) follows the 3–5 m elevation and had probably replaced Site 93 when it became too shallow. Two features were sampled for charcoal and rendered two dates.

Feature A, situated at 5–6 m above sea level, is a hut and produced one radiocarbon date: St. 11904) 735±120 B.P. (A.D. cal. 1167–1392). Feature B, located just above the 3.0 m shoreline, and rendered (St. 11905) 445±105 B.P. (A.D. cal. 1401–1631). . These dates are consistent with the elevations. The net-drying cairns lie lower than 3.0 m and show the use of this harbor after 1600. These two harbors are very similar to the harbors on Stora Fjäderägg and at Jungfruhamn.

### Conclusions

The investigations on the Island of Snöan focused on three sites: the highest lying area, 10–15 m.a.s.l., and two harbor sites at 5 and 3 m.a.s.l. The sealing huts date with some certainty to the Viking Period. It is clear that from A.D. 1300 fishing was the principal activity on the island. The two dates from a "Russian" Oven are a unique result and show that bread was baked on the island hundreds of years prior to the Russian invasions.

## Stor-Rebben Island

Stor-Rebben Island is located in the Piteå archipelago at 65° 11′ N, 21° 56′ E in the County of Norrbotten, about 5 kilometers from the mainland and 90 km north of Bjuröklubb. The island is

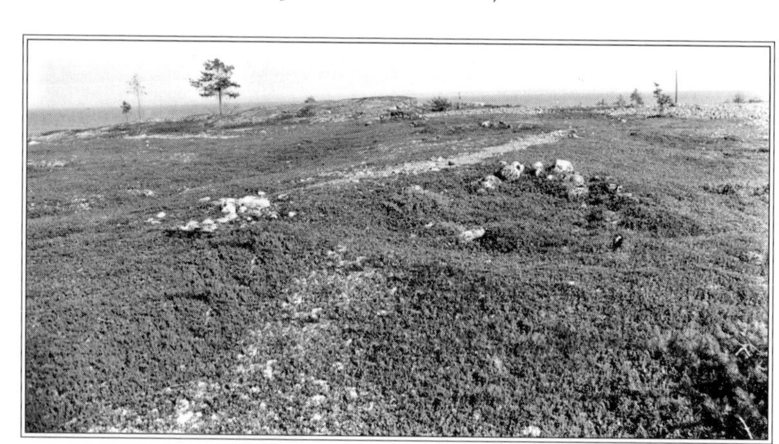

*Figure 126. Photo of Hut A, looking east.*

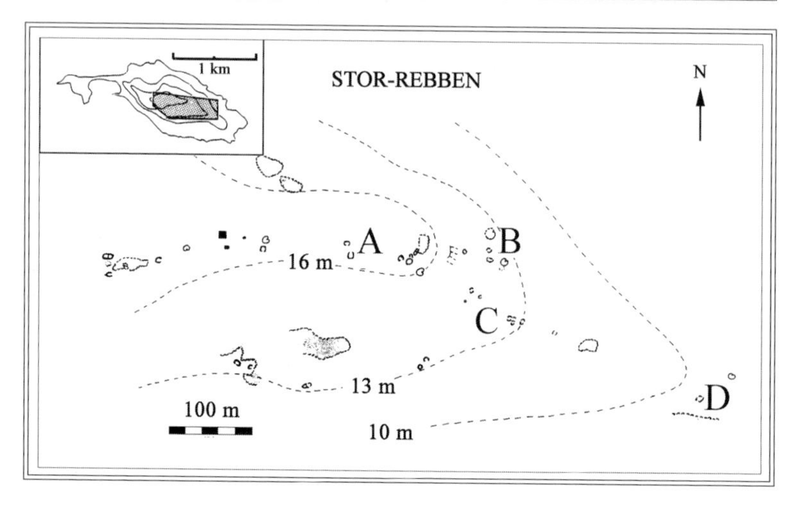


*Figure 127. Map showing investigated huts on Stor-Rebben Island.*

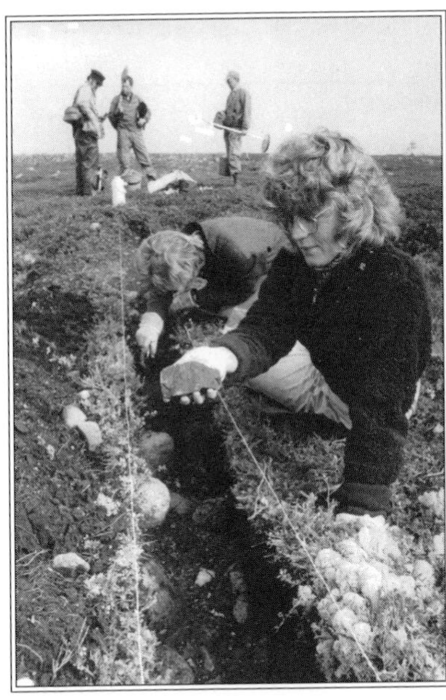

*Figure 128. Ann Wastesson and Ann-Christin Nilsson excavating a trench in Hut A. In the background, left to right, the author, Sture Berglund and Rabbe Sjöberg. Photo by Nils Ögren.*

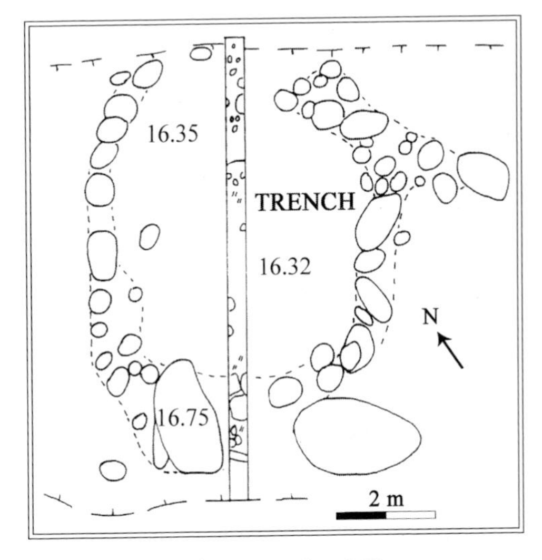


*Figure 129. Map of Hut A on Stor-Rebben.*

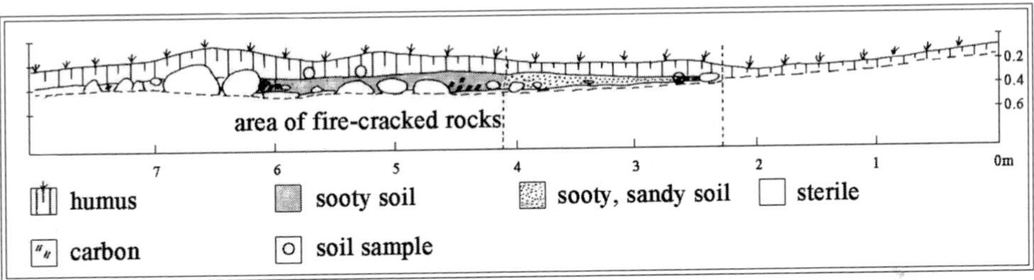


*Figure 130. Profile of trench through Hut A.*

rectangular in shape, 1.6 km long and 0.85 km wide. A sandy spit fans out toward the mainland (Figures 45, 127). According to Swedish historian Birger Steckzén the name *rebben* probably derives from the Saami words *ruebpe* or *riebpe,* which means a stony overgrown hill with brushy vegetation. Reference is also given the term *ruobba* which means a rocky hilltop (Steckzén 1964:232). This is certainly an accurate description of Stor-Rebben Island (Figure 126). This site was chosen for comparative purposes and is the northernmost of these hut localities to be investigated. The island rises up to 17 m above sea level and dwellings are found on beach terraces at three main levels: 16 m, 13 m and 7 m above sea level.

Claes Varenius had described the island in two articles in connection with archaeological surveys in the 1960s and 70s (Varenius 1964, 1978). He identified 27 huts, four of them double huts, and 11 huts with central hearths. He also recorded six labyrinths and a compass rose. Five of the labyrinths occur together with 3 hut groups: two of them at the 16 m level, two at the 13 m level and two at the 7 m level. There are four clusters of huts consisting of two to four structures each, just above the 16 m contour. At about the 14 m contour there are seven clusters, consisting of two to three huts and three labyrinths. Finally, at the 7 m level are the remains of a dwelling with

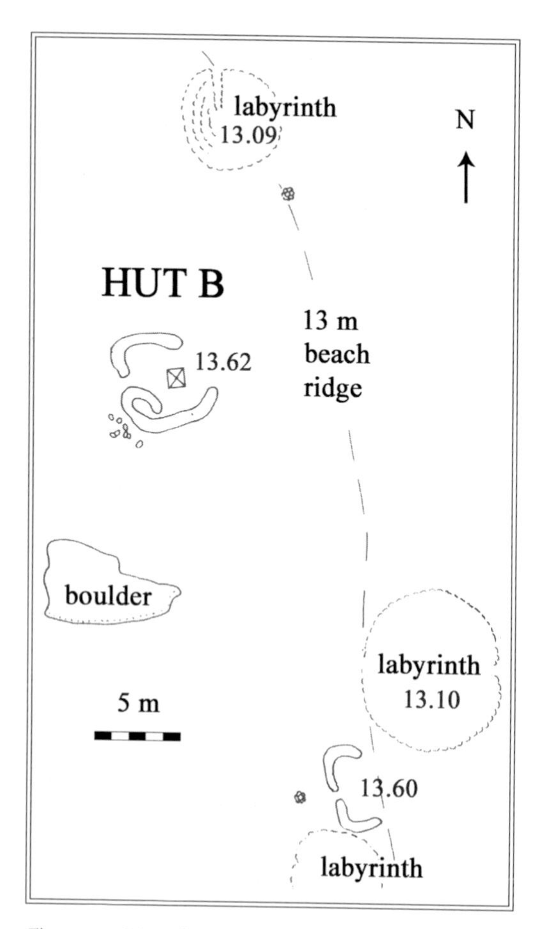


Figure 131. Map of Hut B and three labyrinths.

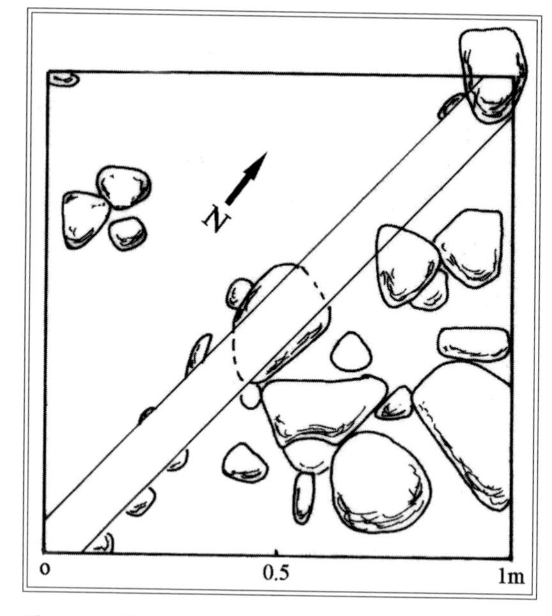


Figure 132. Excavation unit in Hut B.

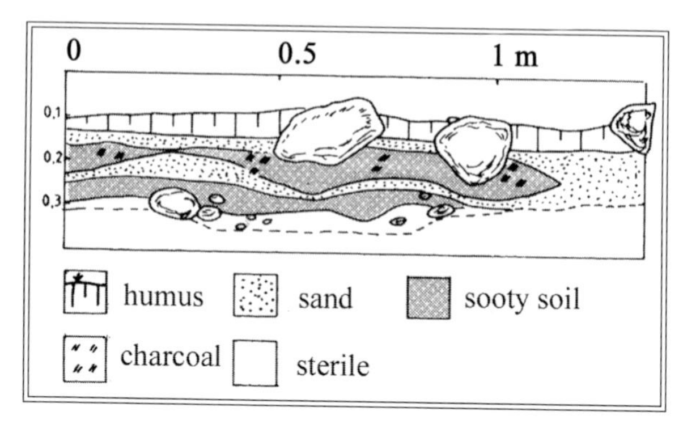


Figure 133. Profile of the hearth in Hut B showing two lenses.

a chimney and steps. Many of these features have only partial walls and are obviously disturbed. The most intact dwellings with archaeological potential, those with charcoal or bones, were chosen for excavation.

### Hut A

Hut A is the larger of two structures at the 16 m level. It lies in a depression between a bedrock outcropping and a gravel ridge (Figures 126, 128, 129,130). The hut consists of an oval foundation measuring 6 × 8 m with a floor area of approximately 5 × 6 m. There are two possible entrances at both short ends of the construction. Although no delimited hearth was distinguished per se, the floor had a thick layer of charcoal and fire-cracked rocks concentrated in the middle of the floor. Two radiocarbon dates were obtained (St. 11910 and St. 11178): (1845±135 B.P. and 1494±70 B.P.). These two dates calibrate respectively to 23 B.C. to A.D. 340 (median A.D. 172) and A.D. 443 to 643 (median A.D. 558). The first date range is the oldest radiocarbon date in the project. Against the

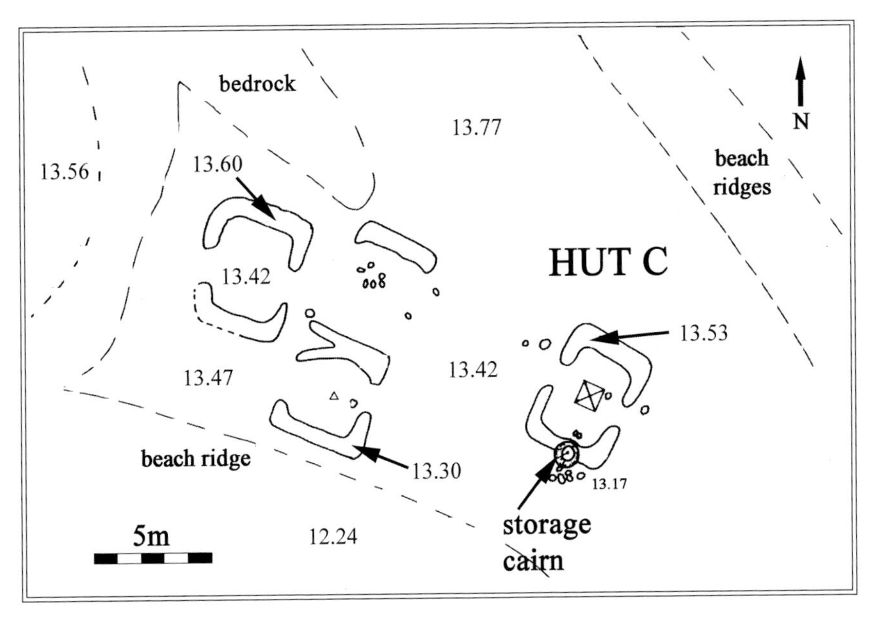


*Figure 134. Map of Hut C.*

background of shoreline displacement at Stor-Rebben, and the calculated age of the 16 m shoreline; the true age for the hut is probably A.D. 200–300. Old charcoal is an obvious risk, but these dates are not totally unreasonable. No bones could be identified from the dwelling. Carbonized seeds were found and identified as coming from crowberry bushes. These berries were also found in hearths at Grundskatan and Stora Fjäderägg. A gray flint chip was recovered, as well as 14 tiny slag fragments. The iron slag is the northernmost evidence of iron working.

***Hut B***

Hut B is one of two structures at 13.5 m above sea level (Figure 131). The form of these huts is rounded-rectangular and they have front and rear entranceways. One wall circles onto a small chamber that was probably a storage space. A central hearth rendered charcoal (St. 11179): 1045±70 B.P. (A.D. cal. 880–1155). The median age is A.D. 985. The hearth displayed two ashy lenses separated by a sterile layer of sand (Figure 133). The radiocarbon date is from the upper level. This evidence shows that the dwelling was not used on only one occasion, and the range of dates from this site indicates – like the dates from Hut A – repeated use over hundreds of years. Iron slag was also found in this hearth, as well as a flint chip from a strike-a-light. Twenty-one bone fragments were recovered, but were small and unidentifiable. Three labyrinths lay within 15 m of these huts, one of which abuts the wall of a dwelling. As will be discussed in Chapter 10, it is not likely that the huts and the labyrinths were contemporary.

***Hut C***

Hut C is one of four structures situated at 13.5 m above sea level. These huts are rectangular in shape and three have central hearths (Figure 134). The huts have entrances through their shortest

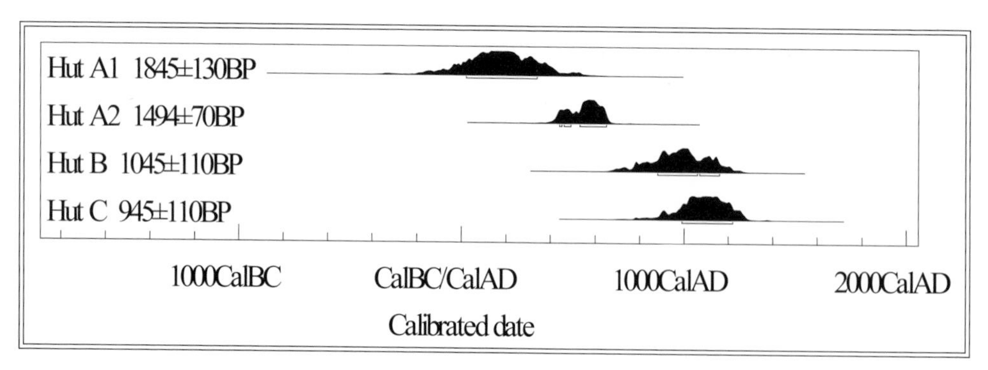


*Figure 135. Calibrated radiocarbon dates of huts on Stor-Rebben Island.*

walls and at right angles to the shore. The floor areas are 3.0 × 4.0 m. There is a small storage cairn in one of the walls. The hearth in the most intact of the three huts was excavated. It produced charcoal and 230 burned bone fragments. One bone was identified as coming from a reindeer or goat/sheep. The radiocarbon date (St. 11180) is: 945±110 B.P. (A.D. cal. 999–1212). The median is A.D. 1092. Two grey flint chips and a steatite piece with a groove and five slag pieces measuring 10– 32 mm were found.

***Hut D***

This dwelling differs completely from the others, and is of medieval or historic date. It has the base of a brick chimney and stairs. In addition to burned bone, there were flint fragments and old iron nails. A possible tripod leg of pottery was also found. The bones derived from goat/sheep, reindeer and an ungulate. The 7 m elevation renders a maximum date of ca. A.D. 1200. This coincides with the thirteenth century colonization of the region and founding of parishes in Piteå (Axelson 1989).

*Chronology*

The location of this island is consistent with many other Bothnian Iron Age sealing sites, such as Stora Fjäderägg in Västerbotten. Four radiocarbon dates were obtained and the period of site use ranges from A.D. 200 to 1200. The oldest dwellings cluster between 13 and 16 m above sea level. The huts are also comparable by size and form to the Västerbotten material, and also include storage facilities and cairns.

The frequency of labyrinths on Stor-Rebben is comparable to Snöan and Stora Fjäderägg. Unfortunately, none of them could be lichen dated. It is also likely that stones from the hut walls were used to build the labyrinths and this can best be seen in the area of Hut B. A partial hut is actually abutted by a labyrinth, and a second labyrinth lies just below it. There is an excellent

Table 49. Stor-Rebben: Unburned bones by fragment.

| SPECIES | HUT C | HUT D | TOTAL |
|---|---|---|---|
| Sheep/goat | | 2 | 2 |
| Reindeer | | 1 | 1 |
| Ungulate | 1 | 1 | 2 |
| Indeterminate | | 4 | 4 |
| Total | 1 | 8 | 9 |

Table 50. Stor-Rebben: Anatomical breakdown of bones.

| ANATOMY | ELEMENT | SHEEP/ GOAT | REINDEER | UNGULATE | TOTAL |
|---|---|---|---|---|---|
| Rib cage | Costae | | | 1 | 1 |
| Front extremity | Humerus | | | 1 | 1 |
| Rear extremity | Femur | 1 | 1 | | 2 |
| | Tibia | 1 | | | 1 |
| Total | | 2 | 1 | 2 | 9 |

example of the relationship of older prehistoric features, in this case a Bronze Age grave cairn, and labyrinths at the nearby mainland site of Jävre. The largest lichens on the labyrinth stones measure 155 mm and date to A.D. cal. 1299±30 (refer Chapter 10).

*Finds*
Hut A: A gray flint chip, 14 tiny slag fragments, crowberry seeds (*Empetrum*)
Hut B: Iron slag, a flint chip
Hut C: Two grey flint chips, and a steatite piece with a groove and five slag pieces measuring 10–32 mm.
Hut D: Flint chips, as well as iron nails and a possible unglazed tripod leg of pottery.

Gray flint chips were found in all four huts and were probably the byproducts of strike-a-lights. Iron slag was found in Huts A, B and C. The frequency of iron slag in these coastal huts suggests that iron working was a common practice. The steatite piece from Hut C could be associated with metallurgy, and has a parallel in a find from Site 138 at Jungfruhamn.

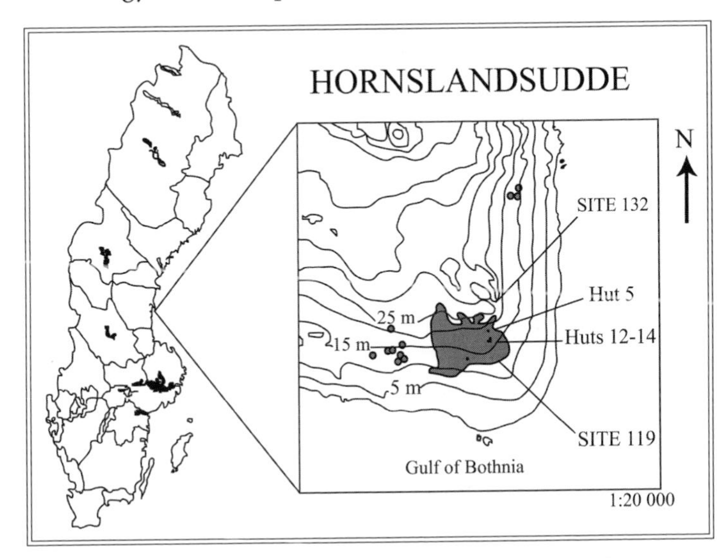


*Figure 136. Map showing location of Hornslandsudde, Sites 119 and 132.*

*Osteological Material*
The bones from the Stor-Rebben hearths emanate from sheep/goat, reindeer and an unidentified ungulate. All of these were unburned. Only one bone could be identified from Hut C, a humerus from an ungulate, presumably reindeer or sheep/goat. The size and shape is most consistent with that of a sub-adult reindeer. All the rest of the identifiable material came from Hut D. In Hut D, a femur of an adult and relatively large reindeer was identified together with a thigh

bone and a fibula of a sheep/goat. There are also rib bone fragments. It appears as though meat-rich body parts had been brought to the island as food. While preservation of the burned material is poor, it is surprising that not one seal or fish bone was identified. But, because of the location, sealing and fishing had to have been the primary reason for these huts. Equally remarkable are the finds of sheep/goat and reindeer bones. These sealers may have had brought food with them, although animals could have also been grazed on the islands.

**Summary**

In conclusion, Stor-Rebben is fully comparable to the other sites in the project. The island reveals both an older hut-based hunting economy, dating to circa A.D. 200–1100, and a younger fishing-based economy from ca. 1300. John Kraft cites some evidence that Bothnian labyrinths could have been associated with Saami magic, but he also noted most were associated with fishing sites and of younger date (Kraft 1977). The Saami place-name *Rebben* coincides with the oral histories at Stora Fjäderägg/Holmön and Hornslandsudde that identify these places as Lappish/Saami camps. The Stor-Rebben investigation, although limited in scope, has provided important data regarding the chronology, technology, economy and place-name context of these Iron Age sites, including the transition to the historic period.

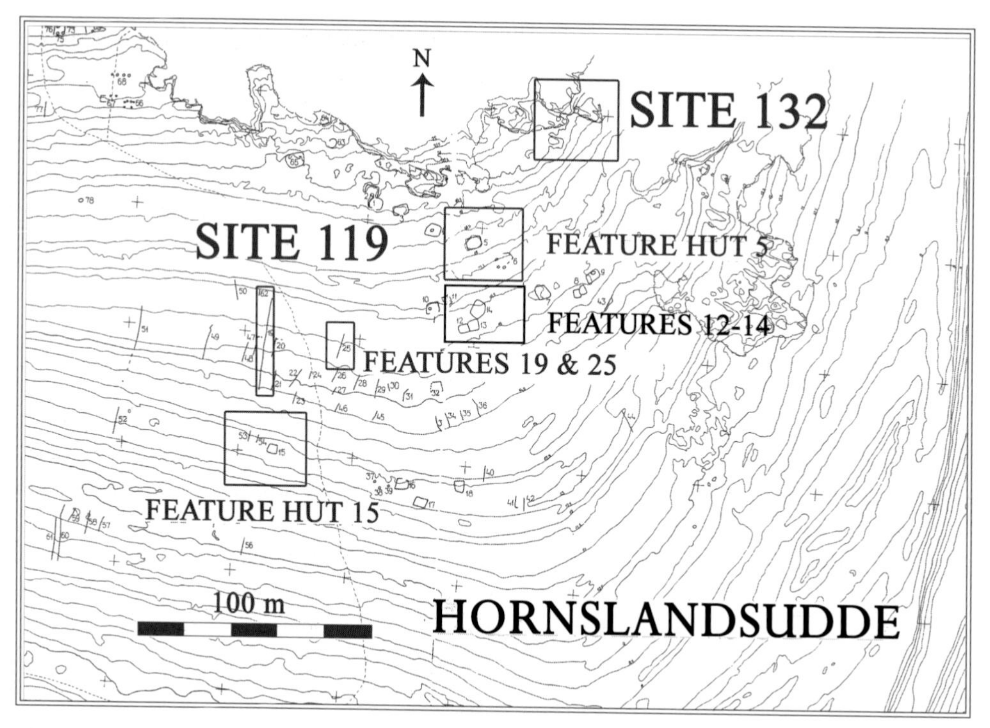


*Figure 137. Site area based on photogrammetry (Eriksson 1975). Investigated areas in 2005 are shown in boxes. The archaeological features (hut foundations) are situated between 12 and 25 m above present sea level. Huts were sampled at 13m, 16m, 18m, and 20m above sea level.*

## Hornslandsudde

Hornslandsudde (Site 119) was chosen for comparative purposes and is located only about 300 km north of Stockholm (Figure 136). The investigated region is in Gävleborg County, Hudiksvall Municipality, Rogsta parish in the province of Hälsingland at 61° 37′N, 17° 29′ E. The site is located in an area of largely exposed wave-washed moraine beaches up to 25 m above sea level. The beaches have distinctive terrace formations. Shoreline displacement is currently 0.75 mm per year. Vegetation consists primarily of pine heaths with dry blueberry (*vaccinium*) type ground cover. Lichen vegetation is abundant, especially reindeer lichens, and a large herd of reindeer were brought to the area during the harsh winter of 2006–2007. Hornslandsudde has stands of very old pine showing traces of burning from a forest fire in 1888. The Hornslandsudde site was first published by Westberg (1964). Björn Ambrosiani (1971) excavated some hut foundations and stone alignments in 1966. Photogrammetry-based mapping was carried out in 1966 and 1973 (Eriksson 1975). A new site survey was reported by Jönsson (1985) (Figure 137). Westberg relates the oral history of the Hornslandsudde area as follows:

> *According to tradition, which is still preserved among the older population who practiced fishing at Hölick's fishing village ca 2 km west of Hornslandsudde, the dwelling sites on the point derive from a fishing people of Lappish (Saami) origin. (1964:24)*

It should be noted that sealing was referred to as "seal fishing" in the Bothnian region (*själfiske*). The place-names *Lappmon* and *Lappmoberget* (Lapp Sand and Lapp Sand Mountain) are very close to this site (Westberg 1964:24). Westberg identified Hornslandsudde as a historically documented sealing place, which is also indicated in the place-name *Själlhällorna* (Seal Rocks). According to a map for Rogsta parish from 1799, a fishing site on Hornslandet was named *Lappbäck*. Westberg has provided an excellent overview of the history of fishing sites in the area and the islands of Kuggörarna, Bålsön and Hästholmen (Westberg 1964). The provincial law, "Helsingelagen," stipulated that one-tenth of all fowl, wild game, fish, moose and bears were to be paid in taxes, as well as every fifteenth salmon and fifteenth pound of herring, seals and gray squirrels. The priest and the Church would divide this equally (Westberg 1964:36). In 1545, Gustav Vasa initiated taxation of all fishing on the Bothnian coast. In the late 1500s, fishermen from the newly founded town of Hudiksvall established many fishing places in the region, although Agön was an exclusive herring fishery of the highly organized Gävle (i.e., urban) fisherman. The fishing harbors and labyrinths dating to the 1600s and 1700s at Kuggören and Bålsön are close parallels to those of, for example, Bjurön in Västerbotten. Salmon and seals were caught using net systems on poles at a number of locations and seals were also hunted on the ice.

The Hornsland Peninsula had formerly been an island and although some lakes provided freshwater fishing, agriculture was extremely marginal. Westberg suggested that this provided a coastal sanctuary for hunter-gatherers in an otherwise Germanic- settled region. Wennstedt Edvinger and I have documented several Saami circular sacrificial features on Hornslandet, one on Yttre Bergön that is similar to an enclosure on Stora Fjäderägg and another by Arnöviken (Wennstedt Edvinger and Broadbent 2006). Neither was associated with harbor basins. Both sites are near Iron Age graves and hut areas.

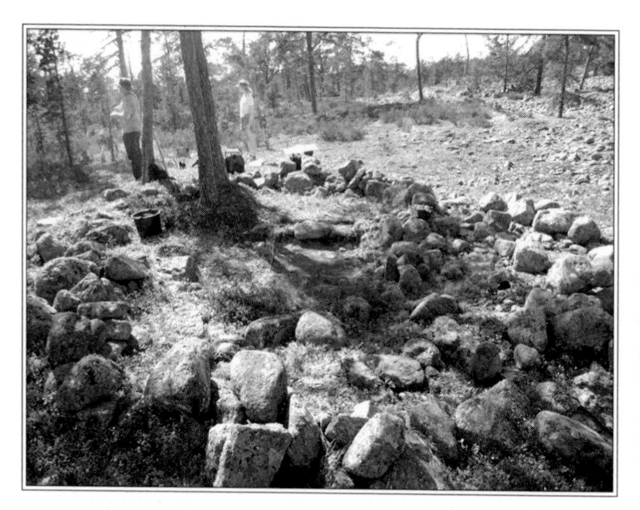

*Figure 138. Hut 5 from east showing double wall-lines.*

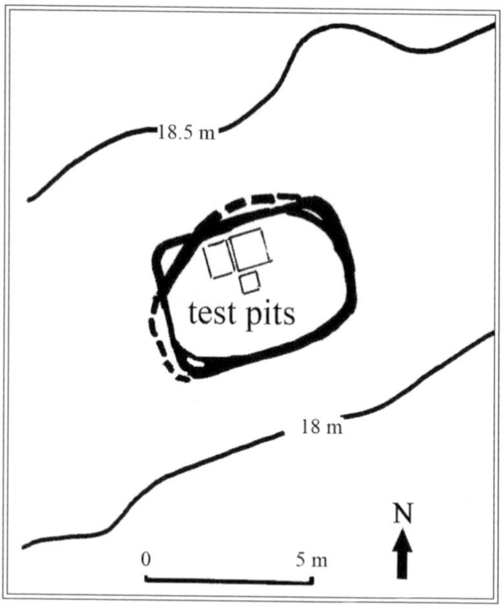


*Figure 139. Excavated area in Hut 5 (Jackelyn Graham).*

The excavations by Ambrosiani in 1966 did not produce any artifacts, radiocarbon samples or osteological results. New excavations were therefore undertaken in 2005 to better determine the ages of the huts and recover any organic remains. According to Jönsson (1985), Site 119 at Hornslandsudde has 48 hut foundations and some 60 stone alignments. The alignments are very distinctive long and low walls of stones with openings that were probably used to catch forest birds using snares. In 2005, we investigated two alignments and four hut foundations at 20 m, 18 m, 16 m and 13 m above sea level (Figure 144). A second site area about 75 m to the east of Site 119 was also sampled. This site (Site 132) consists of three features: two hut floors below a rocky cliff to the north, and a circular storage cairn. They lie at about the 20 m elevation. Finally, 11 storage caches and cairns have been registered at the two sites.

**Feature 5, Hut**

Feature 5 is a rounded-rectangular foundation measuring ca. 3.5 × 6 m and walls measuring 0.2–0.3 m height (Figures 138, 139). The hut is situated at 18 m above present sea level. This hut shows secondary walls indicating re-use. A hearth deposit with charcoal, burned bone and slag was found in the middle of the floor and investigated. The hearth was ca. 1 m in diameter and lacked a stone circle or any demarcation. The hearth is less than 1 m in diameter and, as seen by the profiles, less than 20 cm deep. The soil in the hearth was brown in color and the surrounding area had differing shades of brown. Some charcoal was found in and around the hearth, and samples were taken for radiocarbon dating. An abundance of highly fragmented bones was also found within and around the hearth. Fire-cracked rock (ca. 1 liter) was also found.

*Finds*

Iron slag (120 g)
Six red clay pieces (furnace walls) (0.6 to 1.2 cm)
One iron fragment (1.0 cm).

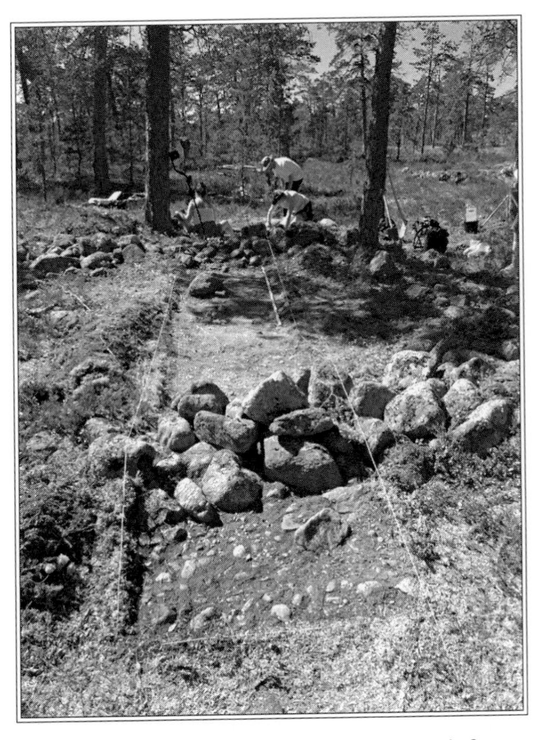

Figure 140. Trench through Feature 13 (foreground) from the east. (See Figure 154.)

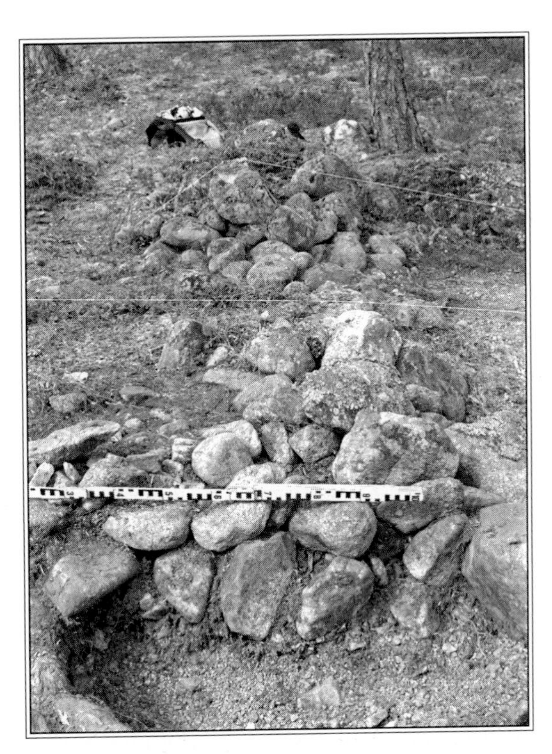

Figure 141. Section through connecting wall between Huts 12–13 where ruminant tooth fragments were found.

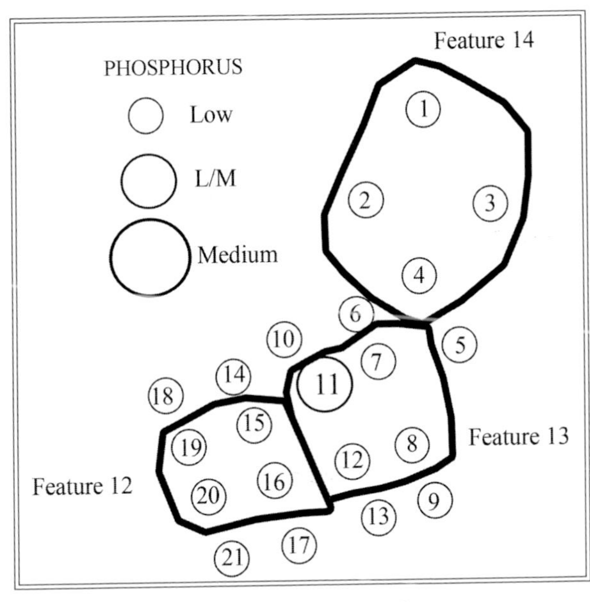


Figure 142. Features 12–14 showing soil samples 1–21.

*Osteological Material*
375 bone fragments (60 g)

The bone material could only be identified as long bones from mammals.

*Chronology*
Charcoal from the deepest part of the hearth was radiocarbon dated, but had nevertheless been contaminated: 140±40 B.P. (Beta 217790). This error is undoubtedly due to the forest fire of 1888. Because of this problem, a bone was submitted to the Svedberg Laboratory in Uppsala for an accelerator dating (Ua-32857), which produced an age of: 1390±30 B.P. (A.D. cal. 623–664).

*Conclusions*
Hut 5 dates to the seventh century, although double walls suggest it had been rebuilt. Of special interest is the fact that iron slag, fired clay and an iron piece, indicative of iron working, were found. This material is described separately, including analysis results by Andersson (2007), in Chapter 7.

**Features 12–14, Double Hut and Enclosure**
Features 12 and 13 are a double hut situated at 16 m above sea level. Feature 12 is rectangular in shape and measures 3.5 × 4.5 m with walls 0.1 to 0.2 m high. Feature 13 is approximately rectangular and measures 4 × 4 m with walls 0.3 to 0.5 m high. Feature 14 is an irregular enclosure with lower walls measuring 5 × 7 m (Figure 142). As far as could be determined, it probably was an enclosure. Only slight traces of burning were found in the Feature 13 hearth, not enough for a radiocarbon date. Adjacent to the hearth was a large cobble, which could have been used as a seat or as an anvil. A possible whetstone was found adjacent to it. A trench was run to cross-cut both hut floors and the wall between them (Figure 141). In addition, the south end of the foundation, which protruded out about 30 cm, was sectioned (Figure 142). Fragments of a tooth from a ruminant (sheep/goat or reindeer) were found at a depth of 20 cm. Hut 12 was found to have a much more uneven floor littered with a number of medium-sized cobbles. A hearth was found up against the north wall, and this feature was full of of iron slag and furnace clay. A magnet produced quantities of iron scales and sphericals that were by-products of iron smithing. In addition, a channel penetrated the wall on the right side of the hearth.

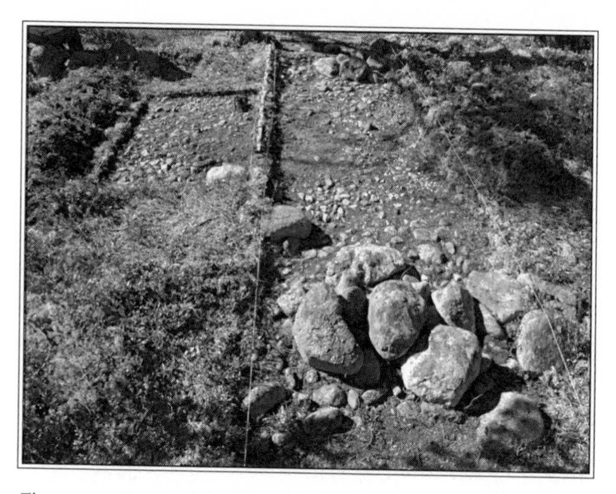

*Figure 143. Excavation of Hut 15, from south.*

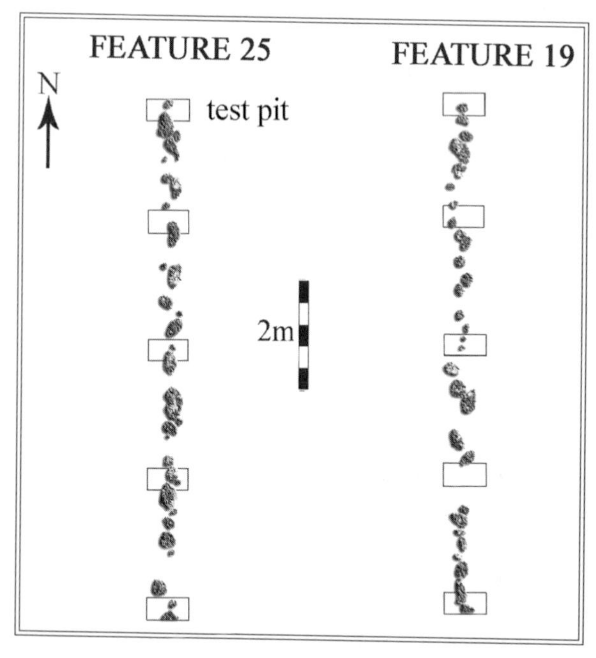


*Figure 144. Map of sections of two stone alignments (Jacquelyn Graham).*

*Finds*
Iron slag, ca. 20, 1–5 cm (1.1 kg)
Iron scales, ca. 100, < 1 cm, (60g)

*Osteological Material*
Tooth enamel from a small ruminant (sheep/goat or reindeer); (numerous fragments (22g) from the same tooth, from maxillary).

*Chronology*
Two AMS dates were obtained: (Beta-209908) 1570± 40 B.P. (A.D. cal. 434–537), and (Beta-207939) 1820±40 B.P. (A.D. cal. 136–236).

The hearth in Hut 12 was clearly used for iron working. The hearth measured ca. 1 m in diameter and lacked a stone circle. The channel-like opening through the wall next to the hearth was probably an air duct for a bellows and is a parallel to the wall opening documented at Bjuröklubb Site 67. No bones were preserved in the hearths of either Huts 12 or 13, although enamel from a ruminant tooth was found in the wall between the huts. Twenty-one soil samples taken across the area of these huts showed very low levels of phosphorus enrichment (0–50 P°). The only high phosphorus level is sample 11 from the corner of the dwelling, Hut 13. This is most likely a consequence of very poor preservation conditions and the shallow deposits at the site. The three features, 12, 13 and 14, form a unit consisting of a smithy, a dwelling/workshop and a possible enclosure for livestock.

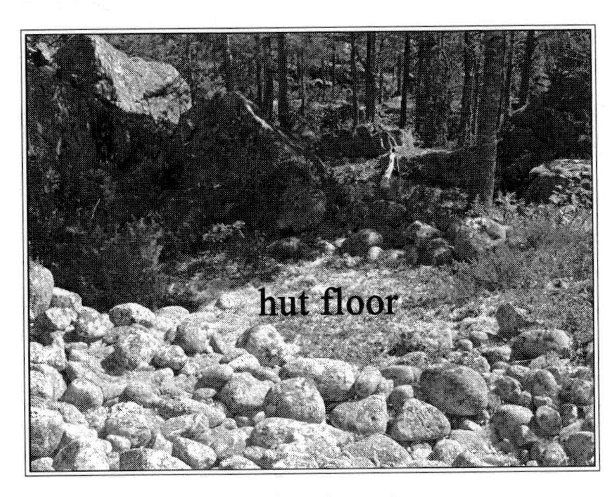

*Figure 145. Site 132 Hut A, from the southwest.*

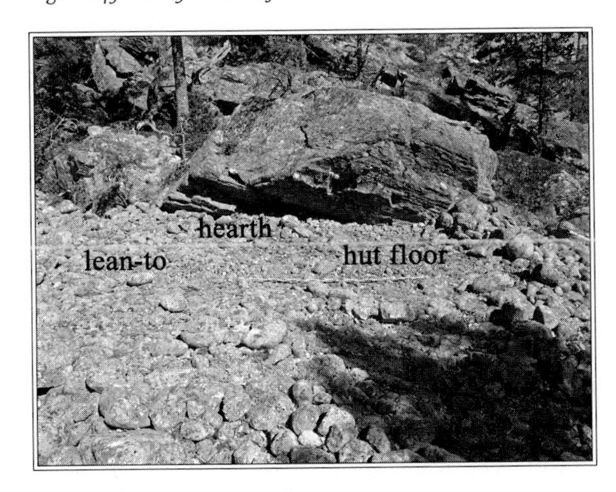

*Figure 146. Site 132, Hut B, from southwest.*

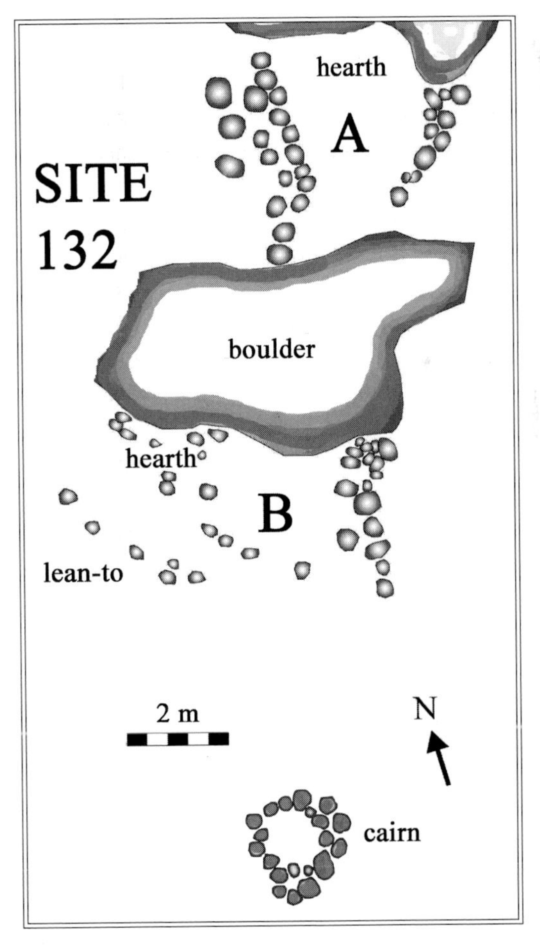

*Figure 147. Map of Site 132 showing Hut A, Hut B and a cache.*

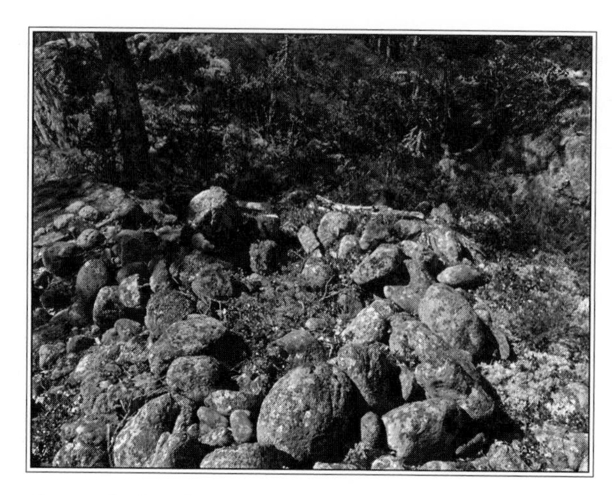

*Figure 148. Cairn by Site 132, Hut B.*

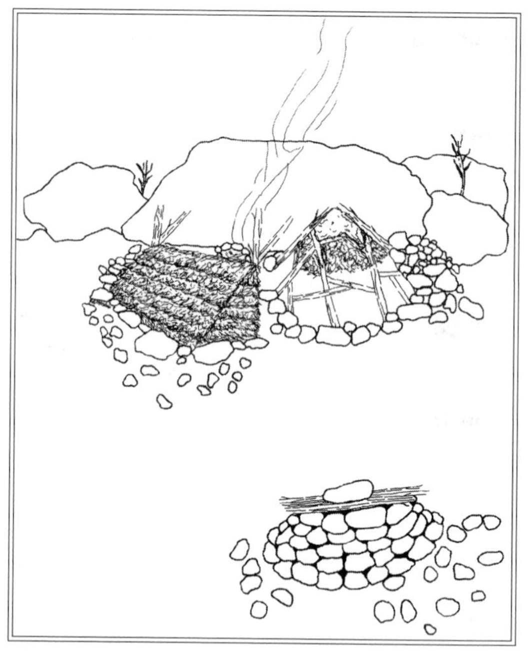

*Figure 149. Reconstruction of Hut B, lean-to and storage cairn at Site 132 (Jacquelyn Graham).*

**Feature 15, Hut**

Feature 15 is a rounded-rectangular hut, measuring 4 × 5 m and with walls 0.2 m high. It is situated at an elevation of 12.5 m above present sea level. Hut 15 was trenched across its midline in order to expose the hearth (Figure 143). A shallow ashy deposit was subsequently found in the center of the floor. An additional 1.0 × 0.50 m unit was excavated to expose this feature. The trench was dug down to 35 cm below the surface across the floor. Only tiny bone chips and small carbon pieces were found in this hut. Even this carbon sample (Beta 210237) proved to be contaminated: 260±70 B.P.. This hut was examined because of its elevation above the 12 m shoreline. No animal bone was obtained for analysis. It is the lowest-lying dwelling we investigated and is adjacent to the area of stone alignments.

**Features 19 and 25, Stone Alignments**

Ten soil samples were collected beneath cairns along two stone alignments, Features 19 and 25 (Figure 144). All the phosphorus samples were low (0–50 P°). Potassium levels, suggestive of burning, were high in all the test pits. This probably reflects the forest fire that had burned over the area in 1888. No reliable charcoal samples were obtained.

**Site 132**

Two hut floors with small hearths and a storage cairn lie approximately 75 m to the northeast of the main hut site. The elevation is ca. 20 m above present sea level. According to a footnote in the survey records from 1982, a local informant believed these were connected with the military signal station that had been established nearby in World War II. Both huts, although not overgrown with lichens or vegetation, had small hearths with charcoal that could be collected among the loose beach stones. Burned animal bone was found in Hut B. Hut A, the smaller of the two huts, is located up against an outcropping and is bounded on the west by a wave-washed cobble beach. This

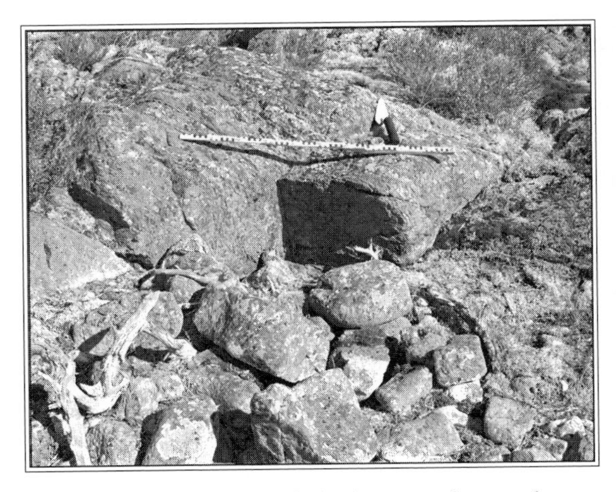

*Figure 150. Cache #4 next to bedrock outcrop, from south.*

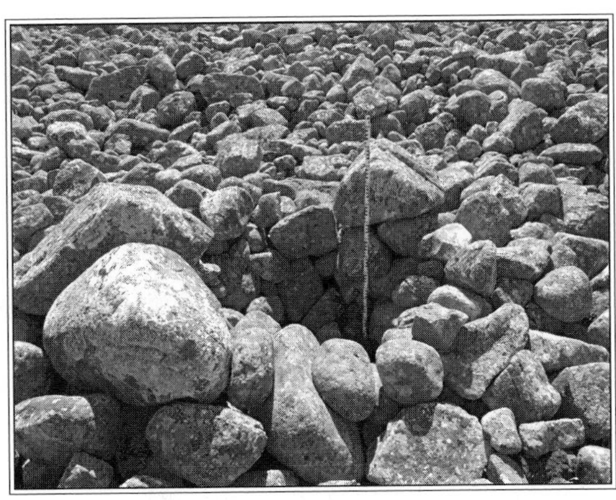

*Figure 151. Cache #1 in wave-washed moraine field, from west.*

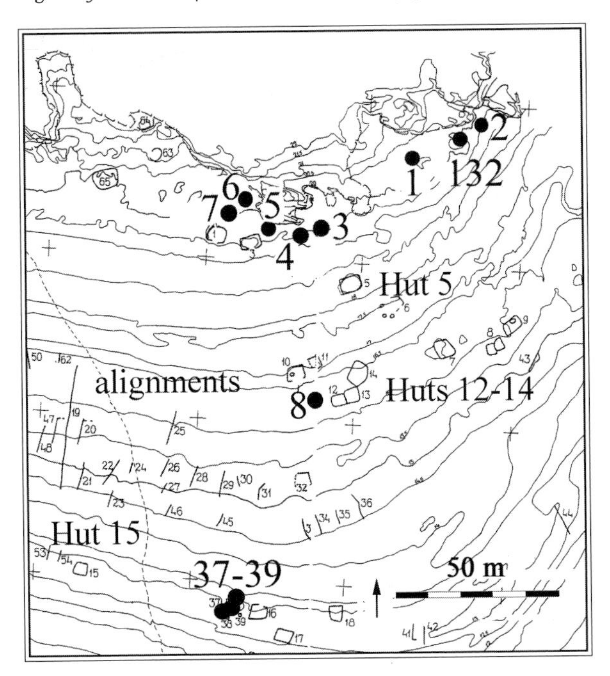


*Figure 152. Map of cache locations, Sites 119 and 132.*

hut measures ca. 4 × 4 m and contains a hearth (Figures 145–147). Charcoal was submitted for analysis but was only partially carbonized and was the by-product of later site use. This proved to be the case (Beta-217789): 210±40 B.P. Hut B is larger than, and located to the south of, Hut A. It measures ca. 6 × 4 m. The northern walls for both huts are bedrock/boulder outcroppings. The stones from Hut B form a pattern suggesting that two structures had stood there. One is an ovoid form with a cleared floor surface and was probably a bent-frame hut. The hearth was outside of this hut and up against the boulder. A second line of stones marks the line of a possible lean-to (Figure 149). An open cairn measuring ca. 2 × 2 m in diameter lies

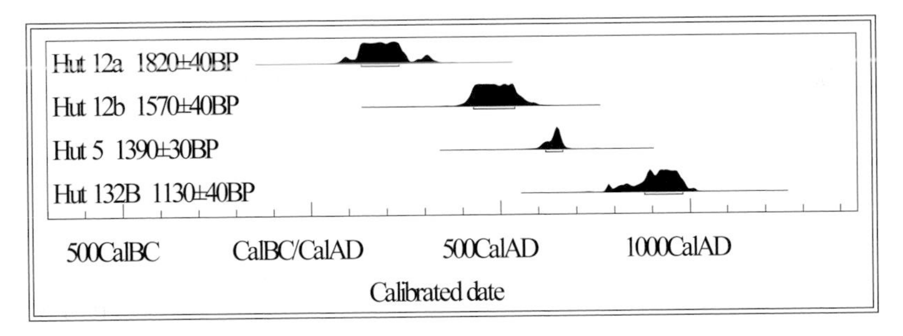


*Figure 153. Calibrated dates from Hornslandsudde.*

ca. 3 m to the south of Hut B. Its proximity to the dwellings implies that it had served for storage and is interpreted as a meat cache.

*Chronology*
Charcoal was found in Hut B (Beta-210238) and dated to: 1130 ±40 B.P. (A.D. cal. 881–980).

*Osteological Material*
Hut B also contained bones that were found to be the proximal epiphysis of the second metatarsal bone from a large seal, probably a gray or harp seal, and a long bone fragment.

Site 132 dates to the Viking Period. The seal bone found in Hut B is consistent with the interpretation of the site as a place for marine hunting. The cairn is interpreted as a storage cairn. This locale was well protected from winds and had good access to the former shoreline.

**Caches**
Five small stone caches were identified at the foot of a rocky outcropping less than 10 m to the north of the upper dwelling area (Huts 1–5) (Figures 150–152). These features appear as small pits and niches by the bedrock outcrop. A larger and deeper cache was found in a boulder field (Cache #1) in an area 60 m to the east of Hut 5. This well-constructed cache measured 1.0 to 1.5 m across and was 1.2 m deep. Additional caches were also documented on the site.

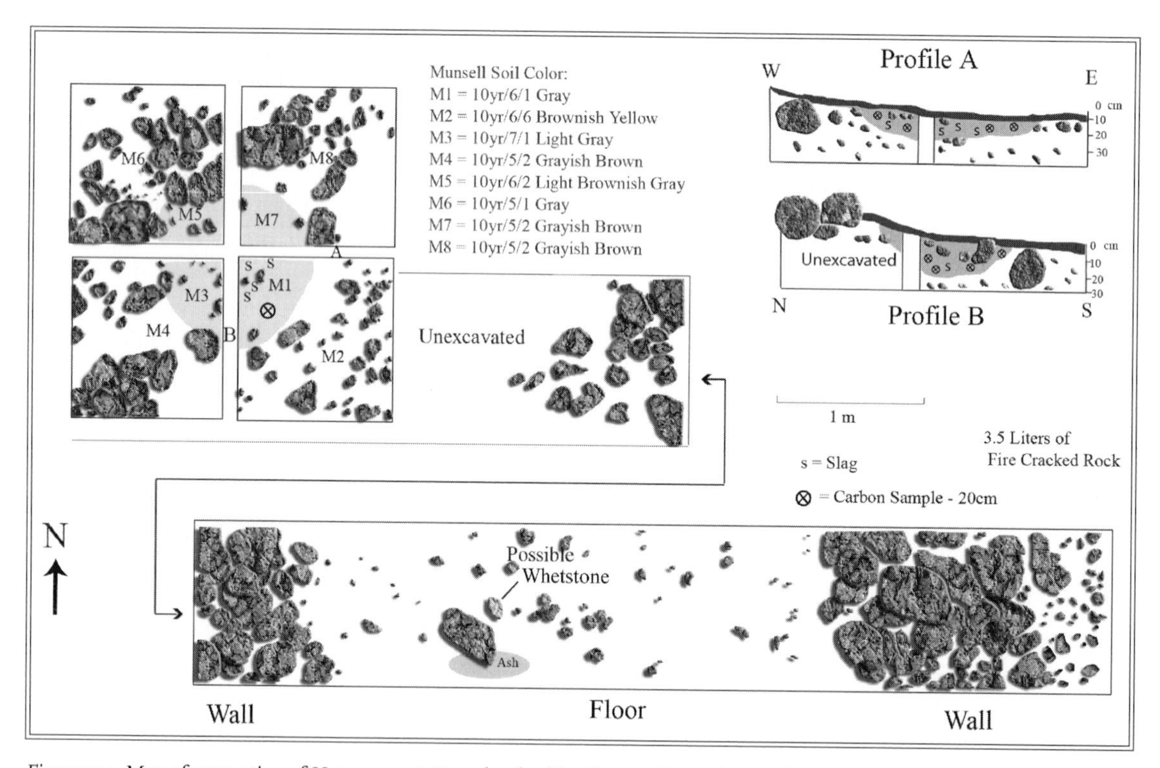


*Figure 154. Map of excavation of Huts 12–13 at Hornslandsudde, Site 119 (Jacquelyn Graham).*

**Summary and Discussion**

The results of the investigation show that the oldest huts at Site 119 date to the Early Iron Age. Site 132 dates to the Viking Period. Most of the bones recovered appear to be seal bone, although this material is very fragmentary. The identification of an adult gray or harp seal at Site 132 is interesting and corresponds to finds from the island of Stora Fjäderägg in Västerbotten. This suggests open-water hunting.

The huts are similar in size and form to the Västerbotten material. Width is fairly uniform, 3–5 m, and length, 3–8 m, is more variable. The huts lie in roughly four groups ranging between 12–25 m above sea level and form loose clusters aligned parallel with the shorelines and facing south and south/southeast. Seven huts cluster along the 12 m level, four to five huts at the 14 m level, seven to nine huts at the 16 m level, five to seven huts at the 17 m level and two to five huts at the 20 m level and higher. It is not certain that the highest lying features are the oldest; net drying post cairns at the highest elevations suggest medieval or historic fishing.

Site 132, Hut B, consists of three elements: a small hut, a hearth outside of the hut and a windbreak. Near the hut is a storage cache. A reconstruction gives an impression of what this dwelling site looked like (Figure 149). The distinctive storage caches are another close parallel to the Västerbotten material. Some caches are adjacent to huts while others could have been more communal. The numerous stone alignments run at right angles to the shoreline and have been interpreted by others as net-drying features or boat slips (cf. Westberg 1964:28). While these lines extend from 8 to 17 m above sea level, they lie in an area west of the main hut clusters and are not necessarily contemporary with them. Two stone alignments (19, 25) were sampled, but unfortunately the forest fire in 1888 left carbon over the whole site surface, thus contaminating superficial cultural layers. Soil samples indicate high levels of potassium on the site, probably a reflection of this fire.

There are many similarities to the Västerbotten region sites by chronology, function, clustering, storage, and even by ritual (cf. Wennstedt Edvinger and Broadbent 2006). On this basis, this archaeological material, together with the place-name evidence, speaks in favor of the theory that these had been hunter-gatherer (Saami) sites. But unlike Västerbotten, there is a parallel Early Nordic Iron Age complex of house terraces, grave mounds etc. in the region (cf. Liedgren 1992). These settlements in Rogsta parish were situated ca. 15 km to the north and above the 15 m level. Interestingly enough, this complex seems to have disappeared around A.D. 600. This raises the fascinating issue of the co-existence of two groups in the region, one a hunter-gatherer/herding/trading group of Saami and the other an agrarian-based/trading Germanic community. The Saami may even have been especially drawn to this region because of Germanic settlement, and offered their hunting and healing skills and even specialized iron working. Conversely, the two groups could have occupied different ecological niches in the coastal zone with long-term Saami interactions in two familiar forms forms, first as hunter-gatherers and later as reindeer herders, but were probably also living in ways analogous to the Germanic farmers and fishermen.

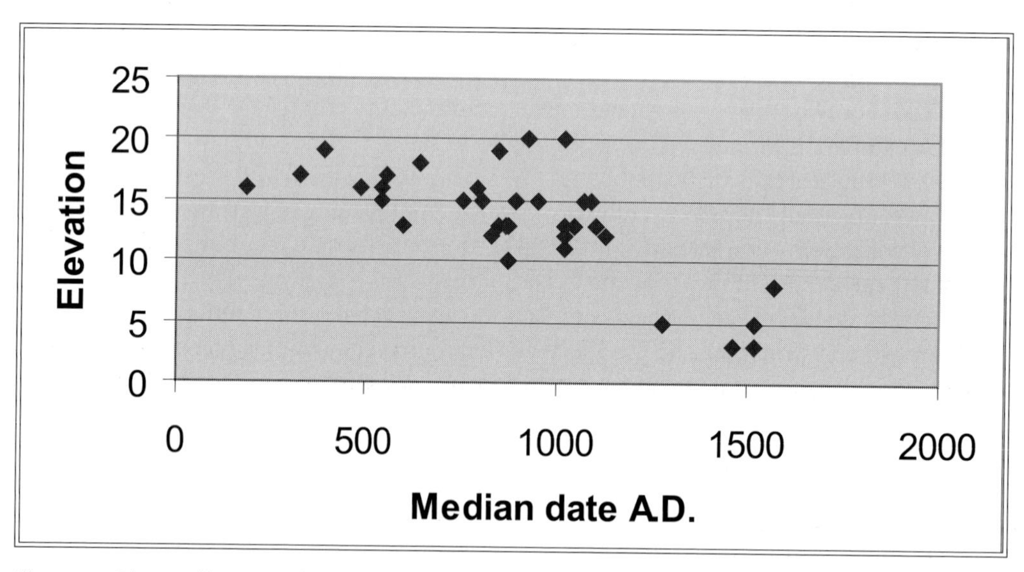


*Figure 155. Diagram illustrating the elevations of radiocarbon dates on the Bothnian shores and the gap between Iron Age sealing sites and medieval fisheries.*

# 6

# Chronology and Culture

This chapter provides an overview of the radiocarbon and AMS dates from huts between 20 m and 3 m above sea level. As noted earlier, this material encompasses 31 huts at 9 locales and 12 elevations. This sampling facilitates comparisons at different elevations above sea level at the same locales and comparisons between regions. There are five major questions:

1) When were these huts first used?
2) When were these huts last used?
3) Were there differences between regions?
4) What is the chronological relationship between the sealers' huts and medieval fisheries?
5) Are there patterns of use reflecting economic or environmental cycles?

Although one standard deviation (68% probability) was used for the descriptions of individual site dates, the following analysis is based on two standard deviations (95% probabilities) of 44 dates.

## Source Criticism

There is always a risk that samples have been contaminated by old wood or recent forest fires. Charcoal analysis has indicated that pine was the most common fuel, although birch and alder were also burned. The Hornslandsudde site area has stands of some of the oldest pines in Sweden, and even dry pine branches can be several hundred years old. This said, elevations above sea level can be used to reject dates that are clearly older than their contemporary shorelines. There are only two potential dates in this latter category: Stor-Rebben A1 and Jungfruhamn C, although they still fall within one standard deviation of their elevation dates. They are therefore considered as probable. In the case of Hornslandsudde, the shoreline association of Hut 12 is confirmed by the fact that the slag found in the hearth had been water-rolled (Andersson 2007). Two recent dates were obtained from carbon samples collected in 2004 from the partially disturbed cairn in Hut 4 at Grundskatan. These are so recent they must be rejected. A sample that was improperly stored from Snöan 49B is also suspect, but is perhaps evidence that the hearth had been re-used during historic times. Three dates from Huts 5, 15 and 132A at Hornslandsudde were clearly contaminated by recent forest fires and unusable. Finally, due to the earlier limitations on charcoal amounts necessary for dates, some results have very large standard deviations, namely Stora Fjäderägg B

(±315), Grundskatan 14 (±185) and Grundskatan 15 (±245). These are not terribly useful except within the framework of the material as a whole. A related question is whether or not the huts had been built no more than 1–2 m higher than their contemporary shorelines. This depended on the topography of each site, but a correlation coefficient of 0.73 between elevation and oldest median date shows that this assumption is largely true.

While radiocarbon dates have a high correlation with elevation dates, the re-occupation of older hut areas during the tenth and eleventh centuries is also evident. Huts from this period lie as much as 20 m above sea level. Huts by harbor basins are much more shore-bound, as can be expected, although these huts can also lie on higher ground. For instance, a hut dating to the seventeenth century on Stora Fjäderägg Island lies 5 m higher than the harbor basin at Gamla Hamnen. In spite of these concerns, consistent results have been obtained from different localities and elevations along the transect.

## Site Comparisons

The individual calibrated dates were sorted by increments for each site in order to see how they were spatially distributed (Table 51). This does not show how many dates were obtained at a given site, but which time periods are represented. Three periods dominate: A.D. 100–400, A.D. 400–600 and A.D. 800–1000. Together these horizons comprise 81% of the total.

Looking at the material as a whole (Figure 156), the dates appear to cluster in four successive steps. The oldest cluster ranges from 1845 to 1660 B.P. The next cluster is from 1570 to 1390 B.P., the third is from 1300 to 1110 B.P and the fourth is from 1045 to 880 B.P. The weighted averages of these clusters and their ranges within two standard deviations are shown in Table 52. The two final age groups are separated by only 55 years and correspond to the early and late Viking Period. This gap is probably not significant. There is a significant gap of 170 years, however, between the second and third groups, or between A.D. 608 and A.D. 778. Groups 1 and 2 are separated by 105 years, which is also significant. These numbers support the conclusion that the clustering is real.

Table 51. Chronological horizons by site.

| SITES (N–S) | 100–400 | 400–600 | 600–800 | 800–1000 | 1000–1200 |
|---|---|---|---|---|---|
| Stor-Rebben | X | X | | X | X |
| Bjuröklubb; Site 70 | | X | | X | |
| Jungfruhamn | X | X | | X | |
| Grundskatan | | X | X | X | X |
| Stora Fjäderägg | X | X | | X | |
| Snöan | | | | X | |
| Hornslandsudde | X | X | X | X | |
| | 19% | 29% | 10% | 33% | 10% |

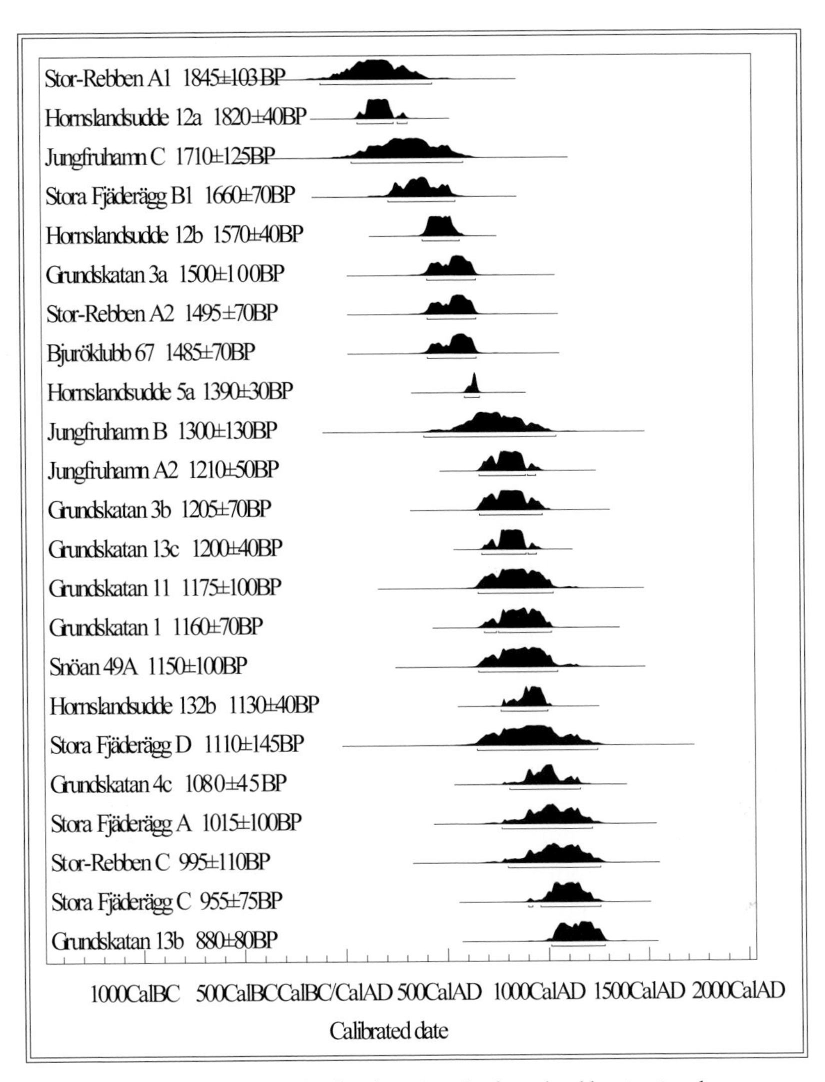


*Figure 156. Representative sample of 24 dates in order from the oldest (top) to the youngest. The dates form a step-like progression.*

Table 52. Clusters of hut dates (weighted averages).

| C-14 CLUSTERS | AVERAGES | (2 S.D.) |
|---|---|---|
| 1) 1845–1660 B.P. | 1776±33 B.P. | A.D. 134–334 |
| 2) 1570–1390 B.P. | 1513±26 B.P. | A.D. 439–608 |
| 3) 1300–1110 B.P. | 1175±20 B.P. | A.D. 778–941 |
| 4) 1045–880 B.P. | 979±30 B.P. | A.D. 996–1154 |

### The Start Dates

The numbers of dates by century show that this form of hut-based sealing began in the early second century A.D., had a peak in the sixth century, a slight decline in the seventh and eighth centuries, reached its greatest peaks in the ninth through eleventh centuries, and declined sharply in the twelfth century.

### The End Dates

The youngest dates at the five main sites range between 1130 and 880 B.P. One of the Grundskatan dates has a large standard deviation, but even discounting this, four dates calibrate to the thirteenth century at the latest. The year A.D. 1279 (discounting St. 11174) can be taken as the best measure with 95% probability for the *terminus ad quem* of this North Bothnian hunting system. The difficulties of obtaining uncontaminated dates at Hornslandsudde have led to only one date from this latter period.

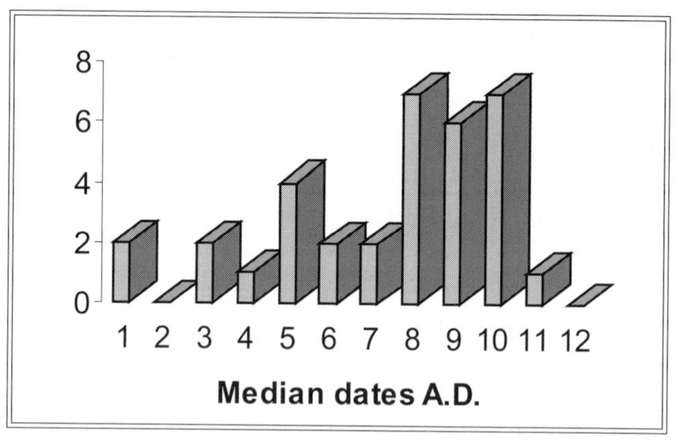


*Figure 157. Numbers of dates of Bothnian sealing huts (median values of calibrated dates).*

### Summary and Discussion

Hut-based Bothnian sealing began in the late first or early second century A.D. and all sites had been abandoned by A.D. 1279, although most sites came into disuse in the late twelfth century. Comparisons along the north to south transect show the same occupation trends. There are few differences between sites or between regions; they were part of the same phenomenon. Clusters of radiocarbon dates fall into three main periods: A.D. 100–400, A.D. 400–600 and A.D. 800–1000. There were peaks in the sixth and the ninth through eleventh centuries A.D., and declines in the seventh and the late thirteenth centuries A.D. that correspond to widespread settlement regressions in the Nordic region and the Little Ice Age.

The Stalo hut sites in alpine areas of Sweden and Norway (Manker 1960; Kjellström 1974; Storli 1991; Mulk 1994; Bergstøl 2004; Liedgren et al. 2007; Bergman and Liedgren et al. 2008)

Table 53. End dates of the sealing sites.

| SITE | DATES | RANGES (2 S.D.) |
|---|---|---|
| Stor-Rebben | 945±110 B.P. (St.11180) | A.D. 886–1278 |
| Jungfruhamn | 985±70 B.P. (St.11176) | A.D. 886-1214 |
| Grundskatan | 1000±185 B.P. (St.11174) | A.D. 656–1305 |
| Grundskatan | 880±80 B.P. (St.11172) | A.D. 1013–1279 |
| Stora Fjäderägg | 1015±100 B.P. (St.11181) | A.D. 788–1221 |
| Hornslandsudde | 1130±40 B.P. (Beta-210238) | A.D. 779–994 |

offer interesting parallels to the Bothnian sealing sites. Both were based on the specialized exploitation of marginal environments. The ecology of the alpine regions is remarkably similar to the outer coasts, especially in regard to vegetation. The Stalo huts are found from the Torneträsk area of northernmost Sweden to Frostviken in Jämtland in South Lapland. There are some 500 registered huts in Sweden, about the same number as the Bothnian huts. They vary in size and shape from oval to rectangular and often occur in clusters of three to seven sod foundations, frequently aligned in straight or bowed lines. Bone caches, hearths and pits are common. Their hearths are often indistinct but can have a *passjo/boassjo* stone by the hearth. There are few artifacts, mostly flint or quartz chips, whetstones and iron slag. These huts were associated with seasonal reindeer hunting and/or herding, although some appear to be more permanent. Radiocarbon dates have ranged from A.D. 400–1600, but a recent source-critical analysis of 22 huts at 12 sites shows them to mostly date to A.D. 640–1180 (Liedgren et al. 2007). These dates overlap with the main period of the Bothnian huts and were probably results of the same historical and economic processes affecting larger regions of the Nordic North. Radiocarbon dates of oval and rectangular Saami hearths in the forest lands of Southern Lapland add a further dimension to this discussion (Hedman 2003). These date to as early as A.D. 1, but mostly date to the Viking Period. They were associated with Saami *kåta/goahte* huts or tents. Rock-filled hearths were associated with the more permanent *kåtas*. These hearths occur in alignments of up to 10 hearths, probably accumulations of two to three tents or huts at a time representing *sijddas*, or family hunting groups (Bergman 1991; Bergman and Liedgren et al. 2008). During the Viking Period there was a change in site locales from the river valleys, where they coincide with Stone Age sites and finds of asbestos pottery and transverse-based projectiles, to reindeer grazing areas by bogs, springs, streams and small lakes. This is interpreted as a change from a hunting-, gathering- and fishing economy to a semi-nomadic herding economy, and a shift from collective to individual forms of property and animal ownership (Hedman 2003; Bergman and Liedgren et al. 2008). There are a number of artifacts with parallels in Saami offer sites, including coins, hack silver and weights. There is also iron slag indicative of forging (Hedman 2003:161–189). While these finds confirm the associations of the hearths with Saami metal offer sites, the hearths did not disappear in the fourteenth century, but instead increased in numbers. This can mean only one thing: Saami population density increased in the interior. This is probably the beginnings of larger winter villages as described by Tegengren for Kemi Lapmark (cf. Tegengren 1952; Bergman 1991; Mulk 1994).

This material reflects a number of trends of relevance to the North Bothnian coastal material. The first is the fact that this manifestation of Saami settlement within the *sijdda* system goes back to A.D. 1, and that this pattern coincides with Stone and Early Metal Age settlements, which is reflective of long-term continuity. The second is the expansion of this system, including linear alignments of hearths that relate reindeer pastoralism, trade and the accumulation of wealth during the period A.D. 700–1100. And lastly, there was an increase in hearth density in the interior from A.D. 1300. As discussed in the following chapters, these patterns are a result of larger-scale changes in the Nordic region relating to state formation.

### What Do the Artifacts Tell Us?

Inga Serning (1956, 1960) has discussed the Iron Age artifact material of Upper Norrland within the context of Saami offer sites and these studies constitute major points of reference for understanding coastal chronology. Inger Zachrisson (1984) has published additional material in this Iron Age context, as has Thomas Wallerström (2000), Lillian Rathje (2001) and Sven-Donald Hedman (2003). Coastal artifacts from the period before A.D. 600, including the Storkåge find (that can be an offer site) from ca. A.D. 350 and the Jävre grave find, a wheel-shaped ornament from a grave cairn in southern coastal Norrbotten (Broadbent 1982:154–255), are mostly of East Baltic, Finnish or central Russian (Volga-Kama) origin.

The chronology of the Germanic longhouse settlement at Gene at the northern limit of Germanic settlement on the Bothnian coast shows it was occupied continuously from ca. A.D.100/200 to 500/600. This settlement was abandoned around 500/600 along with a widespread regression in the cultural landscape, which is also seen in north and southwest Norway, the islands of Öland and Gotland, Östergötland and the Mälar Valley (Ramqvist 1983:194). In Medelpad and in Hälsingland (and the Hornsland region), there is an almost identical pattern with farmsteads from the second century A.D. (Broadbent 1985) and widespread settlement and landscape abandonment at ca. A.D. 600. Although the region still had farmsteads, population did not rebound until Late Viking and medieval times, A.D. 1100–1300 (Liedgren 1992:191–219). Trade was intense during the Early Iron Age especially when the Germanic chiefdoms of the Mid-Nordic region (Ångermanland, Medelpad, Jämtland, Trøndelag and Österbotten) reached their peak. This trade brought Roman goods northward and trapping pits were dug by the thousands in the interior to harvest reindeer and moose (Selinge 1974; Spång 1997).

Artifacts dating to A.D. 800–900 that are of Scandinavian origin are few in number in the northern coastal zone, but a pair of round brooches was found in a grave containing the bones of an adult and a child at Obbola near Umeå. These objects derived from southern Scandinavia but the use of these types in pairs was more of a Finnish custom and the grave form is typical of the Västerbotten coastland. A contemporary find from a grave from Luopa in Österbotten contained buttons/bells of the same types found on Stora Fjäderägg Island (Christiansson 1969:197–210).

During the period A.D. 1000–1100, the artifacts were mostly of eastern origin. This is also the main period of the Saami metal offer/deposition sites in the interior. As offerings, these beautiful and rare objects sanctified the relationships of northern peoples to their own gods, and to the Nordic gods, when this seemed expedient. The 1200s mark a major change and Western European finds became more common, presumably because of German (Hanseatic) trade. The 1300s were the effective end of the metal offerings, although some sites contain objects from later periods (Serning 1960: 67–94: Zachrisson 1984:119).

The main period of Bothnian seal hunting sites conforms well to the main period of the metal offer sites and the Stalo huts, ca. A.D. 800–1100, and declines at the same time, ca. A.D. 1250–1350. The coastal connection to the enormous geography of Saami trade, including the goods found in Saami graves throughout the Nordic North and in local graves on the Bothnian coast, entails that Bothnian seal hunting must be viewed in the same super-regional context. Most authors (e.g., Serning 1956, Fjellström 1985, Hansson and Olsen 2004) have related the changes in eastern and western trade items to middlemen from Finnish Karelia, Russian Novgorod, Birka and Sigtuna in Sweden, Gotland until 1361 (when Gotland fell to the Danes), the rise of Hansa fisheries, particularly through mercantile centers such as Bergen and Vågen in Norway, and the fur market in Torneå on the Finnish border. Lars-Ivar Hansen (1990) and Thomas Wallerström (1995, 2000) have expanded the documentation of these historically known forces in northern trade and mercantilism, including hack silver, a primitive from of currency. Hack silver and part of a scale were found at the Saami offer site of Unna Saiva (Serning 1956). These middlemen groups were undoubtedly important, but Serning proposed a different perspective. She suggested that the Lapps, "who had lived by Lake Ladoga and on the shores of the White Sea and far down in southernmost Finland with all the natural connections to the east from whence many of these objects came, had surely passed trade goods directly from Lappish to Lappish hands" (Serning 1956:105). Serning also discussed the circumpolar shamanistic context of this material, including evidence of Saami drums during the Viking Period. The fact of the matter is that the east-west bands of metal artifacts and metal offer sites in northern Sweden track along the same valleys and eskers as sites from earlier periods (cf. Figure 192). The constellations of objects, technologies and ideologies are remarkably parallel to those of the Stone and Bronze Ages, including connections to Finland, the Baltic and southern and central Russia. In other words, this network and redistribution pattern of goods and social obligations was not new but had been an established network among local societies for hundreds if not thousands of years.

The chronological results from the Bothnian coast add an entirely new dimension to the narrative of the Saami trade: direct and independent involvement by the North Bothnian Saami now seems highly probable. The rise to power of Finnish/Kvennish and other middlemen and tribute collectors is actually one reason why the coastal Saami sites were abandoned, as argued by Steckzén (1964), not the other way around. But the political power of emerging states and the consolidation of that power through the Christian Church are what ultimately changed the balance of trade and social relations. Grundberg (2006) describes this as the Europeanization of the north. According to resilience theory, the thirteenth century was a period of release of social, cultural and economic capital, and the fourteenth century was the reorganization of these northern societies into the forms we have today. This convergence of social, political, religious, economic, epidemiological and climatic factors made this one of the major turning points in North European history. This further entailed the formation of new polities within Saami society itself, and new sources of internal competition for limited resources.

## The Medieval Transition

An important question is that of the relationship between the establishment of the North Bothnian fishing sites and the abandonment of the seal hunting sites. While they occupy completely different places in the coastal landscape, they probably overlapped in time. Although I have previously argued that the sealing sites were largely abandoned by then (Broadbent 2006), there was a transition of sorts between these two kinds of economies. The dates of harbors on Snöan and Stora Fjäderägg indicate that these were established during the period A.D. 1200–1300. This agrees with the chronology of other harbors and centers along the Bothnian coast, in particular the harbors of Kyrkesviken in Ångermanland (A.D. 1220–1300), Saint Olafs hamn in Hälsingland (A.D. 1300–1620) and Kyrkudden in Norrbotten (A.D. 1300–1620) (Grundberg 2001, 2006). Another interesting aspect of this medieval material concerns the labyrinths that were closely associated with fishing sites. The lichenometric datings obtained in the project bracket them into the time period A.D. 1300–1850. The labyrinths and compass roses on Stora Fjäderägg Island date to A.D. 1456–1660. The lichen-dated labyrinths from Snöan Island date to A.D. 1388–1816 (Broadbent and Sjöberg 1990).

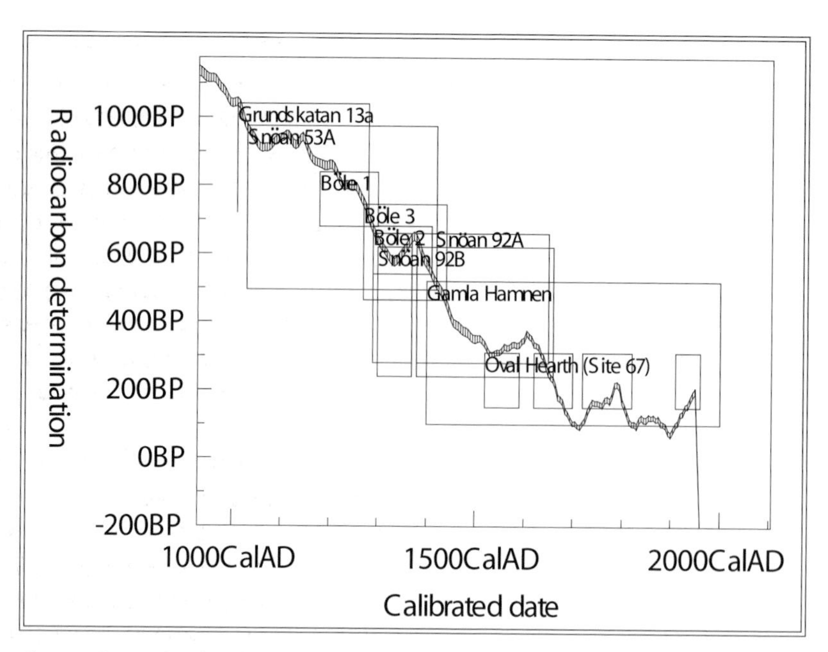


*Figure 158. Graphic distributions (2 s.d.) of the latest sealing hut at Grundskatan, a farmstead locale and a Saami hearth from Bjuröklubb.*

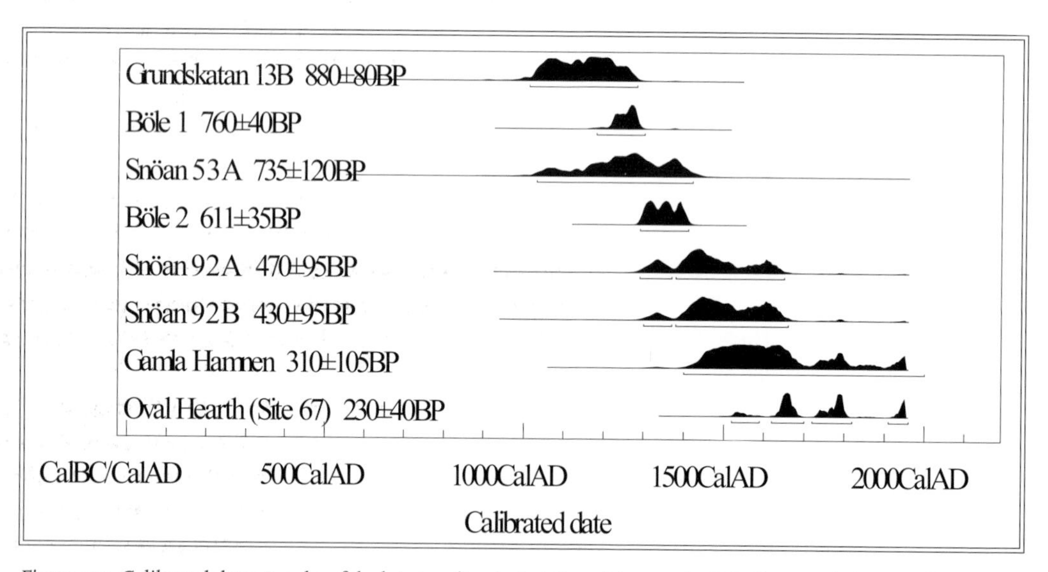


*Figure 159. Calibrated dates (2 s.d.) of the latest sealing hut at Grundskatan, the Böle farmstead site, Gamla Hamnen on Stora Fjäderägg Island and a Saami hearth on Bjuröklubb.*

The youngest date from Grundskatan 13 statistically overlaps the oldest harbor date from Snöan Island. Rathje (2001, 2005) excavated farmsteads with brick fireplaces and field stones at Böle in Lövånger in Västerbotten and obtained three dates that are shown in Figure 159. They overlap with Snöan 53A. The place-name evidence also speaks in favor of this interpretation. The frequency of "Lapp" place-names on the coast is presented in Chapter 9. Even the oral histories of places like Holmön and Hornslandsudde speak of the Saami transition to permanent farmsteads and probably to fishing (cf. Sandström 1988).

## Cycles of Change

The material presented here shows cyclical changes, and although it is not possible to relate these variations solely to temperature, the fluctuations in sealing sites coincide with global and European climate and environmental cycles. The cold and wet Sub-Atlantic period at 600 B.C. ended about A.D. 270, which is a Global Climate Boundary according to Lamb (1977). From A.D. 270 to 450, the global climate became warmer and drier and between A.D. 600 and 690 the climate cooled considerably (Lamb 1977; Stuiver and Kra 1986; Denton and Karlén 1973). This was marked by agrarian settlement regressions throughout the Nordic region. The climate started warming again in the eighth century and reached a maximum (the Medieval Warm Period) around A.D. 1100–1150, but it started to cool by A.D. 1200. It also became wetter and glaciers started expanding, as did sea ice around Iceland (Granlund 1932; Lamb 1977; Stuiver and Kra 1986). The Little Ice Age (LIA) began around A.D. 1300 and lasted until 1850. Starting in 1315, there were widespread crop failures and famines in Europe. From 1300–1350, fishing replaced cereal crops as the main food source in Iceland, and 1408 was the last record of Norse settlement in Greenland (Grove 1988; Fagen 2001). Warmer and more stable temperatures certainly facilitated farming and animal husbandry, and lessened ice conditions may have created exceptional opportunities for sealing. The finds of harp seals on Stora Fjäderägg show that such was the case during the Viking Period. Other ice-dependent seals, such as the ringed seal, may have been highly concentrated in near-shore areas. The Bothnian hut sites were, nevertheless, completely abandoned in the late thirteenth century with the onset of the LIA. Using tax records, Kvist (1988:89) has documented the dramatic declines in Bothnian sealing during even later LIA periods in Österbotten. As in Iceland, fishing became much more important than farming and the Church mandated fish as a necessary part of household economy. For many Saami, reindeer herding took on new significance, and the colder climate was probably in their favor; as for the Christianized Saami/Swedish coastal settlers of Norrland, fishing likewise gained in importance.

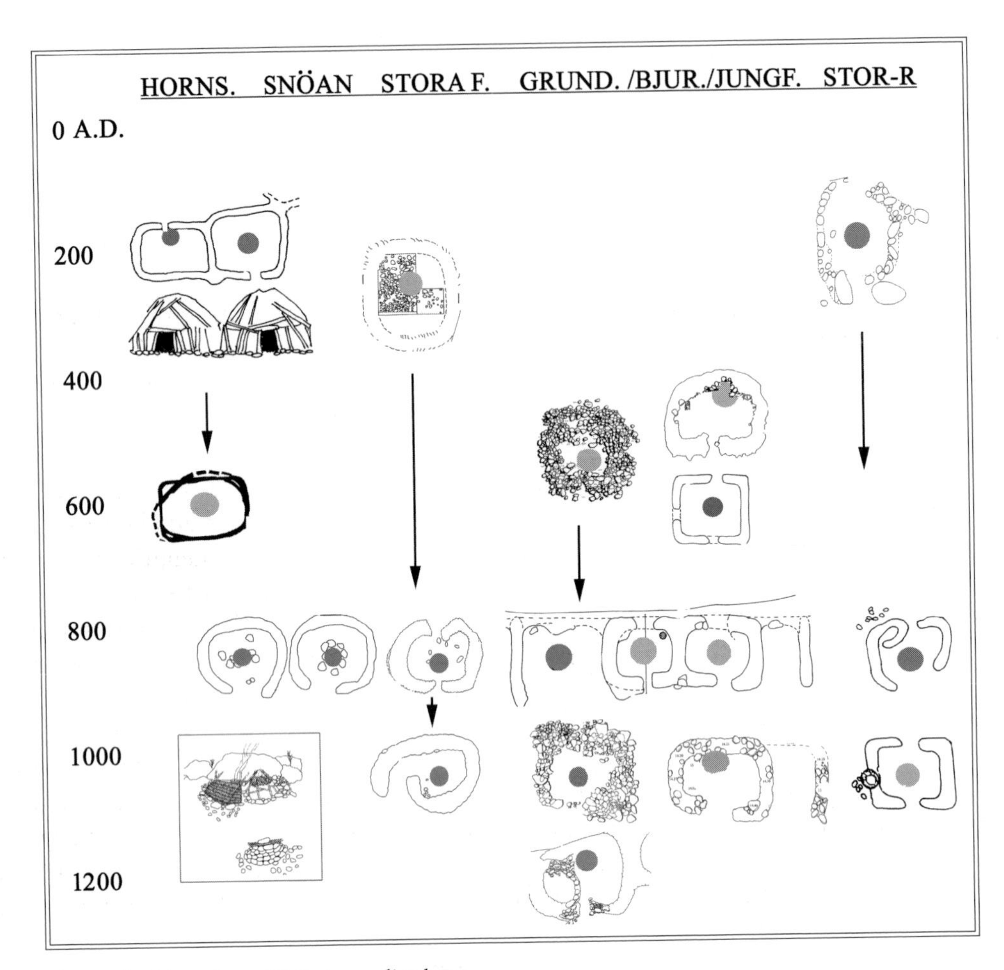


*Figure 160. Chronology of Bothnian sealing huts.*

# 7

# The Archaeological Roadmap

## Architecture

Bothnian hut foundations occur in a variety of forms and varied configurations. Except for huts with iron forges, hearths were centrally placed. These fireplaces often have one or more larger cobbles near them, but are generally without stone fillings or rings. Huts without hearths were probably not dwellings and were rather used for storage of equipment, food supplies, etc. A special type of hut measuring on average 3 × 3 m has been interpreted as a shed and is usually found near dwellings. They are comparable in size to *get-kåtas* (goat huts) among the Forest Lapps of Sweden (Manker 1968:204; Stoor 1991). These small huts lack hearths but have doors and were intended to keep animals warm and safe from predators at night (Figure 163). A sample of 61 dwelling floors on the coast indicates that floor size varied between 3.5 and 6.1 m in length and between 2.9 and 5.0 m in width. Mean length is 4.7±0.57 m and mean width is 3.73±0.47 m. Length was more variable than width (Figure 161). This is logical as structural size could be most easily expanded on either short end, as opposed to broadening width (cf. Liedgren et al. 2007). In only one instance has a posthole been identified and this was too small to have been a roof support. The roof and wall supports therefore probably consisted of internal frames lodged against or set into the stone foundations. Except for the smallest temporary dwellings that might have had skin coverings, walls and roofs were probably constructed of timber, grass sod, skins, birch bark and combinations of these materials. Drift timber was readily available on the coasts because of the continuous outflow of rivers through the forested interior and into the Gulf of Bothnia. The use of timber in constructions has been documented very early in coastal Finland (cf. Ranta 2002) and in northern Sweden at sites such as Lillberget (4200 B.C.) in coastal Norrbotten (Halén 1994). Timber huts are also well documented among the Forest Saami (Manker 1968). It must be assumed that this building tradition has a long indigenous history in northern Sweden.

Bothnian coastal foundations range in shape from round to oval, and square to rectangular. When viewed in terms of the elevations above sea level, the oval forms are the highest lying, and their antiquity is borne out by the radiocarbon dates from Stora Fjäderägg, Stor-Rebben, Hornslandsudde and on Bjurön (A.D. 200–600). The oval huts are, nevertheless, found at all levels. Rectangular and square foundations are not as frequent at the highest elevations and are most commonly found at levels dating to A.D. 700–1200. There is a greater variety of forms after A.D. 700, including "inverted Gs", row houses and dwellings with internal chambers, platforms, porches or lean-tos. Row houses consist of both rectilinear and curved-wall constructions with up to nine

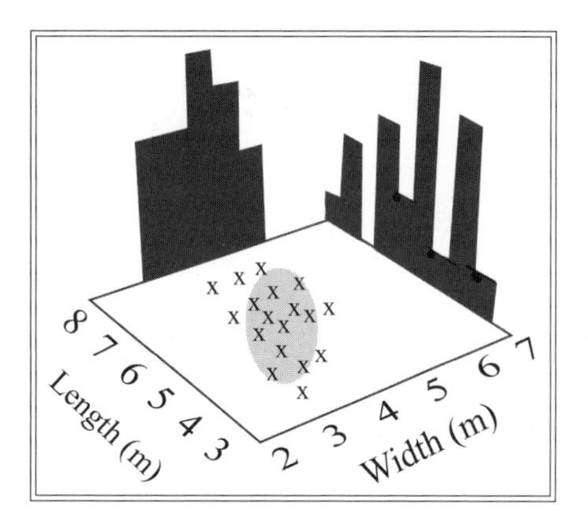

Figure 161. Lengths and widths of Bothnian huts.

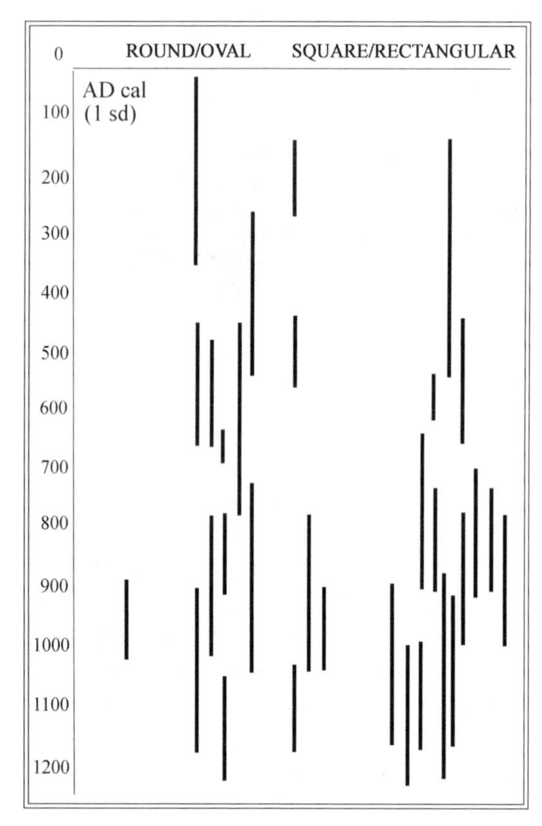

Figure 162. Hut form by calibrated radiocarbon date. The oval/round huts and the rectilinear huts overlap by chronology and are often found together. The oldest lying huts are oval in form and their antiquity is confirmed by radiocarbon chronology. The rectilinear huts were most common during the Viking Period. Tent rings are frequently found at the lowest levels.

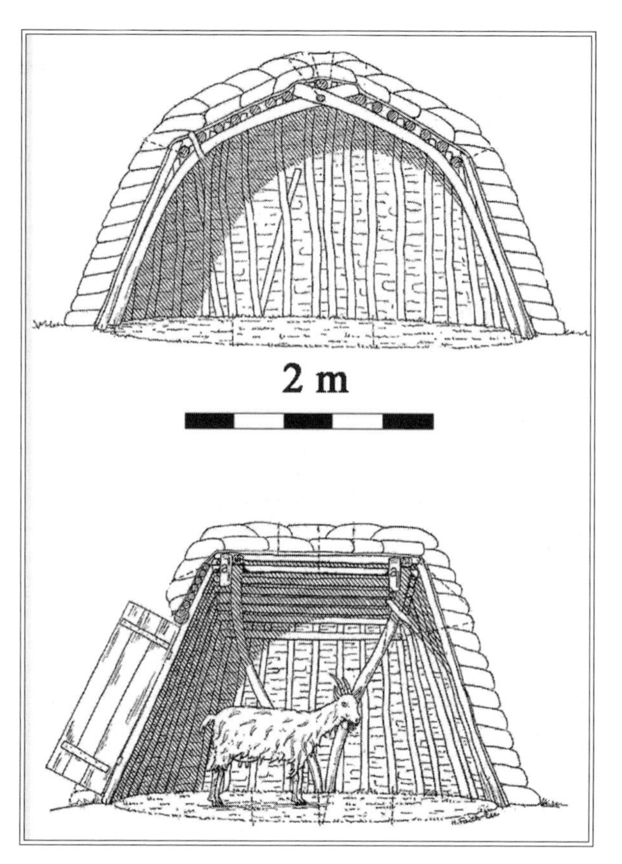

*Figure 163. Saami goat hut used to keep both goats and reindeer safe during the night (Manker 1968). Several foundations for these small huts were documented at the Grundskatan site, one of which was attached to a storage cairn with a central chamber.*

separate rooms (Figure 160). A final category of dwelling is that marked by simple stone circles with evidence of hearths (tent rings). These circles are also found at higher elevations but are most frequent below the 10 m elevation. Following interpretations from North Norway, oval and round huts are of Saami design, whereas the rectilinear constructions could be the result of interactions with non-Saami. Grydeland has characterized the shift from oval to square dwellings as the transition from a hunter-gatherer/pastoralist economy to a farmstead/fishing economy at Kvænangen in North Norway, a fjord with three coastal *siidas*. These changes occurred during the period A.D. 1200–1700. The settlements nevertheless go back

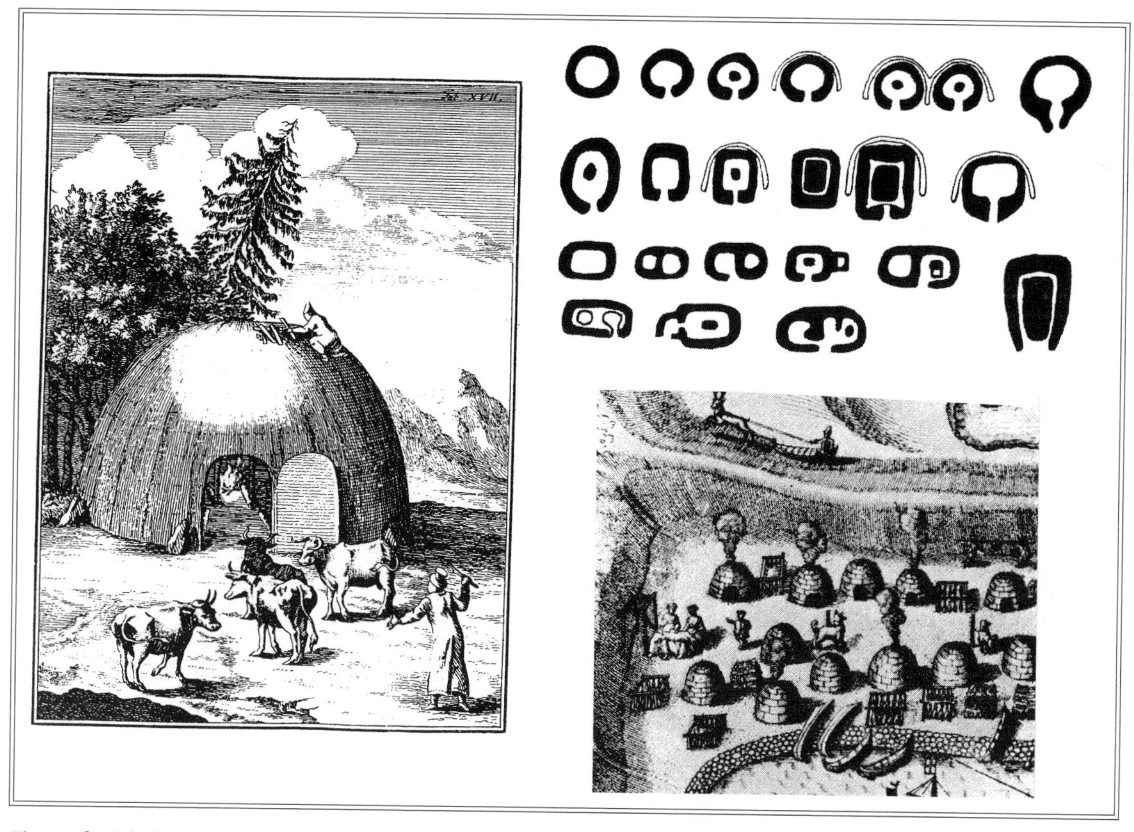

*Figure 164. (clockwise from left) Saami hut with cattle in North Norway (Leem 1767); coastal hut foundations at Kvæangen, North Norway (Grydeland 2001:25); Saami fishing village of sod huts on Kildin Island, Kola Peninsula (Jan Huyghen Linschoten 1594–1595).*

to A.D. 700 (Grydeland 2001:65). These huts are very similar to the North Bothnian huts, including the inverted "G" forms (Grydeland 2001:25) (Figure 164). Odner (1992, fig. 47) has documented similar kinds of forms and arrangements of dwellings in Varanger that are contemporary with the Bothnian sites. Sheep/goat bones have also been dated to A.D. 1000 in Varanger (Schanche 2000), and comparable settlements have been documented by Andersen farther south at Ofoten dating to the Late Iron Age. Even the cultivation of barley has been demonstrated at Ofoten (Andersen 1992: Hansen and Olsen 2004:197). Grydeland (2001:61) has seen this change in hut forms as a shift from collective to individual property ownership, a change that was formalized by the church and state, and there are even implications regarding gender relations; women lost status, and there were dramatic population increases.

## Site Structure

Since North Bothnian coastal features were constructed over a long period of time, some dwellings and areas were inevitably re-used. In spite of this, rough clusters of structures are still visible at the same elevation levels. Although somewhat impressionistic, the huts can be grouped into shore-level clusters at the larger sites.

1) At Stor-Rebben there are clusters at ca. 13 m and 16 m.
2) At Hornslandsudde there are clusters at ca. 12.5 m, 14.5 m, 16 m, 18 m and 20 m.
3) At Stora Fjäderägg Island there are clusters at ca. 11 m, 13 m, 15 m and 20 m.
4) At Grundskatan there are clusters at ca. 12 m, 14 m and 15 m.

At Stor-Rebben there are four clusters of two to three huts at the 16 m level and six clusters of two to three huts down to the 13 m level. At Grundskatan there are five groups of five to seven dwellings; at Stora Fjåderägg there are five clusters of five to nine huts each, and at Hornslandsudde there are five to six clusters of two to nine huts at each level (Figures 165–167). While there is good reason to believe that these clusters represent repeated visits over time, the overall pattern suggests that they consisted of contemporary household groups of 15–25 people. A cluster of three to five households was probably the norm and this is, in fact, the most commonly seen number of huts at the smallest locales (cf. Figure 168). Some of these dwellings could have also been occupied year-round, such as Hut B on Stora Fjäderägg Island. Based on the organization of historically known sealing expeditions in the North Bothnian region, each hunting team consisted of the male members of households, and the teams ranged in size from five to eight households. In the fall and winter, teams of up to eight men in two boats would use 20–30 nets for catching ringed seals (Hämäläinen 1930). Saami seal hunting on the Kola Peninsula, salmon fishing on the Tana River in North Norway and even bear hunts were similarly organized (cf. Fellman 1906; Ekman 1910:252; Grydeland 2001:79). Collective efforts can also be assumed regarding the use of trapping pit systems on land that required a good deal of labor to dig and maintain. As will be discussed regarding tax records from the sixteenth century and the organization of church towns in northern Sweden (Chapter 9), this clustering offers a blueprint of territorial organization as well.

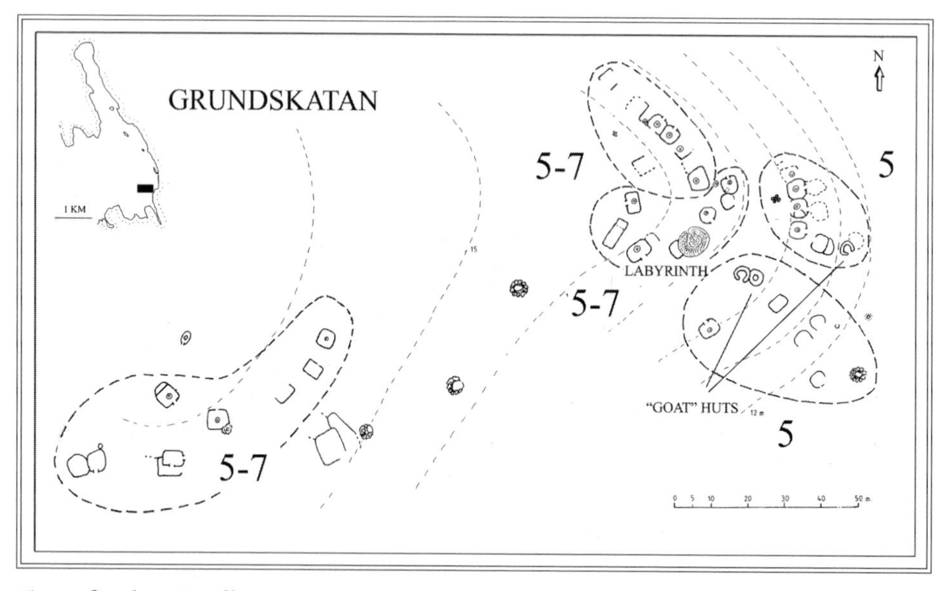


*Figure 165. Clustering of huts at Grundskatan.*

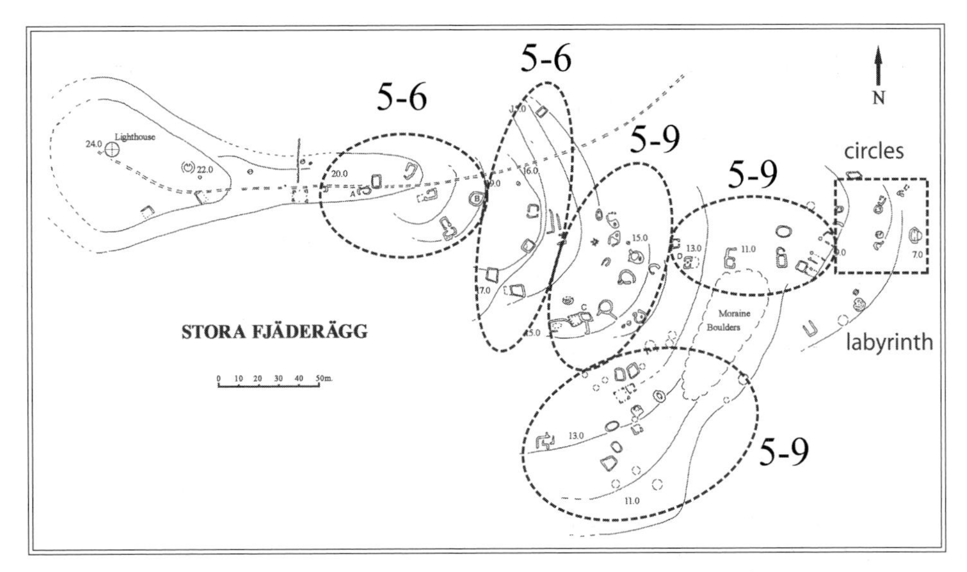


*Figure 166. Clustering of huts at Stora Fjäderägg. Square indicates area of circular features.*

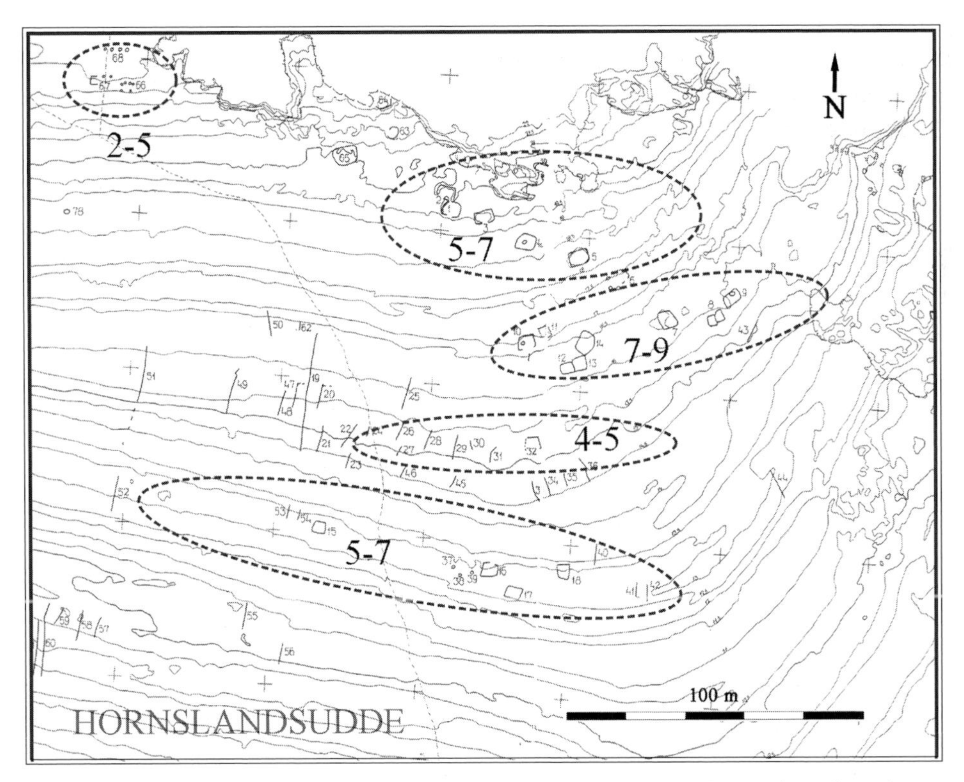


*Figure 167. Clustering of huts at Hornslandsudde. Numerous stone alignments lie at right angles to the shorelines in the center and southwest corner of the mapped area.*

## Storage and Surplus

Storage pits were identified at all sites. They range from small lined pits in hut floors to chambers measuring a meter or more across. Large cairns or pits were observed near dwellings at most sites, often with piles of stones that had been removed to empty them and to subsequently cover supplies or foodstuffs. The largest of these cairns were documented at the Grundskatan site. They consist of stone constructions measuring up to 4 m in diameter and run in a line between two clusters of dwellings (Figures 85, 86). These types of arrangements can be assumed to have been communal facilities. A large well-made pit in a moraine boulder field between Sites 119 and 132 at Hornslandsudde was also probably a shared storage facility of this kind (Figure 169). Historic Saami storage features are well known and consist of above-ground structures, earth cellars, cairns and stone chambers used for storage of milk products, fish and meat (Manker 1968:203; Ruong 1969:128–130; Valtonen 2006:64–74). There were also different types of wooden constructions, including small huts, as well as out-buildings and sheds. Foundations of these types of sheds or storehouses, huts without hearths, are common on the Bothnian sites. While reindeer domestication has been given great significance regarding northern societies, the significance of storage has been little discussed. Both activities in many respects represent the same goal of securing and controlling the distribution of resources. The environment itself was a storehouse for immediate returns and pastoralism was "storage on the hoof." Caches represent the social appropriation of these resources (Ingold 1983). Storage can consist of household supplies, emergency stores and fixed-point storage, but larger depots imply community investments. Caches are thus important expressions of shared social space, access and distribution. They are a form of "resource husbandry." Storage also fosters sedentism and was a precondition for trade and the integration of local hunter-gatherer societies into wider systems of exchange and redistribution (Ingold 1983). Collective hunting and storage efforts further generated a need for leadership and

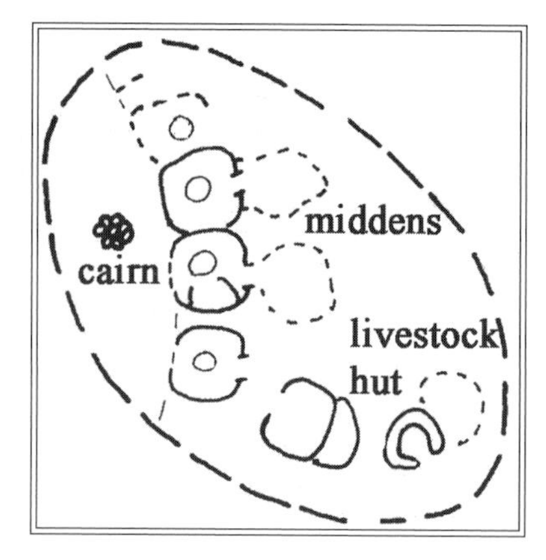


*Figure 168. A small cluster of dwellings, middens and associated features dating to the period A.D. cal. 800–1200 at the Grundskatan site. This constellation corresponds to the Saami sijdda, a group of households living and working together.*

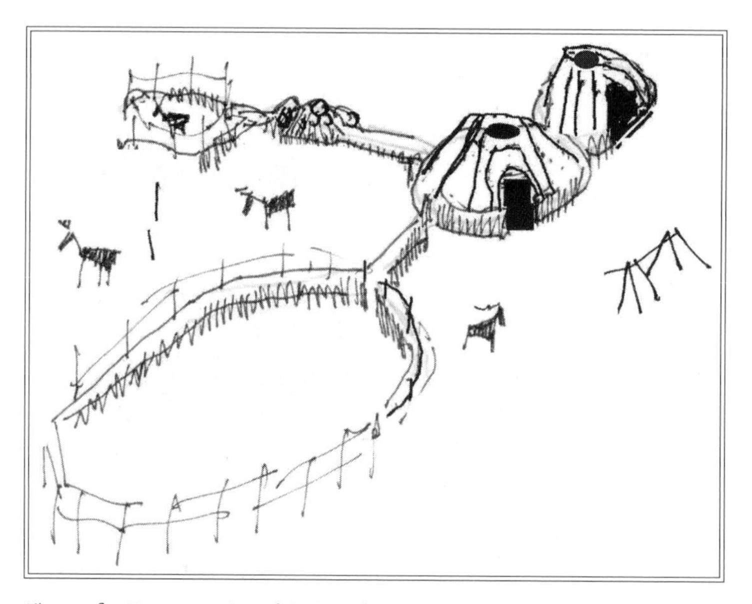

*Figure 169. Reconstruction of site complex near Site 70 on Bjurön.*

coordination. The abundance of large and small storage facilities at the Bothnian sealing sites should therefore be considered as one of the most significant socio-economic indicators at these locales. The osteological results from Stora Fjäderägg show that large numbers of seals were taken and processed beyond immediate consumption needs. A substantial pit (measuring 10 × 12 m) at Grundskatan (Figure 9) is interpreted as a large-scale blubber-rendering basin analogous to those known from the White Sea region (cf. Tegengren 1965). Taken together with the dwellings, the caches and blubber-rendering pits are evidence of the extensive exploitation of resources and the appropriation of these resources by local communities for systematic intercourse with the outside world.

## Corrals and Fences

Stone alignments were documented at Site 70 and Grundskatan on Bjurön, on Stora Fjäderägg and at Hornslandsudde (Figures 84, 106, 142, 169). These walls were all attached to dwellings or were near to them and bear a resemblance to the field, corral and pasture walls (Swedish *stensträngar*) known from Gotland, Southwest Norway and elsewhere (cf. Lindqvist 1968; Myhre1972; Carlsson 1979). Phosphate testing of these features at Grundskatan and Hornslandsudde did not reveal any enrichment as compared with surrounding areas; in fact at Grundskatan there were higher values outside the enclosure. Based on ethnographic accounts of Saami settlements, fences could be erected as corrals, as well as to keep reindeer off huts and out of garden plots (Ruong 1969:130; Kjellström 2000:88). They were also used for milking and as temporary holding (marking) compounds. Obviously, most of these were seasonal hunting sites and not suited as permanent farmsteads, but they do reveal the existence of animal husbandry in the region, and place-names provide valuable clues as to where the more permanent settlements were located. Unfortunately, the likelihood of actually finding preserved wooden structures and fences is small but not impossible in boggy areas.

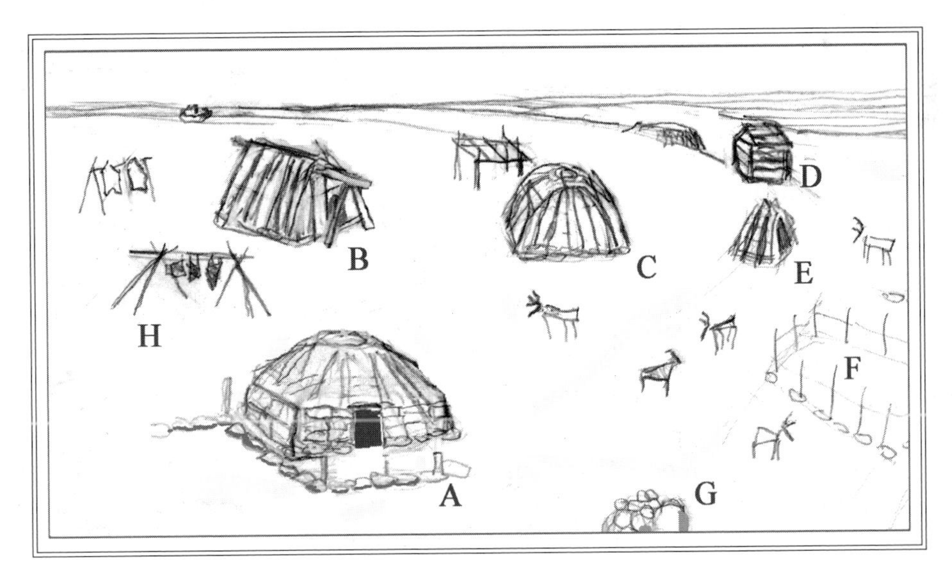


*Figure 170. Various possible hut forms and constructions at Grundskatan: (A) sod construction, (B) beam and timber construction, (C) bent-frame construction, (D) timber storehouse, (E) goat hut, (F) corral/fence, (G) stone cache, (H) meat rack. Based on Kjellström (2000:88–115).*

## Seals, Seasonality and Animal Husbandry

The finds of animal bones and teeth from the individual sites are presented in Chapter 5. From this material it is possible to discern general patterns relating to seasonality, hunting and animal husbandry. Preservation conditions were very poor and varied considerably from site to site, therefore this material only represents what happened to be preserved in hearths rather than what may have been a much more varied array of activities. Based on the numbers of identified specimens (NISP), a total of 4,539 bones were identified from two species of seals, a brown bear, sheep/goat, reindeer, cattle, hare, ducks, birds and large ungulates, probably moose. Ninety-eight percent of the bones are from seals. Of these, only 3% could be identified to species: 52% were from harp seals, which were found at two sites, and 48% from ringed seals, which were found at three sites. The harp seal bones were mostly from Hut B on Stora Fjäderägg Island. This material has been discussed in detail by Jan Storå in Chapter 5. His conclusions are: 1) North Bothnian sealing during the Iron Age was more varied than previously believed, and 2) Hut B has to be regarded as a more or less permanent structure in a well-organized hunting complex.

Seal bones were found at all sites except Stor-Rebben, which can only be explained as the result of poor preservation. The seal bones display considerable variability as regards anatomical representation in different huts. Of 4,439 bones, 34% derived from the cranium, vertebrae and rib cage, and 55% were from the extremities, particularly the flippers. The latter are often considered to be delicacies by seal hunters. The best-preserved seal bones from Stora Fjäderägg Hut B also show selectivity within the dwelling and that large numbers of seals were processed elsewhere. This suggests that the bones from the hearths represent "disposable meals" tossed into hearths, rather than what may have been prepared in other ways. Ringed seals are known to have been hunted on the ice of late winter, although there is also ample evidence that these smaller seals were caught using nets in the dark fall months. Seal skins, blubber and meat were of the best quality during this time of year. Female ringed seals fast in the spring, and unless the goal was to obtain their cubs, they were thin and generally sank quickly. Until firearms were used, ice hunting of ringed seals focused on single breathing holes, required great patience and skill, and the use of dogs to find them in pressure ridges. It can be assumed that this species of seal was hunted during both the fall and the spring, but seal netting in the fall was more efficient and rewarding. The age determinations of the seal bones indicate mostly adults and sub-adults, consistent with seal netting, but this can be biased as younger individuals would not have been as well preserved. Harp seals do not breed in fast ice and are considered an open-water species that was hunted in the summer or fall (Storå 2001b).

Eighteen bones of birds were found at three sites, two of which are from ducks. These animals were probably killed during the summer or fall. Finds of hare bone suggest winter hunting, as they were most easily trapped in the snow (Kjellström 1995:55, 212–273). Bones of larger ungulates, moose or reindeer, were found in several hearths and can reflect fall or late winter hunting. On the whole, the seals, birds and small mammals indicate site use during the late winter, spring, summer and fall. The bear bones derived from one individual, and based on what is known about bear hunting, this animal was most likely killed in late winter (Zachrisson and Iregren 1974:79–83). Some dwellings had apparently been occupied year-round. In spite of this, not one fish bone was identified from any site.

Seventeen bones and one tooth fragment derive from large and small ungulates (cattle, sheep/goat, reindeer and moose). These bones were found at five different sites from the northernmost to

Table 54. Finds and dates of domesticated animals.

| SITE | LATITUDE | FIND | DATE (B.P.) |
|---|---|---|---|
| Stor-Rebben A,B | 65°N | reindeer/sheep/goat | 945±110 B.P. |
| Jungfruhamn, A,B | 64°N | sheep/goat | 985±70 B.P., 1210±50 B.P., 1300±130 B.P. |
| Stora Fjäderägg B | 63°N | sheep/goat, cattle | 1660±70 BP, 1235±315 B.P. |
| Hornslandsudde 13 | 61°N | ruminant (tooth) | 1820±40 B.P., 1570±40 B.P. |

the southernmost locales. The presence of domesticated animals agrees with the evidence that there were livestock enclosures of some kind associated with the dwellings. The anatomical representation of these bones shows that 94% derived from meat-rich cuts, primarily the legs. This can mean that meat was brought to the sites for consumption rather than having been slaughtered there. The evidence of corrals and the place-names relating to reindeer corrals in the coastal region suggests that these animals had not been kept on sealing sites as sources of meat, rather as sources of milk products or possibly even as transport animals. Islands are also ideal places for keeping livestock; there was access to good fodder, including reindeer lichens, and the animals could never roam far from the settlements. This practice was used extensively by northern farmers who routinely transported their animals to islands during fishing seasons. Evidence of heavy grazing can still be observed on Stora Fjäderägg Island.

As a general conclusion, sealing was the main focus of these sites during both the spring and fall hunting and netting seasons. These activities were probably organized by households from local communities. The presence of domesticated animals suggests that there were more than men living at these settlements. The hunting and processing activities were relatively large-scale and well organized. Flotation of hearth soils from two huts at Grundskatan revealed that berries had been collected, including raspberries, bilberries, blueberries, crowberries and bearberries. Additionally, goosefoot and stitchwort were identified. These finds are clear proof of late summer–fall activities. This is further evidence that women were present on these sites and all of these plants are known to have been used by the Saami (Viklund 2005).

## Place-Name Evidence of Reindeer Husbandry

The frequency of place-names referring to reindeer husbandry in coastal Västerbotten is both noteworthy and useful from the archaeological perspective. As early as the 1940s Holm (1949:143–145) had drawn attention to the Lövånger parish place-names *Rengårdtsjärn* (Reindeer Corral Lake) and *Rengårdsmyr* (Reindeer Corral Bog) and commented on the frequency of the place-name *rengård* in the region. He quoted Israel Ruong, a well-known Saami scholar and reindeer expert who commented, "the information that the word *rengård* occurs in the coastland is . . . of great interest, and implies that reindeer husbandry and its intensive Forest Saami form . . . occurred there" (Holm 1949:145). There are, in fact, 74 place-names referring to reindeer in Skellefteå Municipality, 37 of which refer to *rengård* of which 16 are the place-name *Rengårdsmyren* (Reindeer Corral Bog). The Swedish word *ren* means reindeer and *gård* means an enclosure, a yard or a farmyard. In this context, like the word *rengärde*, it probably refers to a reindeer corral.

Reindeer herds belonging to the Vindel and Ume Saami villages still graze in the Västerbotten coastland, including Bjuröklubb. Several nomadic herding routes lead directly to Bjurön. *Cladonia rangiferina*, the main winter fodder of reindeer, grows abundantly on the outer coast and along the eskers leading there. Mixed small-scale intensive reindeer husbandry survived into historic times among the Forest Saami people in Norrbotten, Vasterbotten and Ångermanland. These Saami were not nomadic and based their settled existence on a mixture of fishing, hunting and the keeping of reindeer, goats and even cattle (Manker 1968). They were speakers of the Ume Saami language in Västerbotten. They are remarkably similar to the Bothnian Saami 700 years earlier, and linguistically the Ume Saami language they speak, which has words for seals, is hard to explain without having once extended down to the coast. Interestingly enough, Olaus Magnus' map from 1539 (Figure 7), not only shows a Saami woman milking a reindeer upstream from Umeå, but includes the captions *renaval* (reindeer husbandry) and, just north of Lövånger, *rensby* (reindeer village).

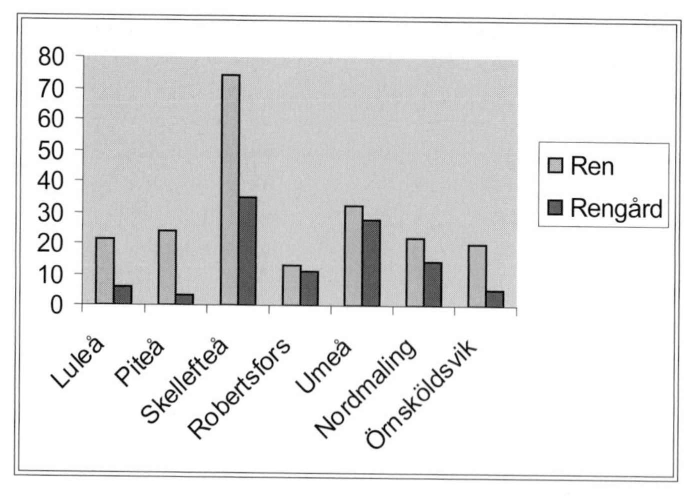


*Figure 171. Numbers of place-names with the prefix* ren *(reindeer) and place-names with* rengård *(reindeer corrals) by municipality between Norrbotten and northern Ångermanland.*

## Pastoralism and Heterarchy

The archaeological evidence has shown that the Bothnian dwellings occur in groups together with storage cairns and caches, fence lines and stone circles that are interpreted as ritual features. Northern huts and doorways normally face south, although this varied depending on topography. On the coasts doorways most often faced shorelines. It should be noted that the actual cardinal directions of north and south, as expressed by most indigenous informants, often had more of a symbolic significance than a magnetic reality, however, and "north" also referred to the area behind the dwelling and opposite the front entrance. According to the Chukchi this orientation was important ". . . in sacrificing, the odor of the hearth of the house standing in the wrong position might reach the sacrificial fire of the preceding house and taint its fire and fire-tools" (Bogoras 1909:613).

Saami settlement clusters, *sijddas*, corresponded to the basic unit of most hunter-gatherers, the band, or a small group of nuclear families living and working together. Such a unit was mobile and less vulnerable than a single family and yet not large enough to overtax local fuel and game. The Saami *sijdda* was a flexible system typical of hunter-gatherer subsistence groups, although it was not incompatible with small-scale herding (Graburn and Strong 1975; Ingold 1978; Storli 1991). Annual *sijdda/siida* territories were roughly circular in inland areas, but changed into long ribbons running parallel with the river valleys with the transition to nomadic herding (Vorren 1968).

Norwegian coastal Saami *siidas* were more like circular inland territories and enveloped coastal fjords and islands (cf. Bjørklund 1985; Grydeland 2001:18). Numerous archaeologists have proposed that the Saami *siida* or *sijdda* was the basic unit of prehistoric settlement, and that the clustering of dwellings in the alpine and forest regions reflect this (cf. Bergman 1991; Mulk 1994; Hedman 2003). This settlement arrangement is described in detail by Mulk (1994:216–221). The dwellings were arranged in rows or bowed groupings of three to five huts. A "courtyard" (*sjallo*) lies in front of and to the "south" of the huts. Directly behind the huts were domestic features, such as earth ovens and caches, and to the north of them were offer sites. Each dwelling represents a family and two to five families generally lived together. These families were not necessarily related and membership was flexible. Larger gatherings of *sijddas* into winter villages, which seem to have originated in the sixteenth century, are called *vuobme* or *dalvadis*. Each *sijdda* also had its sacred ground, a mountain or an unusual stone called a *seite*, a name that probably derives from the same root as *sijdda*. The Stalo huts in the alpine regions and hearths that have been connected with Saami *kåtas* in the forest regions of northern Sweden, Norway and Finland have been described as either single *sijddas* or groups of *sijddas*. Settlements in the forested interior of Finland (cf. Tanner 1929; Tegengren 1952), as well as the coastal Saami sites of north Norway (cf. Bjørklund 1985; Odner 1992; Grydeland 2001), follow the same pattern.

Bogoras (1909:612) described analogous settlements among the reindeer herding and maritime hunting Chukchi of northeastern Siberia. The Chukchi camp usually included two to three families, and the whole number of inhabitants was 10–15 people. Camps of four, five or six families formed a slight minority, and a camp of ten houses was almost impossible except for special reasons, like the temporary camps at trading places. Bergman and Liedgren *et al.* (2008) have recently discussed the kinship and residence pattern of the Swedish alpine regions ca. A.D. 1000 with a particular focus on the linear alignments of huts that became quite distinctive during the period A.D. 640–1150. In their study of historically documented dwellings in the Arjeplog region, huts 6.5 m in length could house up to 10 people [comparable to the large oval Bothnian huts], and the smallest documented hut, measuring 3.2 m in diameter, housed an elderly couple. The *sijddas* consisted of two to six households (Bergman and Liedgren et al. 2008:104). Although there is a clear understanding that *sijddas* were not strictly based on kinship, the authors argue that these linear alignments of huts were an expression of lineages under "great stress" (Bergman and Liedgren et al. 2008:107). The stress factor is identified as the transition from hunting to pastoralism and the need to affirm the security of the "core social unit," the *sijdda*. The main forces of change were internal, according to the authors, although they also assign significance to trade. Comparable linear alignments of huts are, in fact, described by Bogoras and these lines of huts are indeed related to herding (1909:612–614). Reindeer husbandry quite simply created a need for aggregating both herds and herders. Poor herders with only a few animals kept together for a few months and dispersed just as easily. Wealthy herders needed more than their family to manage their animals and distant relatives or strangers camped together with them. *These huts were arranged in lines based on hierarchy.* The "chief" of the camp was referred to as the "one in the front house" among other references, including "the strongest one." The other tent occupants were called "camp neighbors" or "that of the rear house." The eldest of the brothers, or his son, had preference over the others in this lineup. The position of the front house is the first on the right side of the line of houses (Bogoras 1909:613).

The owner of the herd, or largest part of it, was in charge of the pastures, the days of slaughtering, ceremonies and sacrifices. This hierarchy was socially enforced as no one could join a camp without permission, even at temporary camps (Bogoras 1909:614).

Comparable alignments of dwellings, and during the same time period, are seen on the North Bothnian coast (refer Figure 160) and can relate both to the organized labor of herding and to collective hunting (cf. Tanner 1979:73–107). This was a time of exceptional prosperity within Nordic society. The Saami elites, "Finn-Kings," are referred to by Snorre and in other sagas, and 21 curious defensive Mangerom type "manors" are found along the Finnmark and Kola coasts (Hansen and Olsen 2004:214–220). According to Storli (1991) and Urbańczyk (1992:213–215), there were alliances between Saami big men and Norse chiefs, and most relationships were mutually beneficial. The long lines of hearths in the interior and alpine regions of Sweden almost certainly coincide with the acquisition of wealth through intensified trade and the consolidation of labor. Metal objects were given as offerings at numerous locales in Swedish Lapland, and reindeer were sacrificed at hundreds of sites.

Both Mulk (2006a) and Odner (1992) have argued that the offerings of metal objects were intended to maintain internal social solidarity by taking wealth out of circulation. This is reminiscent of the Bergman and Liedgren et al. (2008) argument regarding hut alignments, but as Zachrisson (1984:108, 1987b:61–68) has observed, these offer sites may actually have been inspired by Norse practices. They were expressions of alignment with the Norse gods and Norse society, not attempts to downplay their own social hierarchies. Their cessation might likewise relate to the eradication of Norse religion. Collinder (printed in Manker 1957:51) expressed similar ideas:

> *Lappish heathenism was syncretistic. It took up many Scandinavian beliefs from different times, perhaps as far back as the Bronze Age. As the Saami became familiar with Christianity from the 900s and later, they borrowed from it. Much of their religion was magic, distinguished by crass needs, and their contacts with Christianity could have actually strengthened, but not weakened this in their cults. The Scandinavians were successful and so were their cults. The Saami were wise to take up Scandinavian offer practices without abandoning their own.*

During the period 900–1200, many Nordic and European kings took up Christianity as a way of consolidating power. By the end of the tenth century, Olaf Trygvesson had converted Norway and vowed to put to death all that refused to accept the new faith. Vladimir had converted Russia in A.D. 988, and Boleslav the Brave converted Poland in A.D. 999. In Sweden, Ansgar had spread the faith at Birka as early as A.D. 829, but Sweden took another 300 years to become fully (more or less) Christian, and the Archbishop in Uppsala and the five bishops of southern Sweden were first in place at the end of the 1100s. Erik (later Saint Erik) was martyred in Uppsala over the issue in A.D. 1160. The Church provided the new common denominator of state formation. Needless to say, the Saami seemed to have largely abandoned their borrowed Norse religious practices by the thirteenth century because they were no longer likely to have any benefits for them, spiritually or otherwise, and thereafter quickly aligned with Christianity. Christian symbolism was already embedded in their personal adornments through trade with the west (Vågen, Bergen, Trondheim, Lofoten) and the east (Novgorod, Ladoga) (Urbańczyk 1992). This is, to my mind, the most plausible reason why the metal offer sites, which were inspired by Oden's Law in Norse religion, were so expeditiously abandoned. Interestingly enough, the extended hearth and hut alignments cease at the same time.

The bear rite's distinctive religious expression of social solidarity continued, by contrast, into the nineteenth century.

## Discussion

The *sijdda* system was, as in most band societies, a highly flexible and resilient combination of personal and household autonomy, as argued by Odner (1992, 2000), and social solidarity as argued by many authors (cf. Gjessing 1955; Grydeland 2001:67). It was undoubtedly both of these things, however, and this suggests a heterarchy, different contemporary frameworks of social relations depending on context (Ehrenreich, Crumley and Levy 1995). The egalitarian model, while typical of small-scale societies, does not mean there were no differences in status and wealth (cf. Zachrisson 1997a:144–148). The social obligations within such a heterarchy entailed the responsibility not to dispose of wealth, but to redistribute it, including in the form of offerings on behalf of the community, all of which nevertheless enhanced prestige.

Saami society had been forged from thousands of years of spiritual and economic transactions. The diversity of their graves, perhaps more than any other archaeological manifestation, bears witness to this fact. The impacts of the Christian Church, by contrast, especially after joining forces with the Swedish state following the Reformation in the sixteenth century, were far more disruptive than the beginnings of pastoralism. This was the "end of drum time," as described by Rydving (1995). Sápmi itself was becoming state property.

Nordic linguists have long speculated that the Saami acquired "packages" of knowledge, including terminologies, from Germanic and Karelian agrarians and metal workers. The Saami, it turns out, had borrowed as many as 3,000 Scandinavian words, most of which relate to skill sets. Ingold (2000:312–338) has reasoned that this was not technology in the modern sense, rather skills that were embedded in daily life. Many of the Scandinavian loan words are believed to have been acquired on the Norwegian coast in connection with boat building, fishing and so forth but what is most remarkable is how many words relate to farming and animal husbandry. These are not random words but whole systems of terms, including names for domestic animals, corrals, sheds, farms, fields, animal products and equipment. This list gives some examples of these loans (from Wiklund 1947:57–61; Collinder 1953:53–69): The Norse terms are set in brackets. A cow is called a *kussa* [kyr] in Saami, an ox is called a *vuoksa* [oxi], a calf is a called *galbe* [kalfr], a goat is called a *kaihtsa* [geit] and even cats are called *gatto* [kotta]. The same is true of agrarian byproducts: wool is *ullo* [ull], milk is *mielke* [mjólk], and cheese is *vuosta* [ostr] and so on. The word for "farm" is *garde* [garðr], "sheep byre" is *fiekse* [fāhus] and "field" is *akkr* [akr]. Even the word "tame" was probably borrowed, *tāmes* [tamr]. There are Finnish loan-words as well, such as the word for "flour," *jaffo* [jauho] and "beer," *vuola* [olut].

Based on runic inscriptions it has been possible to document the periods during which these Scandinavian words were acquired. The inscriptions date this process through regular changes in Scandinavian "sound-laws." The oldest runic inscription in Sweden dates to about A.D. 200, the Roman Iron Age (Stenberger 1964:373). Altogether there are about 50 inscriptions of "Urnordic" (Ancient Nordic) age. There are over 3,500 rune stones in Sweden, the northernmost of which is in Hälsingland (Brink et al. 1994).

The first linguistic horizon used by Nordic philologists is called Primitive or Archaic Scandinavian. The theory is that if sound-laws are not observed in the loan-words, the words date to before these changes. The change of *ai* to ā before "h" is seen in the runic inscriptions from the fifth century (Sköld 1979). Another change about the same time is that of *au* to ō before "h". An example of a word supposedly borrowed from Scandinavian includes *sai'vâ* meaning fresh water, water in a river or lake and corresponding to Old Norse *sjár, sjór* (Sköld 1979:108). There are as many as 500 Archaic Scandinavian words in all Saami languages (Collinder 1953:61). Late Archaic Scandinavian ended about A.D. 800 and was followed by Common Scandinavian, in which the Scandinavian languages are divided into western and eastern dialects. The chronology thus spans from A.D. 200 to 800. Most scholars believe that the process of word acquisition by the Saami occurred on the Norwegian coast.

> *From a linguistic point of view, we can come to the conclusion that the forbearers of the Lapps and the Scandinavians met in northern Norway about the time of the birth of Christ, and it's probable that the Lapps were there when the Scandinavians arrived. (Sköld 1979:111)*

Although the Norwegian context is not in doubt regarding linguistic influences, Karl Wiklund suggested that these were not just borrowed words but that the ancestors of the Saami were directly involved in animal husbandry and farming:

> *What we are confronted with is a class of Saami who during ancient Nordic [Archaic Scandinavian] times, presumably around the birth of Christ, in addition to hunting and fishing (possibly reindeer herding), supported themselves through a form of animal husbandry and farming which was at about the same level and in the same region as the Norse. (Wiklund 1947:60)*

Wiklund's ideas were criticized because he had no proof at the time. It is clear today, however, that Wiklund was correct. Archaeological fieldwork in the 1980s revealed that there were Germanic enclaves during the Early Iron Age in both southern and middle Norrland as well; but even more relevant is the fact that we now know that the Saami in these regions practiced husbandry and even cultivation in the ways that Wiklund had proposed for Norway. Aronsson has found this idea plausible even for Pite Lappmark (2005) regarding the many formative connections between reindeer husbandry and settled farming (cf. Khazanov 1984). Recent genetic analyses of Eurasian reindeer show, furthermore, that reindeer herding did not spread to Scandinavia from Siberia but they were domesticated independently in many different regions (Røed et al. 2008). The first Nordic loan words relating to husbandry, herding and farming were undoubtedly acquired much farther south than previously believed, perhaps as far south as Svealand in Sweden, where there were fur markets such as the famous, still-operating *disting* market in Uppsala (Magnus 1555, book 4, ch. 7:182–183).

Saami words were also borrowed by Germanic speakers and these relate to transportation, trade and hunting. Professor Olavi Korhonen (1982, 1988) has examined Saami terms relating to boats and boat building, which was a special Saami skill set, as well as words relating to sealing and the Saami use of dogs for finding ringed seal dens in the ice. The Nordic community, as attested by the Norse sagas, was also highly respectful and even fearful of Saami healing and witchcraft and they borrowed the Saami word *noaidi*, which means "shaman" or "healer." A related phenomenon involves the use of taboo words in connection with hunting. These were words that were used by Swedish hunters to hide their intentions from the game as the animal would never be mentioned

Table 55. Finds of iron slag, clay and iron furnaces.

| SITE | LATITUDE | FINDS | DATE (B.P.) |
|---|---|---|---|
| Stor-Rebben A,B,C | 65°N | Slag | 1845±135 945±110 |
| Bjuröklubb 67 | 64°N | Forge, iron, copper | 1485±70 |
| Grundskatan 3 | | Slag | 1500±100, 1205±70 |
| Grundskatan 11 | | Forge | 1175±100 |
| Stora Fjäderägg B | 63°N | Slag, furnace clay | 1660±70, 1235±315 |
| Stora Fjäderägg D | | Furnace clay | 1110±145 |
| Hornslandsudde 12 | 61°N | Forge, slag | 1820±40, 1570±40 |
| Hornslandsudde 5 | | Slag, furnace clay, iron | 1390±30 |

by its real name. The Saami word *alge* and its variants, including Ume Saami word *alggie,* was borrowed by Bothnian sealers. It means "son" and was also the Ume Saami word for "seal." Another Ume Saami word that was widely adopted by Bothnian sealers as a taboo word is *mårssie* or *morsá,* which means "fiancé" (Edlund 2000).

## Metallurgy

Iron metallurgy was one of the most formative elements of Saami ethnogenesis. Iron slag has been found at five of the sites along the Bothnian coast, from Stor-Rebben in the north to Hornslandudde in the south. Iron forges were documented at Bjuröklubb 67, Grundskatan 78 and Hornslandsudde 119. Slag was found in seven additional hearths, and furnace clay has been documented in four hearths. A forging pit has been previously documented together with Kjelmøy ceramics at Harrsjöbacken in Lövånger (Sundqvist et al. 1992), and the forging sites on Bjurön can be viewed as continuations of these activities. The radiocarbon date of Harrsjöbacken (A.D. 79–245) overlaps those of Stor-Rebben, Stora Fjäderägg, as well as Hornslandsudde. While the detailed technological analyses of this material are important, of equal interest are the shamanistic and symbolic aspects of metal working and, in this study, their connections to Saami bear ceremonialism and offer practices. Fire was the most transformative form of technology available in prehistory. Metallurgy is thus more than a technology, it is magic. Metallurgy is defined as the extraction of metals from their ores and modification of metals for use. It is a form of pyrotechnology, the use of heat for manipulating raw materials (Hodges 1970). In this sense it is an extension of the methods employed by earlier hunters and gatherers to anneal stone to make them easier to flake, or of quarrying using fire and water to shatter rock or to manipulate minerals, as has been documented at the Lundfors site in Västerbotten, 3400/4200 B.C. (Broadbent 1979:99–108).

The oldest documented iron working in Sweden is found in a band across the 60th parallel from the Mälardalen region in the east to the Swedish west coast (Hjärthner-Holdar 1993). This can be connected to early metallurgy in Finland and emanates from the same regions as textile- (Lovozero) and striated ceramics, as well as Mälardal- and Ananino axes, that is, from the Volga bend to the Ural Mountains in Russia (Hjärthner-Holdar 1993:17–29). Iron working was possibly underway in Russia as early as 1800 B.C. (Chernykh 1992; Khlobystin 2005) and spread to Sweden by at least 800–500 B.C. Asbestos-tempered ceramics are closely associated with this technology in north Nordic regions and date to ca. 900 B.C–A.D. 1 in Norway and somewhat later in Sweden (Hulthén 1991; Olsen 1994:101–108).

Iron technology represents a major economic breakthrough because iron ore was readily available locally, especially through bog iron precipitates (limonites) and also because there were vast pine forests that could provide the fuel necessary to produce and manipulate it. Even winter was an advantage as iron deposits could be easily scooped up and transported through the stable platforms of frozen lakes and bogs. Sweden was to later become one of the major exporters of high quality iron from sources in the so-called *Järnbaraland* (iron-bearing land) of southern Norrland, as described in many early texts, including that of Saxo Grammaticus in the 1190 (Hyenstrand 1974). During the period A.D. 400–600, large amounts of iron were produced in the forests of Dalarna and Jämtland, presumably for trade (Hyenstrand 1974; Magnusson 1986). This activity shows the same drastic decline as elsewhere in the Nordic region during the seventh century, but rebounded, albeit on a smaller household scale, from A.D. 1000. This is also where the so-called forest or hunting graves are found and these are most likely Saami in origin (cf. Hvarfner 1957; Sundström 1997:21–27; Gollwitzer 1997:27–33; Zachrisson 1997a:195–200; Bergstøl 2008). Most of the slag has been found on the shores of lakes and rivers and coincide with the distributions of Stone Age settlements.

## Three Iron Forges

### Bjuröklubb 67

Bjuröklubb 67 (Chapter 5) is a solitary dwelling that lies just below the top of a ridge facing west on what was once a small island. The elevation is 17 m above sea level. A radiocarbon date was obtained from charcoal (1485±70 B.P.), which calibrates to A.D. 460–640. The find material consists of 22 pieces of iron slag and clay. This material was analyzed by Lena Grandin, Eva Hjärthner-Holdar and Emma Grönberg at the Geoarkeologiskt Laboratorium of the Swedish National Heritage Board (2005).

A heavily corroded cylindrical piece of iron measuring 28 × 8 × 8 mm and weighing 2.8 g was examined, but its exact composition could not be ascertained. Slag samples were determined to consist of complex combinations of slag and silica, some of which could have derived from melted sand in the soil, and some of which seems to have been added on purpose to improve smithing. Silica reduces oxidation of the metal and helps to weld iron to steel. There were also traces of copper that might have been used to decorate objects (Grandin et al. 2005:5). In general, the slag is homogeneous reduction slag containing both magnetite and wüstite that had been produced in a highly oxygenated environment. It was the result of secondary smithing using billets of the quality of so-called Fellujärn or Kode types (cf. Andersson 2007:6). An analysis of the silty clay furnace wall material shows it had been tempered with sand and had been heated to 1150°C. The hearth soil was swept using a magnet in 2008 and both plano-convex hammer scales and iron sphericals were obtained, both by-products of smithing (Figure 178). At the time of excavation, it was believed that wall stones had fallen into the hut, but these were probably anvils.

### Grundskatan 78, Hut 11

Excavations at the Grundskatan site (Chapter 5) also produced evidence of forging in a hut. The form of the hut was very similar to that at Bjuroklubb, a rounded-rectangular foundation with low

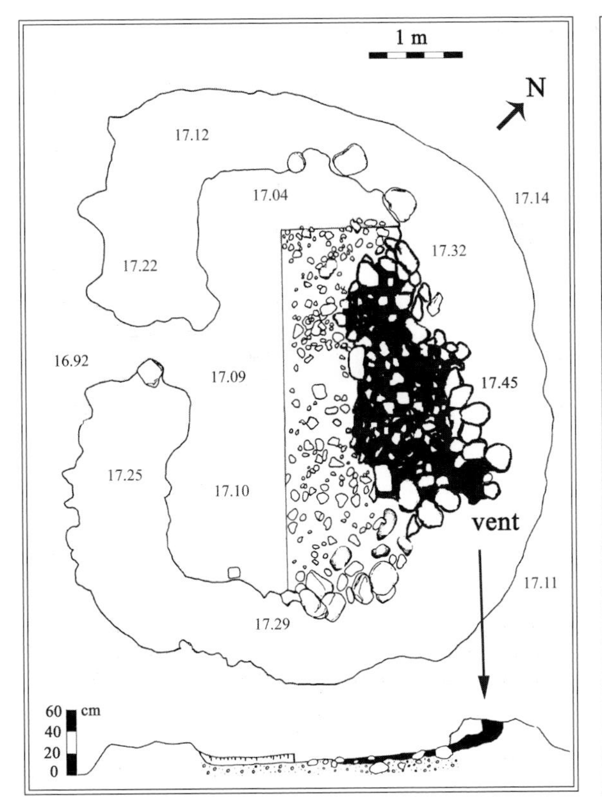


*Figure 172. Bjuröklubb 67 showing area of sooty soil and vent in the rear wall of the hut.*

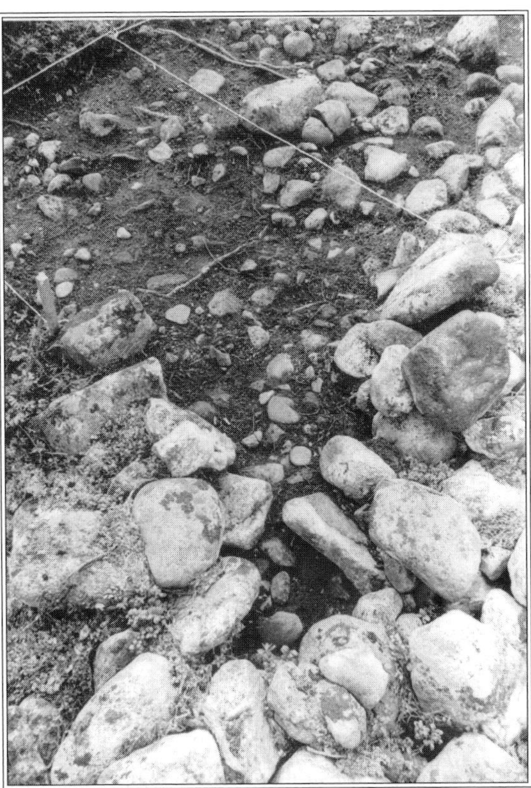

*Figure 173. Close-up of the vent in Bjuröklubb 67.*

cobble walls measuring 7 × 5 m. A radiocarbon date of 1175±100 B.P. (A.D. 720–980) was obtained from the hearth. No animal bones were found and 300 grams of iron slag were collected. This material consists of both homogeneous slag, slag with melted stones, red-burned clay and rusted iron. The slag includes varying proportions of wüstite, olivine laminates and glass. Two pieces derived from the same smithing hearth cake. Fine-grained magnetite and drops of metallic iron occur and the iron content is high. There was a good supply of oxygen. The slag derives from secondary forging (Grandin et al. 2005), and iron scales, the results of hammering, as well as sphericals were also picked up in the hearth using a magnet. Wood charcoal from the hearth was varied and included *Betula* sp. (birch), *Pinus* sp. (pine) and conifers (pine or spruce).

**Hornslandsudde, Site 119**

Features 12 and 13 are a double hut situated at 16 m above sea level. Two dates were obtained: 1570±40 B.P. (A.D. cal. 430–540) and 1820±40 B.P. (A.D. cal. 130–240). The hearth measured ca. 1 × 1 m and was ca. 20 cm deep. Some 1.1 kg of slag was found in or near the hearth and a hundred or more hammer scales (60 g) were collected. Charcoal derived from pine (*Pinus* sp.). Some slag and furnace clay was water-rolled, which confirms the oldest radiocarbon date of this feature (Andersson 2007:3).

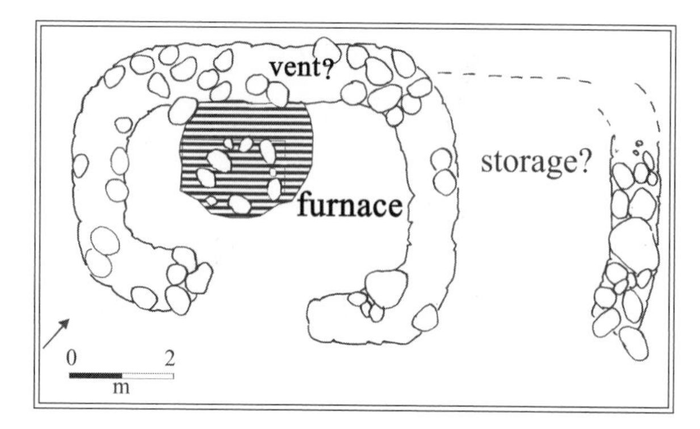


*Figure 174. Map of Hut 11 at Grundskatan.*

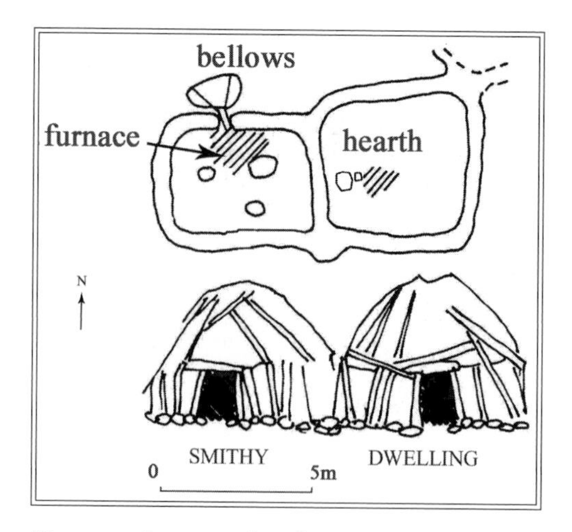


*Figure 175. Reconstruction of Huts 12–13.*

Technical analyses were performed by Daniel Andersson of the Geoarkeologiskt Laboratorium of the Swedish National Heritage Board (2007). The slag derived from smithing hearth cakes that had probably been formed on the bottom and sides of the pit, which is somewhat unusual as they usually only stick to the walls below the air inlet and rest on a bed of fuel. Differences in mineral composition from the same area suggest that both oxygen and temperatures were rather unstable. The hammer scales are generally comprised of iron oxides and the sphericals of glass and dendritic wüstite. High quality iron was found, including one small metallic piece of steel, and three corroded pieces of iron. This find suggests the manufacturing of edged tools. Additional slag, burned clay and a small rolled thin iron sheet measuring 1 × 0.3 cm were found in Hut 5, which dates to 1390±30 B.P. (A.D. cal. 465–779). Feature 5 is a rounded-rectangular hut foundation measuring ca. 3.5 × 6 m with cobble walls measuring 0.2–0.3 m height. No traces of a smithing hearth were found in this dwelling, and it is probable that the slag had been collected from Hut 12. Iron slag (120 g) and six red clay pieces (0.6 to 1.2 cm) were found in the hearth together with 375 bone fragments (60 g) and one iron fragment (1.0 cm). The large number of burned bones and a central hearth supports the interpretation that this hut was a normal dwelling, not a forge.

## Smithing and Shamanism

Three shallow smithing hearths have been identified in huts ranging in age from A.D. 130 to 980. The oldest dated material is from Hornslandsudde and the youngest from Grundskatan. This spread suggests that iron working had been carried out the entire time these sealing sites were used, over 800 years. The three forging sites are very similar and consist of simple huts of comparable sizes and constructions to the dwellings. Bjuröklubb 67 had seal bones and phosphate enrichment indicative of a normal dwelling, and Huts 12–13 were a double hut, a smithy and a dwelling with a livestock enclosure. All three smithies were adjacent to or directly within settlements. The smithing hearths were small and shallow and quite comparable to what is known about clay-lined bowl furnaces, which average 30–80 cm across and 12–45 cm in depth (cf. Martens 1988:70–85; Hjärthner-Holdar 1993:94–101). The floors of the forging huts also have numerous anvil stones.

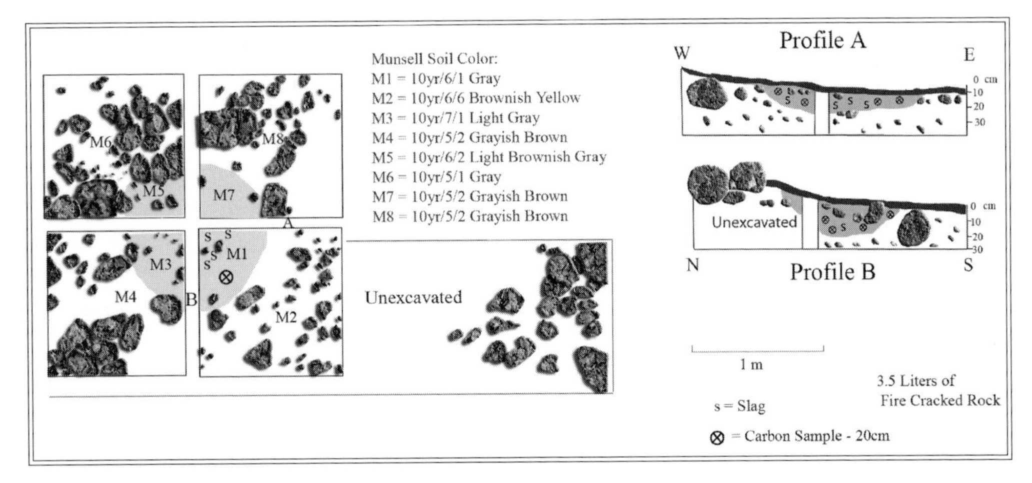


*Figure 176. Detail of forging hearth in Hut 12, Hornslandsudde. S= slag, X=AMS dates.*

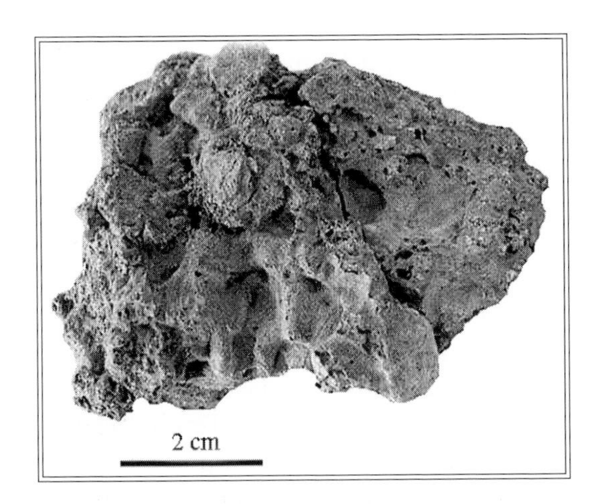


*Figure 177. Slag from Grundskatan Site 78, Hut 11 (Grandin et al. 2005:11).*

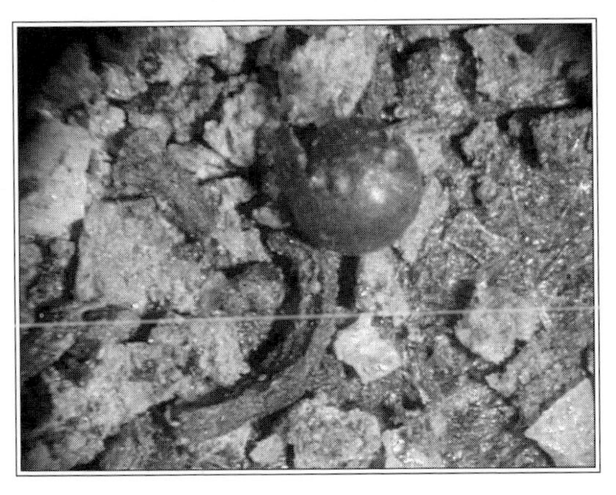

*Figure 178. Iron scales, ropey iron and sphericals from Grundskatan Site 78, Hut 11. Spherical = 1 mm.*

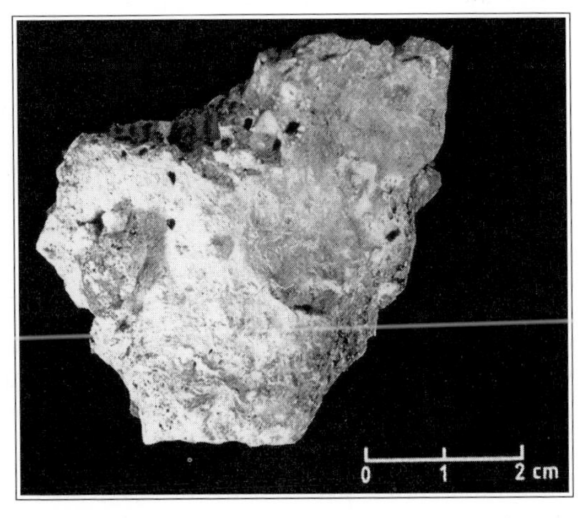


*Figure 179. Furnace clay from Bjuröklubb 67 (Grandin et al. 2005:14).*

This coastal smithing was evidently carried out for domestic uses and the manufacturing of edged tools (Andersson 2007:6). According to Grandin et al. (2005:8–9), the material is not comparable to the site of Lappnäset (Englund et al. 1996) or Kyrkesviken in northern Ångermanland (Kresten 1999), where primary smithing had taken place. It is nevertheless comparable to the material from a smithing hearth at Lill-Mosjön, Grundsunda, Ångermanland, which dates to 2500±65 B.P. (Englund 2000). Although no primary iron production has been found in the Lövånger area, there are sources of bog iron in the Nolbyn-Mångbyn area (Granlund 1943). The iron on the sites came in the form of billets, but only one billet of the spade-shaped type produced in Middle and Southern Norrland has been found north of Ångermanland, and this was in northern Finland (Liedgren and Johansson 2005:290).

The Bothnian sealers were clearly very familiar with the intricacies of small-scale iron working. They could produce high quality objects, including decorated items. To gauge temperatures by color, the smithies were in huts with special venting systems involving channels running through rear walls; one of these was probably for a bellows operated outside of the hut. It is quite possible that they were in use during all sealing seasons, both the fall and spring months for ringed seals, as well as during the summers when harp seals were hunted. It is also notable that slag nodules and even furnace clay have been found in so many hearths without furnaces. For example, 23 small iron slag nodules were found in the hearth of Hut 3 at Grundskatan, which is adjacent to and partly contemporary with Hut 4 (with the bear burial) and the circular sacrificial feature at this site. Slag was also found in Huts A, B and C at Stor-Rebben, Huts B and D on Stora Fjäderägg and the aforementioned Hut 5 at Hornslandudde. Slag was similarly found in oval Saami hearths in Norrbotten (Hedman 2003:161–189) and in the hearths of Stalo huts. Mulk (1994:177-184) has, for instance, recorded iron slag from two Stalo huts at Suollakavalta and a hearth in Singi. These sites date to ca. 1000–1200. Similar sites have been documented in southeast Norway (Narmo 2000). Iron blanks, rivets, tongs and other tools together with iron fragments are otherwise documented from Stalo huts (cf. Mulk 1994). Iron blanks and rods, as well as a crucible and asbestos wares, are recorded at other sites, such as Hälla (nos. 869–870) in Åsele, Lake Överuman, Tärna, Norrvik, Paulundsvallen in Lycksele, Rappasundet in Arjeplog, Landsjärv, Sörviken and Varghalsen (Zachrisson 1976:71). Zachrisson has also observed that slag is found on Saami sites and has analyzed some, including parts of a small plano-convex cake measuring 10 cm in diameter. Four of these pieces were verified by the technical department of the Museum of National Antiquities and two of them, from Gafsele in Åsele Parish and Ställverket on the Ångermanland River (Zachrisson 1976:129). In a more recent overview of the evidence, Zachrisson (2006) describes likely Saami iron working sites in Jämtland, Härjedalen, northern Dalarna, western Hälsingland and Medelpad, as well as iron objects with distinctive Saami markings.

Iron slag has likewise been documented in North Norway, for example in a probable shaman's hut at Vapsgieddi (Grydeland 2001:37–42). While some sites are smithies, most of them are not, and this raises the very real possibility that slag was deliberately put in hearths because of its magical, especially transformative, properties. Metamorphosis was an empirical reality and the hearth was a sacred place (Qvigstad 1926:321). Mats Burström (1990) has argued that slag had been deliberately placed in Iron Age graves in southern Norrland, both as grave goods and as fill. This ritual connection in Scandinavia has been discussed more recently against the background of comparative ethnographic analogies in Africa (Haaland 2004; cf. Haaland et al. 2004).

European and Norse mythology is full of the myths, legends and folktales that build on the magic and rituals of the smith and iron working (Haaland 2004:11; cf. Green 2002). Hedeager (2001) pursued this idea regarding the Norse figure Völundr, who could change shape as a shaman to mediate between humans and the gods. She also discusses Regin from the Volsunga Saga, who is a liminal figure and a dwarf (Hedeager 2001:492). Although a person to be respected and even feared, in Germanic society the smith was nevertheless only working at it part-time, and this was not necessarily a high status profession (cf. Haaland 2004:14).

## Völundr and the North

The master smith Völundr/Weland is described in the *Older Edda* from ca. 1000, which is one of the oldest of the Icelandic texts. He was originally a dwarf or from a family of dwarves or elves, but he was completely human and with human emotions. His tale is prefaced by a brief description of his background: "*The Finn King had three sons, Slagfinn, Egil and Völundr, who traveled on skis and hunted reindeer . . .*" (Bæksted 1970:228). The tale then goes on about how Völundr, having made a magic sword and 700 rings of red gold that he tied to his forge, was robbed by King Nidud and his soldiers, who wore chain mail. Meanwhile, Völundr, on returning home from bear hunting, was captured and tied up. He had his leg tendons cut, but took to the sky using wings he had forged (Bæksted 1970:229).

Most intriguing about this story are the references to the "Finn King," skis, reindeer, dwarves and even a bear. Völundr's forge was on an island. The Völundr allusions point northward, and there are valid reasons for taking them seriously. For one thing, there is now credible archaeological evidence for Finn Kings (Hansen and Olsen 2004:214–220), and the hunting of reindeer on skis could only have taken place in the north. The reference to dwarves, who knew magic and were devious, can refer to the meeting of the Saami and the Norse as proposed by Nilsson's early study of the saga literature (cf. Nilsson 1866) and, of course, the Saami stories about Stalo giants. The shamanistic context in Norse religion is also expressed through the Seiðr rituals, which involves female divination, as seen among the Saami (Dubois 1999:121–138; Price 2002:91–328). Amanda Green (2002) has related the ritualistic value of iron to the Germanic practice of offering weapons and animals in bogs and watery cult places, which we know the Saami practiced. There is likewise a strong gender component to metallurgy in which the forge is seen as a womb and symbolizes fertility (Herbert 1993).

## Conclusions

The chronology, architecture and organization of North Bothnian settlements coincide extremely well with what is known about other Saami settlements and cultural manifestations throughout the Nordic region. Although dwelling constructions differ by region, they reflect comparable social and resource exploitation strategies. They were closely connected with pastoralism, trade and intense cultural interactions. The closest Saami architectural parallels to the North Bothnian material that I know of are in northern coastal Norway. The combinations and even the transitions from oval to rectilinear structures could similarly relate to contacts between the Saami and other groups, or simply reflect different seasonal needs. Technology, it must be assumed, was a shared interest and yet another arena of collaboration between Saami and non-Saami. Ritual behavior, the connection between metallurgy, metal offerings in bogs and shamanism, seems to have belonged to the realm of common ground. As will be discussed in the next chapter, the transformative properties of the bear, and the significance of the bear rites, relate directly to the dwelling, the hearth, fertility and to Saami social identity.

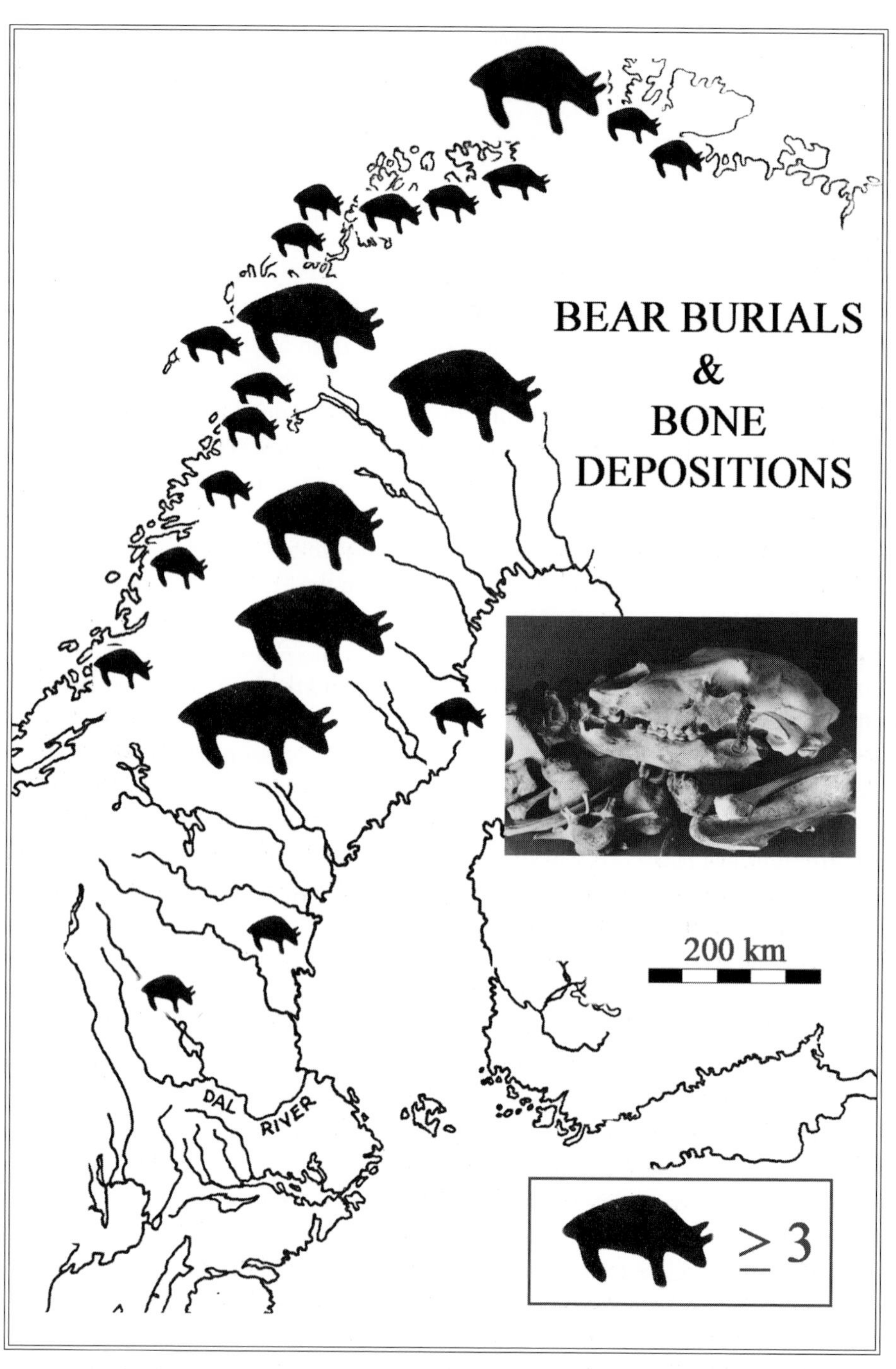


*Figure 180. Map showing general distribution of documented bear burials and bone depositions in Sweden and Norway. Icon based on an image from a Saami drum (Kjellström and Rydving 1988:26). Bear burials in Sweden concentrate in South Sápmi, to which Grundskatan belongs. Bone depositions are more common in North Sápmi. Photo inset of bear skull find from Jämtland. Courtesy Antikvariskt-topografiska arkivet, the National Heritage Board, Stockholm.*

8

# Rituals and Religion

Most religious interpretations of Saami archaeological material are based on written accounts from the 1600s and 1700s. Swedish Lord High Chancellor Magnus Gabriel De la Gardie commissioned studies by Swedish priests who were to then turn over their materials to Johannes Schefferus, author of *Lapponia* in 1673. Priests also collected information on religious practices in Norway. These efforts were intended to define, and then overpower, Saami witchcraft, magic and heathen beliefs and practices (Manker 1957:9).

Information on Saami sacred sites can be sought from many sources: physical traces in the landscape, place-names, traditional knowledge and written accounts. Each source has its limitations, however. Landscape impacts were often minimal and building materials mostly perishable. Most constructions were made of wood, brush, sod and birch bark. Place-names, which once identified locales, have in many areas been replaced by names from the linguistic majority. In other instances, Saami place-names have been lost along with the disappearance of the Saami language and changed land uses. The written sources are relatively recent and were recorded by non-Saami. It is probable that the Saami were loath to reveal the locations of sacred sites, sacred place-names or practices, either because this would shame the sites and weaken the power of their traditions, or simply to avoid punishment, prison and even execution (Lundius 1905:32, Olsen 1910:7 ff.).

Saami sacred sites were often landforms such as mountains, lakes, islands, points and peninsulas, caves, crevices, cliffs, ridges, ledges, water divides, rapids, waterfalls, springs and streams (Qvigstad 1926; Manker 1957). These were places where power was concentrated. These powers consisted of the spirits of ancestors and different categories of helping and protective beings that maintained different classes of animals. Special rules applied regarding the interaction of humans and these powers. It was at these kinds of sites one could seek contact with spiritual forces. According to Saami traditional beliefs, to die was to wander in the underworld (Högström 1747:210). The underworld was also the home of dead relatives (Bäckman 1975). These people lived a parallel existence and even walked upside down with their feet against those of the living (Lundius 1675:6). All of these spiritual entities received offerings at places where conditions for contact were favorable. Offerings to dead relatives could occur near graves or at other locales, especially on special platforms near settlements or in the natural landscape where there were transitions between worlds. Sacrifices and offerings often occurred at places that were associated with game. Offerings were made to *Tjaetsieålmaj*, "the water man," for fishing luck on the shores of lakes or in the water. Offerings were made at a kill site to *Liejpieålmaj*, "the alder man." Inside the hut, offerings were made to the female deities *Maadteraahka* and her daughters *Saarahka, Joeksaahka* and *Oksaahka* – overseeing all that is female, including menstruation and childbirth. Offerings were made daily. Each entity had its own special place in the hut. Under the hut floor resided *Jaemiehaahka,* "death woman," who controlled the distribution of the vital powers between the living and the dead.

Traces of Saami ritual practice have mostly disappeared, but some constructions have survived. These can be graves, stone circles or enclosures, mound-like constructions and different types of sacrificial platforms or cairns. Sacrificial idols were often made of wood, but in some instances were made of stone on or near the offer site. Rich deposits of bone and antler together with blood, fat and flesh gave rise to both lush vegetation and characteristic plant types (cf. Manker 1957:123; Wennstedt Edvinger and Winka 2001:108). Sacred sites were used for both "bloody sacrifices" and metal offerings. Of the bloody offerings, bone and antler could survive, but seldom any other visible indications. Archaeological investigations of offer sites, which were known from oral traditions, have rendered astounding numbers of artifacts (Hallström 1932; Serning 1956; Zachrisson 1984). A single site can contain hundreds of objects from a wide geographic region. The objects consist of brooches, pendants, clasps and buckles of pewter, bronze and silver, silver coins and iron arrowheads. Coins and ornaments are usually perforated. There can also be considerable amounts of bone from many species: reindeer, cattle, horses, sheep/goats, pigs, fish, birds (including swans and roosters), bears, dogs, wolves and cats (Manker 1957:45–46). The most common day-to-day offerings were ordinary items: bits of food, reindeer milk, and tobacco or vodka (Mebius 2003; cf. Jordan 2003).

While Saami sacred sites can consist of a number of different features or none at all, two types are of particular interest in this study. One form is a circular sacrificial feature and the other manifestation is the bear burial. Circular stone features of these kinds have been known for over a century in Norway and have now been documented in coastal Sweden. This new material has been presented by Wennstedt Edvinger and Broadbent (2006). An analysis of the Grundskatan bear burial is based on 42 comparable bear burials and bear bone depositions in Norway and Sweden. The bear burial is one of the most powerful manifestations imaginable of Saami identity and territory. In order to avoid confusion regarding Nordic grave types, the term "burial" is used instead of "grave" to describe the interment of bear bones. The use of this term encompasses the act of covering the remains and the rituals connected with it. An offering is a symbolic gesture, and as most of the animals had been consumed prior to being offered, they are not, strictly speaking, sacrifices. Interestingly enough, the creatures that were not normally consumed, for example fur-bearing animals, were sacrificed with their bones intact. Some animals were obtained specifically for sacrifices, such as house cats and even horses (Manker 1957:46).

Manker (1957:10–11) has defined nine traits of Saami religion:

1) All nature was animated and forces of nature, and even illness and death were personified by gods.
2) Reindeer herding, hunting and fishing had specific gods and guardians.
3) Power and danger were connected with specific locales.
4) Gods were worshiped in the form of unusual stones, cliffs or wooden idols.
5) Cults and rituals most often had utilitarian motives, such as good luck in fishing, hunting, herding and health.

6) There was no priesthood, and every family used sacred drums for their spiritual needs.
7) The drum was the primary instrument of Saami cults.
8) The most distinctive of the Saami cults relates to bears.
9) There were a number of female taboos regarding offer sites, hunting, the handling of the drum, etc., but special goddesses (family or kin spirits) were connected with the dwelling, childbirth and small children.

There are also a number of special terms that applied to sacred sites, three of which are relevant here. The term *seite* and its variants refer in part to an idol, usually an unusual natural stone and also the place of this idol. The South Saami term *bissie* has three meanings: the concept of sacred, a sacred offer site, and the offering itself. The term *ahka or akka* refers to the female goddesses, including the mother goddess *Maadterahka* and her three daughters (Læstadius 1838–1845: Manker 1957:13 ff.). The Saami cosmos had two, possibly three, levels: the upper world (including the heavens) and the underworld. These are, in any case, parallel worlds and their boundaries can also be defined by the land and the sea, or by a mountain top and the sky. These worlds were united through the world axis. Physical representations of the supernatural world, such as idols, were part of everyday life. Human graves, however, were to be avoided (Storå 1971; Mulk and Bayliss-Smith 2006b:25–29).

Acts of communication with *Maadterahka* took place through routine domestic observances, small-scale offerings, larger-scale seasonal offerings and, when necessary, through shamanistic intercession (Mulk and Bayliss-Smith 2006:91). There was also a hierarchy of offer sites and sacrificial sites that related to different social settings. The primary setting was that of the family and the family dwelling; the second setting was the territory used by a local band or the *sijdda;* and the

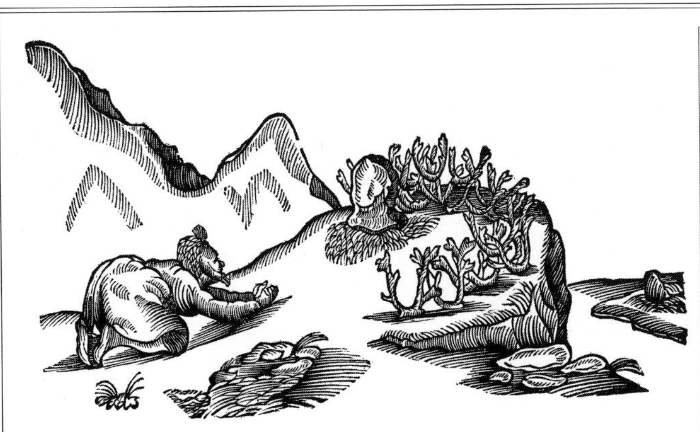

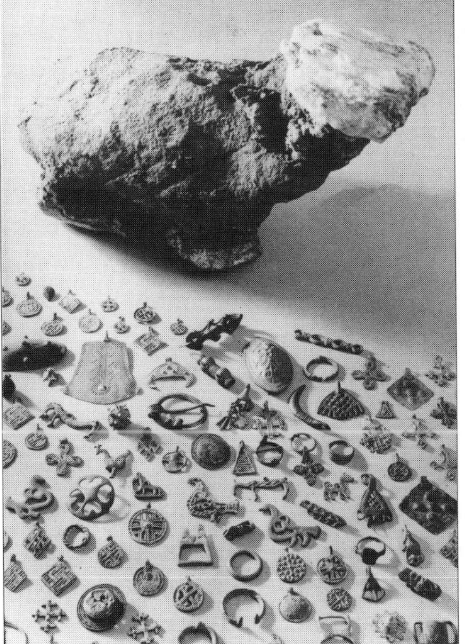

*Figure 181. A Saami at an offer site with a stone* seite *and antlers. Note location on a hill with a wide view of the surrounding landscape (Schefferus 1673:140). A stone seite from Lapland and an assortment of offerings from the Gråträsk site (courtesy Antikvariskt-topografiska arkivet, the National Heritage Board, Stockholm).*

third setting was the region used by related bands, referred to as the *vuobme* or *tjiellde* (Swedish, *lappby*). These units are comparable in size to hunter-gatherer bands; a family normally averages five people, a band 25 people or three to five families, and a viable biological and linguistic group of about 500 people (cf. Lee and Daly 1999). Comparable numbers have been obtained from cameral records for the Forest Saami of Jokkmokk parish (Kvist and Wheelersburg 1997).

Ernst Manker published more than 500 sacred sites in 1957. Eleven of these sites are known for their rich finds of metal objects. A twelfth major site has been added since then (Zachrisson 1984). These sites date primarily to the period A.D. 700–1400, but there are also sporadic finds of quartzite, slate and asbestos-tempered pottery. There is thus every reason to believe that these offer practices did not originate during the Late Iron Age, but have deep roots extending back 4,000 years or more (Manker 1957:52).

## The Wild and the Domesticated

While Saami shamanism related to mediation between hunters and prey, there was also a strong pastoral element that involved tame and domesticated animals, herds and pasturelands. Saami ideology thereby embodied a dualism of dependency and control (cf. Ingold 1986; Hamayon 1996:76–89). Seventy-six percent of the animal bones from offer sites derive from combinations of wild and domesticated reindeer and 8% derive from livestock, especially sheep and goats. An offering is a ritualized form of communication with the gods, and it is evident that Saami gods could be satisfied by this mixture of wild and domesticated creatures. As quoted in Manker (1957:44–45): Randulf (1723) described live sacrifices of horses, goats, dogs and cats at sites with wooden idols in North Norway; Forbus (1727) mentioned sheep or goats being sacrificed to *Beifwe*, the sun god in Swedish Lapland; Kildal (1730) described the offering of spirits, tobacco, cheese, porridge (*Saaraahka*'s porridge), calves, sheep, lambs, goats, pigs, cats and roosters to *Maadteraahka* and her three daughters; Högström (1746) in Lule Lapmark mentioned sheep and goats among other animals sacrificed; Leem (1767), writing of Finnmark, mentioned that sheep and other livestock together with milk and cheese, but seldom seals, were offered. While many of these finds date to the historic period, Manker has presented evidence that livestock had been offered during the Viking Period: goats were found at seven sites and cattle at three sites. Reindeer and goats were, in fact, among the most common offer animals (Manker 1960:46, 76).

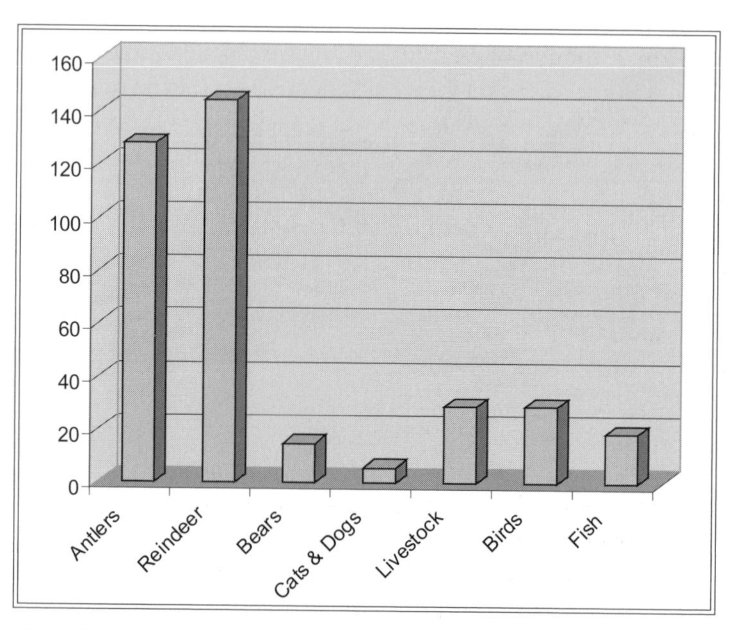


*Figure 182. Animal offerings at 357 sites (based on Manker 1957:52).*

## The Bear Burial

The bear was one of the most important symbols of Saami society. While bears were the largest and most dangerous predators in the Nordic region and were revered as such, their spiritual significance among circumpolar peoples like the Saami related in greater measure to their humanlike attributes, including body proportions, particularly when skinned, their upright and sitting stances, footprints, omnivorous diets, feces, cleverness and even emotional behavior, including crying and masturbation (Edsman 1994:20). Added to these qualities is the bear's ability to hibernate, to survive without eating, and then seemingly rise from the dead in the spring (Hallowell 1926:149). The bear was a sacred animal in all Saami areas and bear hunting was a sacred undertaking (Bäckman and Hultkrantz 1978:83). Saami bear rituals were first documented by Danish, Norwegian and Swedish priests in the seventeenth and eighteenth centuries (Niurenius 1645; Rheen 1671; Graan 1672; Thurenius 1724; Högström 1747; Fjellström 1755; Leem 1767). A comprehensive synthesis and analysis of the large corpus of original source materials, as well as published literature on Saami and Finnish bear ceremonies, is given in Manker (1957) and Edsman (1994).

The brown bear (*Ursus arctos arctos*) was a co-migrator with humans into the Scandinavian Peninsula from the south and east following the rapid deglaciation of the region between 8,000 and 10,000 years ago. Bear figures appear as portable art (Carpelan 1977) and images of bears in early northern rock art, together with figures of birds, fish, reindeer and humans, have close parallels on Saami drums (Helskog 1988). It has been speculated that the drums may have replaced rock art as a shamanistic medium (Helskog 1988:110–112). After reindeer, bears were the most common animals portrayed on these drums (Kjellström and Rydving 1988).

Twenty Nordic sources from 1631 to the nineteenth century describe Saami bear burials. Zachrisson and Iregren (1974) summarize these accounts and describe nine Swedish bear burial finds, as well as 20 finds of bear bones of "special character" (i.e., bear bone depositions, including skulls). The latter are more common in north Lapland and Norway (Zachrisson and Iregren 1974:38). Although of seemingly different character, the motivation for a burial and for a bone deposition was the same, the need to show respect for the bear and for renewal (Mebius 2003:108–110). Mulk and Iregren (1995) published an additional bear burial from a dwelling site at Karats near Jokkmokk in Lapland. A study encompassing 30 finds from North Norway was published by Myrstad (1996), and another about Spildra, an island with nine bear burials/bone depositions in Norway, was published by Bjørklund and Grydeland (2001). Altogether, some 43 burial sites are recorded in Norway and Sweden. An additional find had been made at Onbacken in Hälsingland in 1923 (Liedgren 1985). According to the excavator, Gustaf Hallström, bear bones and a complete skull with teeth were found in the southeast corner of an Early Iron Age terrace house and not far from some graves. This is a "typical bear grave of Southern Lappish type" (Liedgren 1985:340). This parallels the Grundskatan find and shows that the Saami were directly involved in spiritual interactions with Germanic farmers in Hälsingland.

Saami rituals took place at many locations in the landscape and within a hierarchy of space, from the mountaintops to the hearths. Manker sorted 342 offer sites by topography. Forty-four percent were by springs, waterfalls, rapids, lakes, islands and points. He also noted that islands were important because they were isolated and protected (Manker 1957:23–28). A majority of the bear burials/depositions (73%) are also associated with water and had been placed on islands or on points. All but two of the Norwegian finds were on the Norwegian coast.

The construction of bear burials, like dwellings, reflects the availability of local raw materials (e.g., cairns in the mountains and on the coasts and inhumations with earth or log coverings in interior and forested areas). Most bear burials and depositions (48%), especially in Norway, were found in fissures, under boulders or in caves. It has been pointed out that these are the places where bears live, their dens, and also where there were openings to other worlds (Myrstad 1996:66–67). Some 17% were in cists or stone circles, 6% were in earth mounds, and 8% were under cairns. Although not common, the bones could be charred, as seen at Grundskatan (see also Paulson 1963), and a burned surface was observed under a bark layer at the bear burial site at Karats (Mulk and Iregren 1995).

Of the 29 bear burials and depositions with multiple skeletal parts, 22 of them (78%) had some or most of the bones chopped, broken and split. Because of the ritualistic significance of the bear burial, only a selection of bones seems to have been, in practice, necessary. The common lack of phalanges shows that the bear had been flayed with the claws attached. According to Saami tradition, bear claws, which could have been removed as amulets, contained *väki*, the essence of the power of the animal (DuBois 1999:105). Even the bear skull, which was of special significance in bear ceremonialism (Hallowell 1926:135), was not necessarily put into the burials and could have been removed for other purposes: 32% lacked skulls and 31% of the skulls were fragmentary. Only 38% had teeth present. Long bones, by contrast, were nearly always present in both depositions and burials. These bones contained the most marrow, were highly prized as food, and were powerful symbols of the life force of the animal (Edsman 1994:20).

Seventeen radiocarbon dates of bear burials/depositions range from A.D. 200 to 1800 (Zachrisson and Iregren 1974; Mulk and Iregren 1995; Myrstad 1996). There are two apparent spikes: A.D. 800–1200 and A.D. 1600–1800. The first spike corresponds to the Viking Age and the Grundskatan find, and the second to the "end of drum time" during which Lutheran priests cracked down on Saami religion.

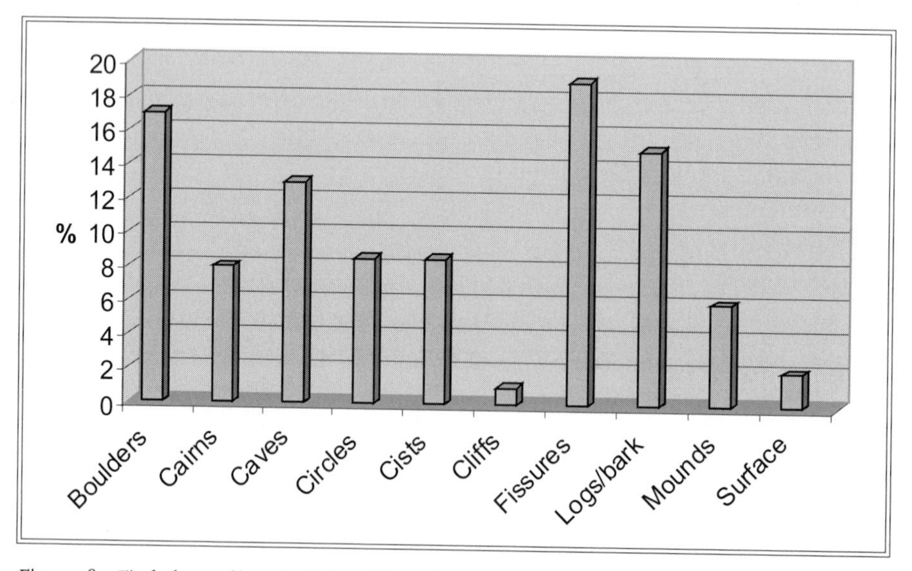


*Figure 183. Find-places of bear burials and bone depositions in Norway and Sweden (N=48).*

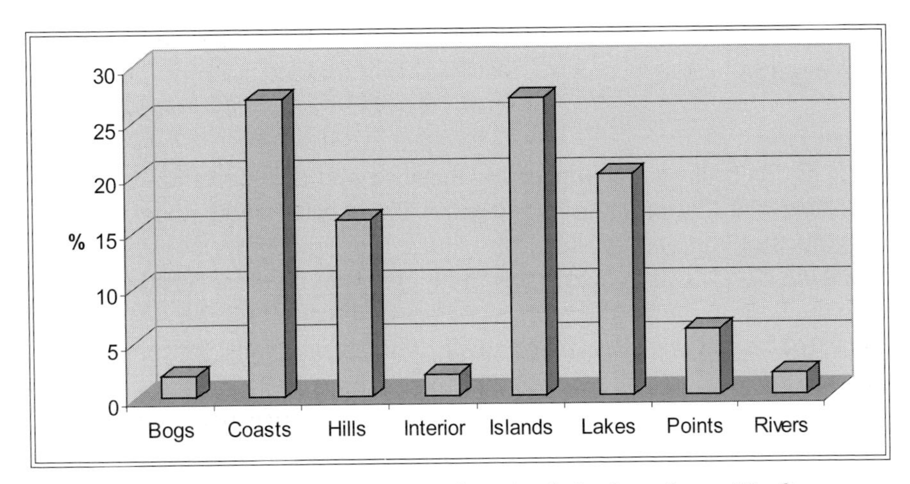


*Figure 184. Percentages of bear burials and bone depositions by landscape feature (N=56).*

Lutheran suppression of Saami religion was at its extreme during the seventeenth and eighteenth centuries (Rydving 1995), and the bear rite had a revival before finally disappearing along with many of the old ways in the nineteenth century. A logical reason for the increased frequency of bear rites during this final period was religious confrontation. This was a direct assault on the underpinnings of the Saami relationship to the spiritual world and to the bear itself as a personification of this relationship. Bear burials span over 1,500 years and represent one of the most ancient and symbolically important cults in the north Nordic region.

Against this background, it is possible to assess the Grundskatan find and contextualize some of its meaning. Religious historian Håkan Rydving (1995) has defined the significant parameters of Saami religious analysis: the setting, the timing, the social context (including gender) and the eco-

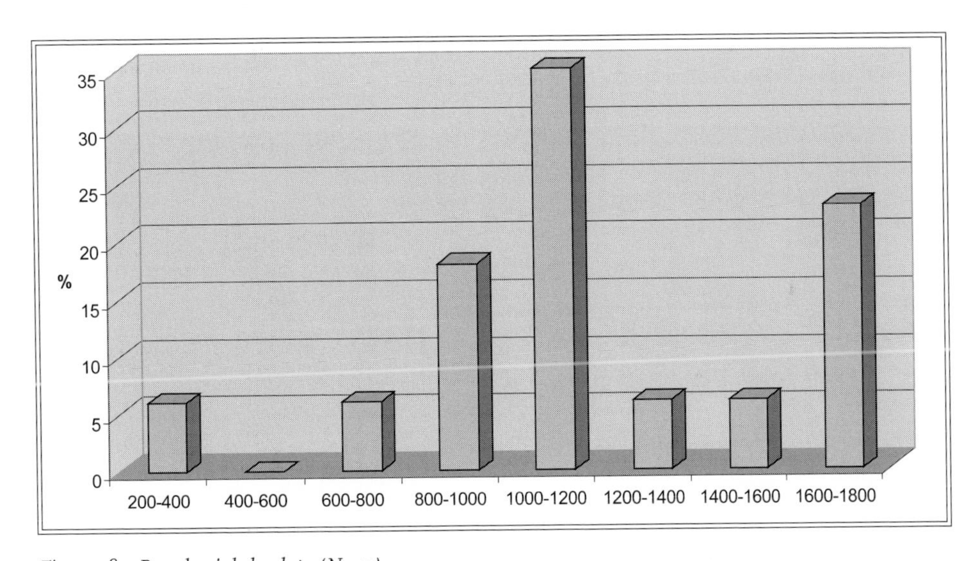


*Figure 185. Bear burials by date (N=17).*

nomic context. The Grundskatan find can be assessed using these criteria although these aspects overlap in many regards.

### The Grundskatan Find

The significance of this find was referenced in Chapter 1 and the excavation is described together with the other features at Grundskatan in Chapter 5. To recapitulate, the burial was found during the routine excavation of Hut 4 at Grundskatan. Hut 4 is a rounded rectangular foundation with a floor area measuring ca. 3 × 4 m. A hearth lies in the center of the floor. The burial cairn had been built directly on the floor in the southeast (rear) corner of the dwelling. An AMS date was obtained for the bear bone: 1080±45 B.P. (A.D. cal. 898–1014). This shows good correspondence to the date of the hearth 1110±110 B.P. (A.D. cal. 780–1020). The medians are: A.D. 958 and A.D. 912, respectively.

The bear bones were found under a cairn. Eight percent of bear burials have this find context. These stones were extensions of the wall at Grundskatan, however. The bones were chopped and broken for marrow. This coincides with 78% of the bear burials. Large pieces of long bones were kept, as were fragments of the skull and teeth. These were among the most symbolically important parts of the bear skeleton and the most anatomically represented in bear burials. The phalanges were missing and this shows that the bear has been flayed and the skin kept with the claws attached. This is consistent with the oral and written sources. The bones were sorted. This is an important aspect of the burial act. There were no other animal bones present in the grave. This is true of most bear burials. There were no artifacts. This is true of the majority of the burials: two of which contained bullets, one a silver leaf, and two that had links of brass chain.

There are two persistent misconceptions in the written accounts regarding bear burials: 1) all the bones were to be buried in anatomically correct position and 2) the bones were to be undamaged (Myrstad 1996:20–22). The archaeological evidence shows that nearly all of the bear bones in both Norway and Sweden had, in fact, been chopped and split for marrow extraction, and this is true of nearly all offer animals that were considered edible. In addition, it is rare that all of the bones were collected and buried, much less in anatomical order. Most burials with complete skeletal material date to the eighteenth and nineteenth centuries, and this was possibly influenced by the tenets of Christianity that prescribed that a body be intact for resurrection.

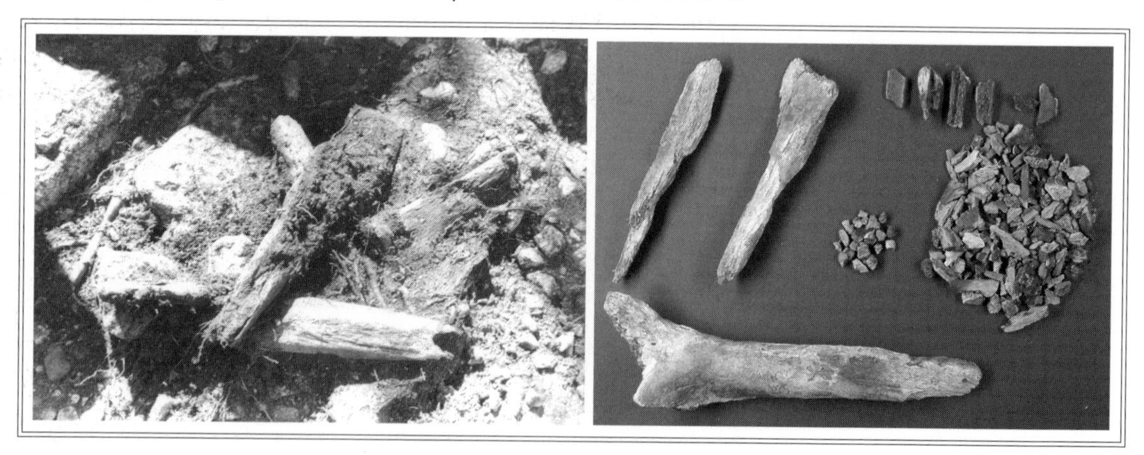

*Figure 186. Bear bones from Hut 4 at Grundskatan, in situ (left) and sorted (right).*

### The Setting and Social Context

The Grundskatan settlement is situated on a point and on an island. As a coastal site it coincides with the majority of Nordic bear burial locations. Its association with an island is characteristic of Saami grave sites, as is its location near water. The bear burial at Grundskatan is directly associated with the dwelling and the deities associated with the bear cult. These female deities relate through their attributes to all aspects of the bear rite: fertility and birth, the hearth, the hunt and rebirth. The hut at Grundkatan has a rear opening corresponding to the *boassjo* area and sacred doorway. The dwelling had possibly been rebuilt for the ceremony and ashes were found spread in a thin secondary deposit around the hearth.

### The Economy and Timing

The local context is that of hunting. The main season for hunting ringed seals on the ice is February through the end of April. Bears were most easily hunted in late winter, February to April, when they could most easily be dispatched in their dens (Zachrisson and Iregren 1974:79–83). The den was located in early winter and involved "ringing them in" by following their tracks in the snow. The hunt was initiated when the crusty snow of late winter supported a skier, but not this large and dangerous prey. The bear hunt sometimes involved some six months of planning.

Although Grundskatan conforms in nearly all aspects to other bear burials in Norway and Sweden, the most unusual aspect of this find is that it was made in a dwelling. This matter becomes less problematic, however, when viewed within the overall circumpolar context of bear rites and their symbolic associations with dwellings.

### The Dwelling as the Saami Cosmos

The bear feast has been characterized as a primeval expression of hunting mentality with associated female taboos (cf. Reuterskiöld 1912), but the setting was neither isolated nor did it exclude women. The bear was brought back to the settlement and the creature was brought into a dwelling. A special hut or ordinary huts were always used or constructed for the feast. In Fjellström's words, the rites and feast were conducted "at home" and then buried at the site where it had been prepared (cf. Zachrisson and Iregren 1974:96). The bear flesh was to be brought into the dwelling through the back door. The hunters also entered the hut through this doorway. The goddess, who allowed the hunt, *Båassjoeaahka*, lived beneath this sacred portal (Mebius 2003:111, 117–122). The hut (*goahte*) was not just a dwelling, however, it was the center of the Saami cosmos (Storli 1991:51–58). Rydving describes this with respect to its place and the perils of the universe:

> *The center of the ritual cosmos was formed by the goahte and the place where it stood (sjalljo). The goahte represented security in contrast to the wilderness (miehttse), where all sorts of perils threatened, both real such as wolves, wolverines and other beasts of prey, and perils we would classify as mythical. (1995:100)*

The dwelling was the realm of the principal female deity, *Maadteraahka*, the creator of human bodies, and her three daughters. The fertility goddess, *Saaraahka*, who lived beneath the hearth, was the most important. *Oksaahka* was the guardian of the doorway, and *Joeksaahka* was the bow woman, who was probably identical with *Båassjoeaahka*. Another goddess in the dwelling was

*Jaemiehaahka,* who was the ruler of the world of the dead (Mebius 2003:117–123, 131). She lived beneath the floor of the hut. Both bears and humans went to her after death.

Blood was also a major theme. Ceremonies employing alder bark juice were performed in honor of the alder man, *Liepieålmaj,* who was the hunter's deity as well as the animal master looking out for the bear's interests. He ruled over the wild animals (Mebius 2003:94–95; Bäckman and Hultkrantz 1978:108). In actual fact, it appears that *Lieipieålmaj* was one of the disguises that the bear could take. The bear was himself "the master of all the other animals in the forest" (Rheen 1671:143). Blood-red alder juice was spit (by the women) on the bear, the hunters, the hunting dogs, the reindeer that dragged the bear, the hut where the bear was skinned, the children who possibly carried the meat to the women and even over the portions of meat that were to be eaten by the women. The red pigment was also rubbed on the posts of the hut for protection from evil (Collinder 1953:199). The Saami word for alder, *lieipie,* means bear blood and menstrual blood (Paproth 1964). All the family members were involved in the sacramental consumption of the bear flesh. The association of the bear and the dwelling underscores its social focus. Through this domestic context the bear can be viewed as a key symbol of Saami society (Wennstedt Edvinger 2001:14).

Although dating to the 1600s, Kvænangen in North Norway is an interesting parallel to the Grundskatan find. Spildra Island is at the nexus of three *siidas* and has nine bear burial/bone depositions, as well as finds of animal offerings in dwellings (Grydeland 2001:37–42). In the rear of Hut 1 at Vapsgieddi, and in the sacred back door area (the "bloody" door according to Saami practices), were offerings of fish, seals, sheep/goats, cows and reindeer. The bones had been sorted and were split for marrow. Fragments of a shaman's drum were also found nearby and the locale is called Noaiddi Point (Shaman's Point). Considerable amounts of iron slag were also found in the dwelling. Bones of a lamb – but missing the pelvis, ribs and leg bones – were buried by the front door. This is similar to reindeer offerings in Västerbotten (Grydeland 2001:37–42). In other words, a young domesticated animal by the front door and game animals by the back door had been offered to the *ahka* goddesses of the hut in accordance with traditional principles of domestic and sacred space. This find manifests the dualism of the hunter and the pastoralist within the principal spiritual setting of Saami society. The bear in the dwelling at Grundskatan, as an even more powerful creature, explicitly connected the whole of the animal world to the Saami world.

The bear ceremonies of the Ainu in Hokkaido and Sakhalin, who had a maritime economy, are particularly close parallels to Saami beliefs and practices with respect to their social and domestic meanings. While there are many potential Eurasian comparisons that could be of interest in these discussions, the Ainu example is particularly relevant because it provides an archaeological parallel to the Grundskatan find. According to Ainu beliefs the bear god offered himself to humans as a gift. His spirit was to be returned through the bear rituals, called "spirit-sending ceremonies" or *iyomanti* (Hallowell 1926:120–131; Akino 1999:248–260). This was a ritual of rebirth (Ohnuki-Tierny 1999:241). The *iyomanti* ceremony, like the Saami bear ceremony, was held at the settlement and in a dwelling. The bear's body and spirit entered the house through the sacred eastern window (God's window). The bear was given fine gifts and was an honored guest. The role of women is emphasized through this context:

> *. . . the rite is held in the woman's domain, inside the house and, most importantly, by the hearth where Fuchi, the female counterpart of the bear resides. (Ohnuki-Tierny 1999:243)*

Cooking and food preparation have the same symbolic purpose as the bear ceremony, human spiritual and physical nourishment (Ohnuki-Tierny 1999:244). The spirit-sending ceremony has been identified in archaeological contexts through depositions of skulls or skull fragments (representative of the species), the systematic arrangement of bones, evidence of processing such as burning and, finally, association with a dwelling. There are three types of sites, referred to as *nusa*, "the sending back place." These sites are: soil-conscious (house depressions), stone-conscious (cairns or rock outcrops), and shell middens (Utagawa 1999:256–260). The skulls were kept near the sacred eastern wall of the dwelling, but the rest of the bones were taken back to be buried in the mountains. The criteria for "sending-back places" coincide well with Grundskatan: 1) the finds in a dwelling, 2) the sorting of the bones, 3) the traces of burning and 4) the placement of rocks (a cairn) over the bones.

The overall goals of Ainu and Saami bear ceremonies, judging by the written and oral accounts, were identical: the renewal of nature, the strengthening of social bonds, and a sense of identity and place in the universe. From the comparative anthropological point of view, this material suggests that the social relevancy of the bear rite was fundamental and widespread.

> *Ainu society is structured by relationships between these ceremonies and families, groups and communities . . .These ceremonies allow the Ainu to maintain their ethnic identity and sense of belonging . . . (Akino 1999:260)*

**The Tree of Death and Rebirth**

Charcoal from under the cairn stones at Grundskatan has rendered some even more remarkable results that align with the ritual context of the bear burial: the wood of the yew tree, *Taxus* sp. (*baccata*), was identified together with birch, alder, heather, conifers and angiosperms (Poole 2005). The local plants are not surprising. The yew tree, however, grows in southern Sweden, mostly as a 2–3 m high shrub. Its wood is very hard, dark and elastic, and was highly prized for making bows throughout Europe (Nitzelius and Vedel 1966:113). The yew tree is an ancient symbol of death and rebirth in Eurasian mythology. The yew was the sacred tree of the Greek underworld, and the Romans used yew boughs at funerals (cf. Davidson 1964; Lindow 2002). This belief derives in part from the way it grows by putting stems into the ground that emerge as new trunks alongside the old. It is also poisonous and was used for weapons. There are also good reasons for considering yew as *Yggdrasil*, the everlasting World Tree that holds all the worlds: Asgard, Midgard, Utgard and Hel (Davidson 1964:26–28). Ull, the Norse god of hunting and son of Thor, used a bow of yew.

There is no other explanation for this wood at Grundskatan except that it had been introduced at the time of the burial. It could conceivably even have been part of the burial rites. In any case, this is an astounding find that adds yet another dimension to the narrative of the bear burial at this site and potential ties to pre-Christian Norse beliefs. Interestingly enough, a Norse cult site, including bear skulls/bones, was found on Frösön in Jämtland showing the proximity of these parallel worlds in northern Sweden (Iregren 1999).

**Conclusions**

The bear burial at Grundskatan was situated in a coastal hunting, herding and trading environment where the role of the hunter and the prey, the herder and his/her animals, the boundaries between land and water, and between life and death, were manifest. Bjørklund (1985) has suggested that bear burials also marked the spiritual boundaries between the Saami and the Norse at Kvænangen in coastal Norway. This concept is reiterated by Bergman and Östlund et al. (2008:1), who regard Saami sacrificial sites as "ethnic and religious demarcations in times of conflict between Swedish society and the Saami." Saami and pre-Christian Germanic societies were, nevertheless, probably closer than previously acknowledged, a fact already evidenced by the combinations of cremation burials and Saami offer practices at Krankmårtenhögen and Smalnäset in interior South Lapland, and the metal offer sites. This syncretism can even be seen through the Christian belief in resurrection and the reassembling of bear bones in bear burials. The bear, however, was a personification of Saami identity that transcended these dualisms. It was the ultimate symbol in a world of increasingly complex and competing cultural, spiritual and economic transactions. The bear burial at Grundskatan could very well have been the most powerful way for the Saami to assert their identity and territory, perhaps through intercession in a shaman's dwelling.

It has been suggested that bear rites were more frequent during times of stress (Myrstad 1996:75–77; Norberg 2000). Although not a necessary part of the bear rites, involvement by a *noaidi*, whose primary function was to deal with crises – hunger, disease, isolation and anxiety about the future (Bäckman and Hultkrantz 1978:42) – may have been called for, and this could very well be the reason for taking the unusual step of burying the bear in a dwelling at Grundskatan (and at Onbacken). The bears were buried there for reasons we can only guess at, but these burials are certainly among the most important evidence for considering this coastal territory as part of ancient Sápmi. The overall chronological and cultural context of the Grundskatan hut and its contemporary circular sacrificial feature, tell us further that this was a Saami dwelling and settlement.

## Circular Sacrificial Features

Circular sacrificial features have been documented in use in North Norway and there is little doubt about their functions: they were used for offerings of meat, blood, entrails and fish. Some sites were still in use in the 1700s and were also being torn down through local initiatives (Olsen [1715] 1934; Qvigstad 1926; Vikberg 1931:88; Vorren 1985, 1987; Vorren and Eriksen 1993; Stenvik 1988). They have been documented in both the interior and coastlands of northern Sweden (Manker 1957; Huggert 2000; Wennstedt 1989; Wennstedt Edvinger and Winka 2001). This chapter is largely based on a detailed presentation and analysis of this material published by Wennstedt Edvinger and Broadbent (2006). Special attention is given to features documented on Bjurön (Lappsandberget, Jungfrugraven, Grundskatan) and Stora Fjäderägg Island. These locales are fully described in the Chapter 5.

Circular sacrificial features consist of stone rings or enclosures. Both single rows of loosely placed stones and solidly constructed circular walls have been documented. There is often a cairn in the center of the enclosures. Most were built on cobble or gravel beaches or on bedrock (Vorren and Eriksen 1993:197). Most of them consist of single rows of stones, but sometimes there are up to 12 rings (Vorren and Eriksen 1993; Wennstedt Edvinger 1989:28). Enclosure walls can stand over a meter in height, but smaller features are much more common. Diameters vary from less than 1.0 m up to 17.5 m. They are often round in form, but can also be oval or horseshoe shaped. There are also examples of square, rectangular and pentagonal features (Manker 1957:204; Vorren and Eriksen 1993:150, 159 ff.). The primary function of the circles was to enclose a sacrificial idol and these idols often occurred in groups (Regnard [1681] 1946:88 ff.; Rheen [1671] 1983:37 ff.). Walls were used to

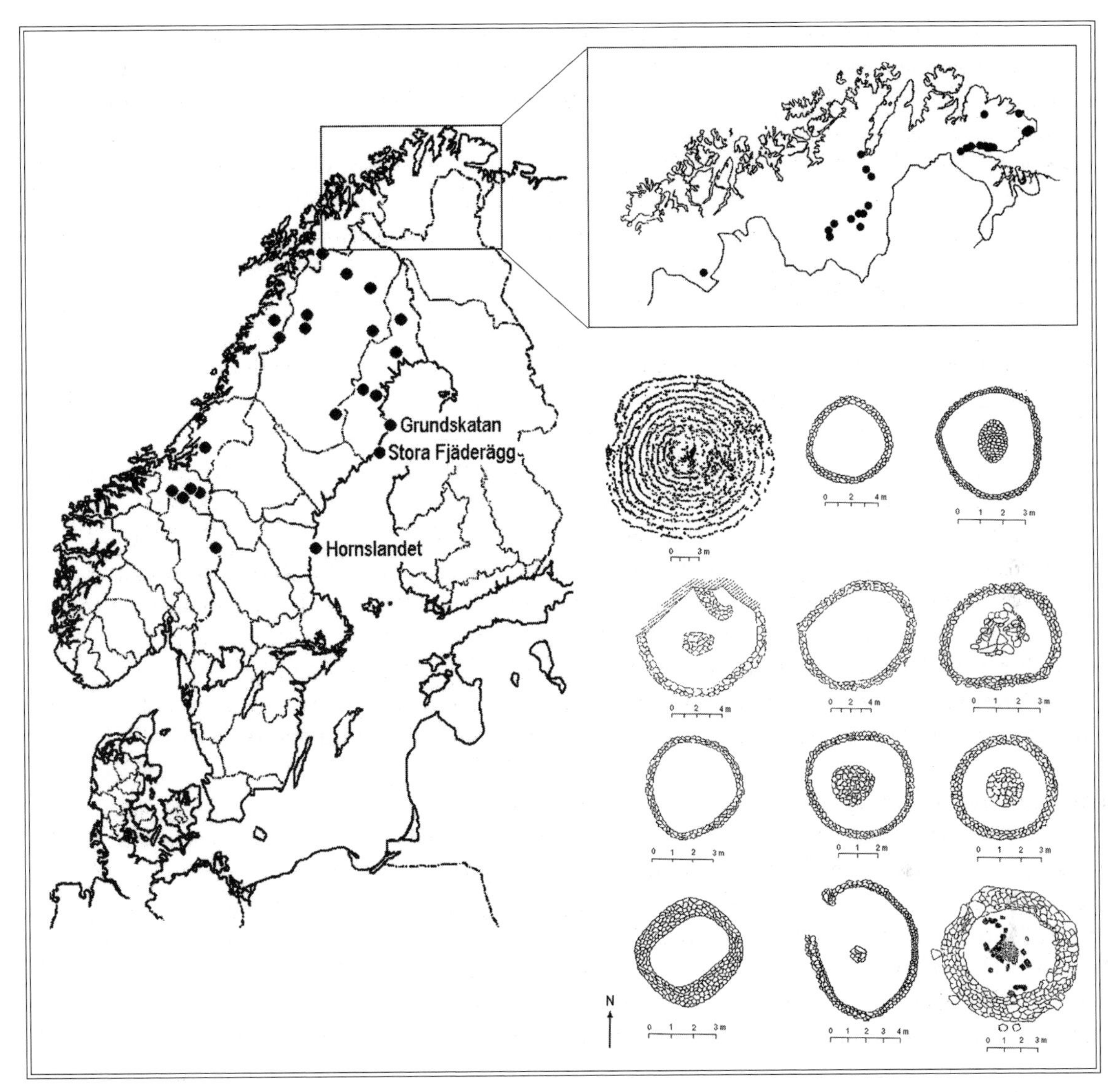


*Figure 187. Map of circular sacrificial sites in Sweden and Norway (Wennstedt Edvinger and Broadbent 2006) and inset of Norwegian features (from Vorren & Eriksen 1993).*

protect offerings or sacrifices of animals. The written accounts confirm that it was important that dogs or other scavengers did not get at the bones or antlers. If this happened, the dogs were killed (Thurenius 1724:392). There are also references to antler enclosures, brush and wooden constructions (Schefferus 1673; Manker 1957:26).

An idol could be of wood or stone and these objects (*seites*) often resembled humans or animals, but preferably birds. There are many references to transformations of people into animals, fish, birds or stones (Qvigstad 1926:321). Powerful beings could themselves choose the form they wished to take. Wooden idols most often consisted of birch trees, which were sometimes turned upside down so the root formed a head depending on which god was represented (Högström 1747:180). Idols could be placed directly in or on the ground or small piles of stones or cairns used to support them. According to the written sources, blood, fat, internal organs, as well as bone and antlers were offered. Most organic traces quickly disappeared, however, and can only be identified today through soil chemistry. Arrowheads or other objects were not offered at these sites, but a metal ring was found at Mortensnes in Varanger (Vorren and Eriksen 1993:198 f.). There are also many references to a *dorga* surrounding an idol (Högström 1747:193; Rheen [1671] 1897:42; Karlsson 1931:83; Mebius 2003:150). To *dorga* was to cover the ground with brush in the same way one covers a hut floor. It is uncertain if special huts were built for the idols, as was done for the bear in the bear ceremony, but some features resemble the floor plans of Saami dwellings and it is conceivable that circular sacrificial features symbolized dwellings.

It was earlier assumed that circular sacrificial features were primarily a North Norwegian phenomenon (Jacobsen and Follum 1997:107; Hansen and Olsen 2004:226), but these features had been constructed in the whole West Saami region (cf. Dunfjeld-Aagård 2005). Altogether, the National Heritage Board has registered some 20 stone circles at 15 different sites in Swedish Lapland. In addition to the sites presented here, we presently know of an additional 30 sites in northern Sweden, but these have not yet been verified in the field. It is very probable that these types of sites can also be found in Finland and northwest Russia.

A number of Saami villages in central Scandinavia have initiated their own cultural- history documentation projects. One such project took place from 1998–2000 in four South Saami village territories on both sides of the Swedish-Norwegian border (Wennstedt Edvinger and Winka 2001). Within this region it had been assumed there were no Saami sacrificial sites, as the Saami were believed to have recently migrated into the area well after Christianity had made inroads among them. The new project demonstrated that the lack of registered sacrificial sites was due to a lack of survey. Numerous and varied types of sites were recorded, two of which were stone circles (Wennstedt Edvinger and Winka 2001:40). But even before these discoveries, circular sacrificial sites had been recorded in the South Saami region. Two examples are known from Forolsjöen Lake on the border between Hedmark and Tröndelag in Norway (Stenvik 1988). The archaeological investigation did not produce any artifacts, but a soil chemical analysis indicated phosphate enrichment. Another example of a circular sacrificial site is Altarringen [The Altar Ring] on Fulufjället Mountain in Dalarna. The original feature was oval, 5 × 4 m in diameter and 0.5 m in height. It had an entrance facing west. It was common that Saami sacrificial sites were interpreted as altars by the majority population and have therefore often been given this name (cf. Huggert 2000; Manker 1957). A coastal locale with three features with concentric rings is situated on a wave-washed moraine outcrop near the village of Gagsmark, Byske parish, in Västerbotten (Figure 188). These features have two to three concentric circles: two ovals and one round, varying between 4.5 m and 7.0 m in diameter. There are also a number of irregular circular arrangements and two pits.

In northern Norway graves have been found near these rings, and they are also associated with hearths and small piles of stones. The hearths can be remnants of ritual meals or burned offerings. Stone piles or cairns in association with the circles often contained offerings of bone, cloth, etc. Circular sacrificial sites are frequently situated on hilltops or on mountain ridges with wide views overlooking lakes or coastlines. Landforms were of great significance for the Saami, but the

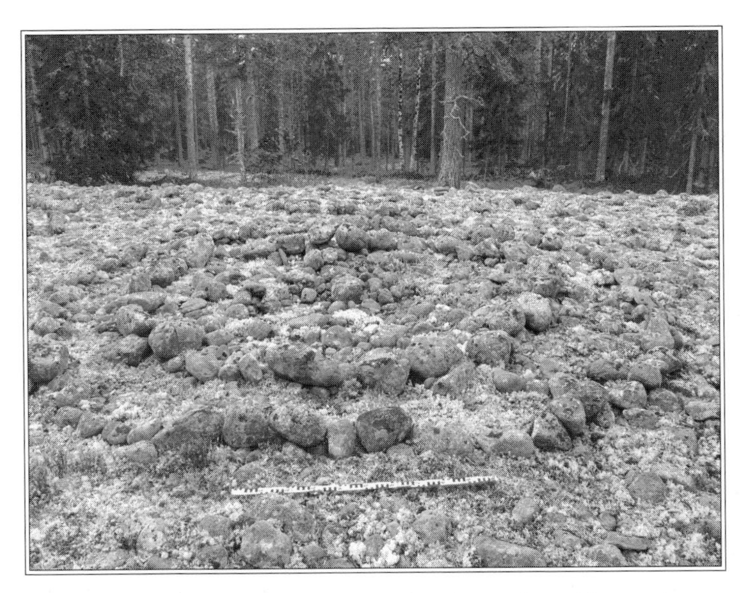

*Figure 188. Photo of a circular feature at Gagsmark in Byske parish, Västerbotten.*

circular sacrificial sites have no obvious connections to unusual geological formations. There is a connection, however, to specific resources. Vorren and Eriksen's studies in North Norway (1993) connect these sites to trapping systems, fishing lakes and seasonal camps.

The most common reason for the disappearance of these ritual features in Lapland was their deliberate destruction by parish priests. The desecration of Saami sacred sites and the "drowning" of idols in lakes or bogs is well documented (Drake 1918:356; Viberg 1931:88; Manker 1957:151; Vorren and Eriksen 1993:201). Following the Reformation in the 1500s, there was a systematic campaign of forced Christianization. The Church used threats and force, carried out executions, collected and destroyed Saami drums and altars, desecrated sacred sites and even nailed shut the sacred *boassjo* doors of huts. Organized raids were carried out into the 1700s (Myrhaug 1997:96).

**Hornslandet and Yttre Bergön, Hälsingland**

Ten circular features of interest in Rogsta parish in Hälsingland are described in the National Registry. Eight locales could be eliminated following our brief survey, but two features could be Saami sites, one on Yttre Bergön in the north of the parish, and one on the Hornslandet peninsula. The first site was registered as a grave (stone setting) in the 1982 Central Board survey. It was subsequently rebuilt and, judging by the original description, substantially altered. It is located near the top of a wave-washed moraine boulder field at about 15 m above sea level. It is quite similar to the largest walled feature on Stora Fjäderägg Island. A labyrinth lies only 70 m east of the circle. Bothnian labyrinths were expressions of Christian hegemony in this region and were responses to the dangers of Saami heathenism and magic. They date to the Medieval Period and later, and can be considerably younger than the Saami features. This interpretation is discussed in more detail in Chapter 10.

The second site in the region to be investigated was undisturbed. It is located in the southwestern part of Hornslandet peninsula. The circle is situated on bedrock on the southeastern tip of a rock outcrop. It is almost round and 2.5 m in diameter (Figure 189). There is no central construction, but there is a thin soil layer with a very high organic content and a few cracked rocks. They are no traces of burning. This circular feature, like the previous find, lies at about 15 m above sea level. The hilltop location is typical of sacrificial sites, a rise facing the south toward the light. The closest archaeological features are grave cairns and stone settings about 270 m away at the 10 m elevation. These graves can very well have been associated with the circular sacrificial site. The closest settlement, a site with hut floors (*tomtningar*), is 4.5 km away. Only a century ago a Saami family is known to have come to Hornslandet to fish every summer. The family lived in a timber *kåta* at Lappmon near Hornslandsudde (Wennstedt Edvinger and Ulfhielm 2004:18).

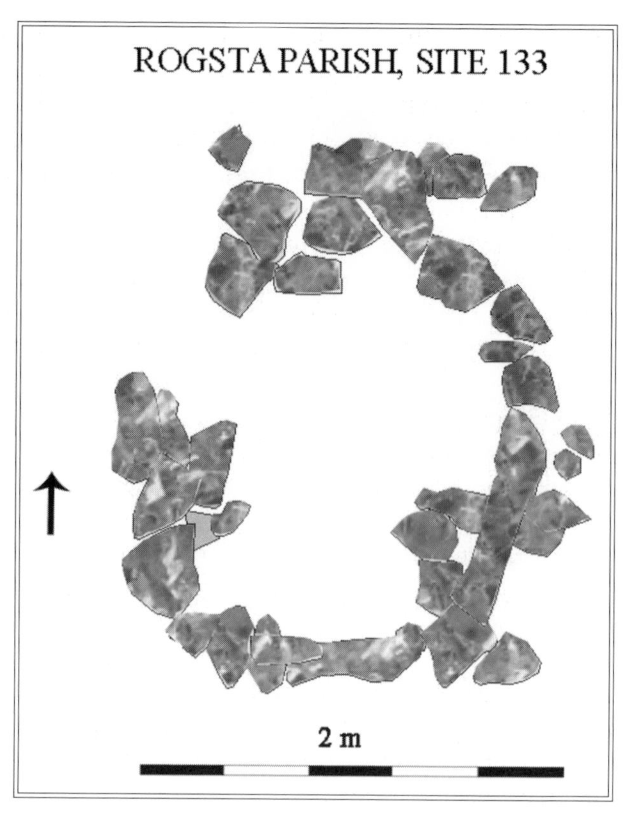


*Figure 189. Circular sacrificial feature, Site 133, Rogsta Parish, Hälsingland.*

**Lappsandberget, Västerbotten**

A circular stone setting was found at 20–25 m above sea level on a level bedrock area just below the highest point on this hill. The stone circle measures 2.70 x 2.70 m. It overlooks the sea toward to southeast (Chapter 5, Site 144, Figures 63–64). Dark brown and thick soil deposits were found in patches within the circle and must represent some kind of organic enrichment. Phosphorus samples support this conclusion as the values were higher within the circle than anywhere else surrounding it. Nitrogen levels were also high within the circle. Charcoal, by contrast, was not found in any of the samples. Three lichens of *Rhizocarpon geographicum* measuring 80–110 mm in diameter were growing on two stones in the circle and on a disturbed stone within the circle. These lichens date to A.D. 1480–1583. An angular pit in the center of the circle indicates plundering using a metal shovel. There is no evidence, such as burned bone, that this circle was a grave and there is nothing to indicate it was a signal pyre. It does overlook the Jungfruhamn basin and sites, as well as two grave cairns near the shore between the settlements. The place-name "Lapp Sand Mountain" suggests a Saami context, as does oral-historical accounts of Saami living on Bjurön (Wennstedt 1988).

**Jungfrugraven, Västerbotten**

One rather mysterious feature of much greater size, the so-called Jungfrugraven or "Virgin's grave," is situated on the north side of Jungfruhamn inlet and just above the 10 m elevation (Chapter 5, Site 79, Figures 51, 52). The site is described locally as having been the burial place of a shipwrecked man and a woman with long hair (Hallström 1942:128–249). A stone with an engraved cross was erected in the middle of the cairn. Lichen growth on the cairn stones show that the cairn had been disturbed before 1827, and that the cross dates to ca. 1910–1917. Jungfrugraven is made up of boulder-sized stones set in an irregular oval with one straight and one curved side. A horseshoe-shaped (plundered) cairn, measuring 7 x 8 m today, lies nearest the northwest opening. A smaller entranceway faces toward the south. Lichens on the surrounding wall suggest a minimum age of A.D.

1480–1605, but the shoreline level dates to the Viking Period. The first association that comes to mind for the site is a chapel enclosure of some kind. The large cairn is incongruous in this context, however, and this is most likely the background to the story of a drowned girl and sailor having been buried there. The name of Bjuröklubb could have originally been *Jungfrun* (The Virgin) and related to the dangers and taboos associated with the place that go much farther back in time (Wennstedt 1988). The site predictably became "the virgin's grave." In view of the other archaeological evidence for this coastal area, including radiocarbon-dated huts and the sacrificial circle on nearby Lappsandberget, Jungfrugraven was probably originally a Saami site. Jungfrugraven is a larger version of the Saami sacrificial sites of Biekkanoi've and Syletevikmoan in North Norway (Vorren and Eriksen 1993:63, 170). They measure over 7 m in width and both have large central cairns.

### Stora Fjäderägg, Västerbotten

A reexamination of a cluster of features above the 7 m elevation (Chapter 5, Site 33), classified in the archaeological survey as "ten tent rings," revealed a complex of varied constructions, one of which is a 1 m high circular enclosure with an embedded stone with an odd eye-like depression and holes. This strange rock could be a sacred stone (a *seite*), but these are not known to have been incorporated into walls. The cobble wall is characteristic, however, and could have been intended to protect the sacrificial contents of the circle and support a roof or covering of some kind. The surroundings have other constructions including circles, depressions, short walls and cairns. These are cache-like and tent-like, and some meters to the south are the remnants of a labyrinth. The lowest elevation of these features suggests a date of ca. A.D. 1200. The oral history and ethnology of these islands refers to these islanders as Lapps, and local informants still believe this interpretation to be correct (oral communication in 2005).

### Grundskatan, Västerbotten

The circular sacrificial feature at Grundskatan measures 3 × 6 m and has a 30 cm high wall (equal to that of dwellings). It is oval in shape and has an 80 cm wide central cairn. A single entrance faces southwest (Chapter 5, Feature 16, Figure 95). It is situated only 10 m to the north of Huts 3 and 4 (with the bear burial), both of which date to the Iron Age. In 2007, a crustose lichen (*Rhizocarpon geographicum*) measuring 220 mm in diameter was observed growing on the inside wall of the sacrificial circle, thus providing an unparalleled opportunity to obtain an age for the feature. On the basis of lichen growth curves specifically developed for Bjuröklubb and Grundskatan, this specimen is calculated as being 916 years old and dates to A.D. 1034±31 (with B.P. = 1950). The linear regression equation used to determine this date is: Y (age) = 153 + 3.47 × (max. diameter in mm). This lichen date is almost identical to the radiocarbon and AMS dates for the bear burial and Hut 4 hearth.

## Overall Chronology

As is the case of most stone constructions, circular features are difficult to date. Stenvik (1988) obtained a radiocarbon date from a circle that calibrated to A.D. cal. 680–1030. Vorren (1985) obtained dates between A.D. 1425 and 1665, and Huggert (2000) dated the Altarberget site near Lycksele to the seventeenth century. Elevations above sea level provide maximum possible dates on the Bothnian shores and rock weathering and lichenometry provide new opportunities for determining the minimum ages of these stone constructions. The Lappsandberget site near Bjuröklubb lies at the 25 m elevation. But this was a mountaintop locale and was chosen for its view of the sea. The nearby Jungfrugraven enclosure, by contrast, lies just above the 10 m elevation, which dates to the Viking Period. Radiocarbon-dated huts on the same shore support this chronological association. The lichens growing on the walls provide a minimum age of A.D. 1532–1604. The ritual circle complex on Stora Fjäderägg Island lies above the 7 m shore level, dating to A.D. 1200. Artifacts from the island also date to the Iron Age and Early Medieval Period. In the most general terms, Jungfrugraven dates to between A.D. 1000 and 1604; Lappsandberget dates from A.D. 1000 to 1583, and Grundskatan to the early eleventh century. The circles on Stora Fjäderägg Island probably date to A.D. 1200 or later. The elevations of these sites, the lichenometric dating at Grundskatan and their respective associations with radiocarbon-dated dwellings makes it highly probable that all these features originated in the Late Iron Age, but these places were known about and used for offerings until the 1600s.

## Social Context

The circular sacrificial features on Bjurön have three find contexts: 1) a settlement, 2) a hilltop and 3) a shoreline (Figure 190). These localities thus correspond to the three levels of Saami societal and ritual engagement, the family, the *sijdda,* and multiple *sijddas* in the region. The proximity of the Grundskatan feature to the dwelling area and its small size suggests that it was associated with daily sacrificial practices at the settlement, as described by Rydving:

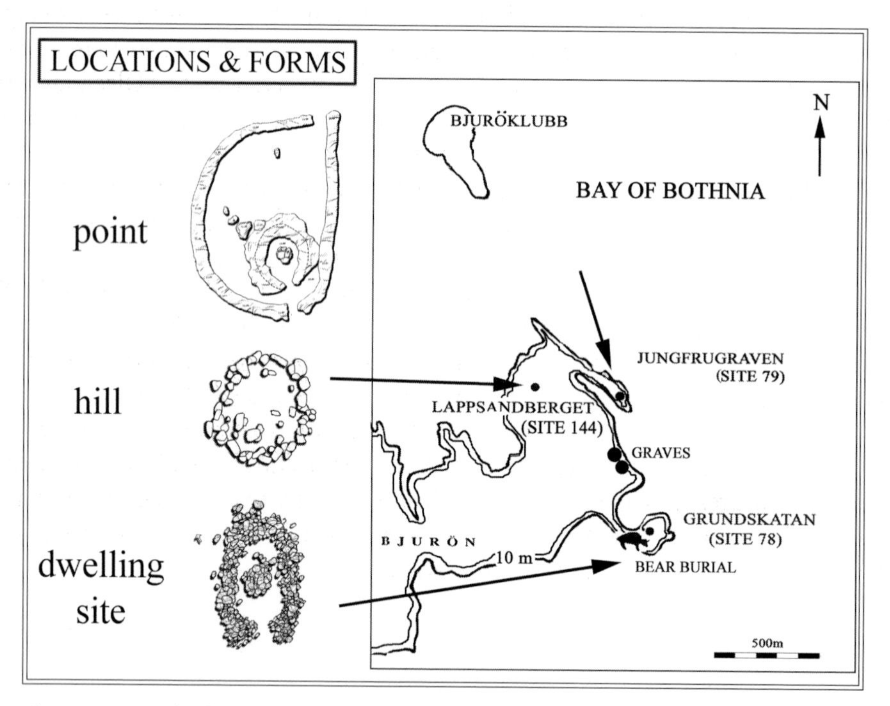


*Figure 190. Circular features in context. These are associated with a settlement, a hilltop, and a point on Bjurön. They can reflect ritual settings of the family, the band (*sijdda*), and multiple bands from the region.*

*At every place where the goahte was pitched, a bench (luovve) used for sacrifices was erected, and in every fireplace (árran) offerings of food and drink were made to the divinities that were believed to rule over the different parts of the goahte. (1995:100)*

These platforms were mostly temporary constructions and very few have been preserved (Bergman and Östlund et al. 2008). These wooden types may have been more common in the forest regions, whereas stone constructions, including cairns, have been better preserved on the coasts, for example in North Norway and the White Sea Island region of Russia (Olsen 2002). Lappsandberget could be the offer site of a *sijdda*, and there are three settlements nearby: Sites 70, 138 and 139. The larger Jungfrugraven site could represent the interests of a number of *sijdda* groups in the region. Like the complex of circles at Stora Fjäderägg, the focus was on the sea and all that it represented to these hunters of marine mammals.

## Summary

The circular features at numerous locales along the Bothnian coast have been interpreted as sacrificial/offer sites used by coastal Saami. By both morphology and location in the landscape, these features are close parallels to Saami ritual sites in the mountain, forest and tundra regions of the Nordic North. Offerings of fish, seal flesh and bones, blubber, intestines, etc. were undoubtedly made. Soil chemistry has provided some evidence that this was the case. Circular sacrificial/offer sites reflect a pre-Christian tradition. Bergman and Östlund et al. (2008) have related wooden altars and idols to Saami social organization and landscape demarcations, and there is every reason to believe that the stone circles functioned in the same ways on the coasts. Bergman and Östlund et al., (2008) also argue that they were erected in times of conflict. Hansen and Olsen (2004: 222–233) and Fossum (2006) have similarly proposed that the circular features were a response to stress during the period A.D. 1200–1600. As noted earlier, bear burials have been seen in the same light. While this might be true to some extent, these practices clearly did not originate in the 1200s. A circular sacrificial feature has now been directly associated with a bear burial at Grundskatan, and bear burials have been found in stone circles, for example at Hanno-oai`vi, Karlebotn, Norway (Myrstad 1996:29, 46). The circles could represent the Saami dwelling and thereby the Saami cosmos itself, concepts that have existed as long as people have lived in the North.

The land was conceived of a living entity by northern peoples, endowed with meaning through their narratives, myths, cosmologies and genealogies. Sacred places can embody these meanings with or without cultural remains and are frequently related to prominent natural features such as mountains, rivers, islands, strange formations, rocks and trees. The bear burial and the circular sacrificial features have given us a rare glimpse of this world. The ecology of place-naming is founded on the same spiritual and human-environmental belief systems, and these sources offer us yet another pathway to understanding where these people lived.

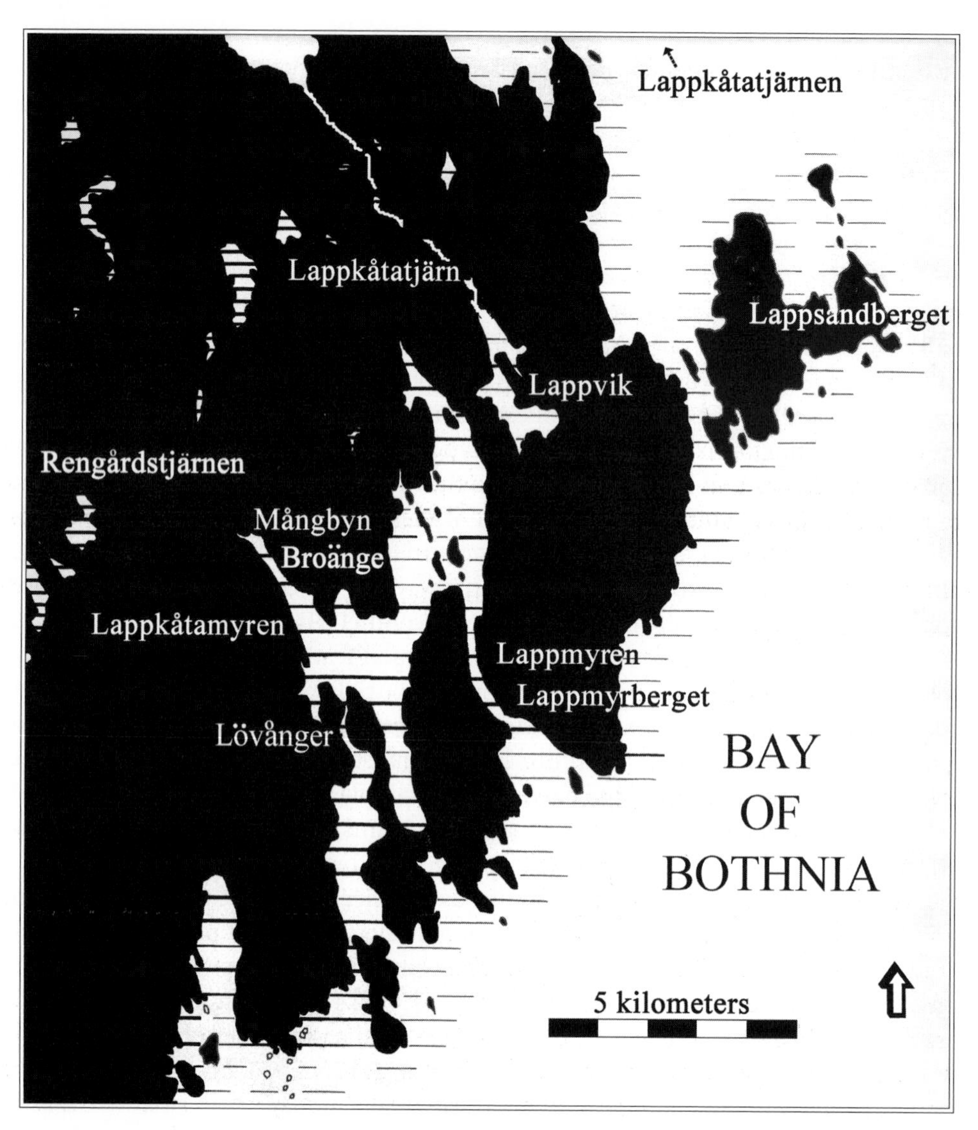


*Figure 191. Late Iron Age coastline (10 m) and place-names referred to in the text. The frequency of Lapp place-names, archaeological features pre-dating Scandinavian colonization and long-term settlement continuity indicate that this region had once supported a Saami population. These people were assimilated as well as driven inland in the late thirteenth century.*

# 9

# Place-Names and Church Towns

> *Places are constellations of past activities, connected by paths and marked by physical features; the landscape as a whole furnishes the basis for social identity, including a point of origin and a specific destiny. The landscape is an enduring monument inscribed with the lives of all who have lived there. (Ingold 2000:54)*

The aboriginal, ethnographic or cultural landscape concept embodies traditional knowledge of spirits, places, land uses and ecology (Buggey 2004). When oral history, folklore or ethnographic data are available, the meanings and memories of these human-landscape relationships can be pursued directly (Krupnik et al. 2004). Depending on the character of the physical evidence, human-ecological, cultural and spiritual relationships can also be inferred from archaeological sites, place-names and even terrain.

## Place-Names

The study of Saami linguistics and place-names, like Saami ethnology and archaeology, has concentrated on the landscapes of the mountains and interior forests of northern Sweden where Saami languages are still spoken. Areas outside of this region constitute an untapped store of Saami place-names and derivatives. The language area in this study is called the Southern Saami region and includes languages spoken by the Forest Saami of Pite Lapland, the Saami in southern Arjeplog, and by all the Saami in the counties of Västerbotten and Jämtland (Collinder 1953:59; Hasselbrink 1981, 1983). Southern Saami languages, which include Ume Saami and Pite Saami, are almost extinct today and are of great interest to this study because of their unique characteristics and their association with the Forest Saami people who once practiced a mixed hunting, fishing and herding economy. It is very likely that the South-, Pite- and Ume-language areas had all once extended down to the Bothnian coast (Figure 9). The river valleys and eskers transected the mountains, forests and coastal plains and connected these people in an east–west highway of information and social relations. Judging by the archaeological material, these were continuous from the Stone Age.

Swedish historian Birger Steckzén (1964) argued for a Saami presence in coastal Norrland based on place-names. According to him the name *rebben,* and the archaeological site at Stor-Rebben Island in Norrbotten, probably derives from the Saami words *ruebpe* or *riebpe,* which means a stony overgrown hill with brushy vegetation (Steckzén 1964:232). Numerous other names in the Norrbotten coastal region are presumably also of Saami origin. The suffix *skatan,* for instance, refers to a narrow point and is of Nordic origin, but the Saami terms *skaite* and *skaido* could also be behind its use (Steckzén 1964:231). Steckzén (1964:234) noted seven locales with this name between the Ume and Åby rivers, and 82 locales from there up to the Lule River. The important archaeological site at Grundskatan has this suffix, but is not otherwise associated with a Saami name. *Avan* is also probably of Nordic origin but could have been borrowed by the Saami and can relate to their words *aappa* and *aavikko* (Steckzén 1964:230). It goes without saying that many of these names could be of much greater antiquity than their Scandinavian derivatives. Although some of Steckzén's interpretations may be speculative, he identified the existence of a non-Nordic place-named landscape in the coastland that needs more study by both linguists and archaeologists.

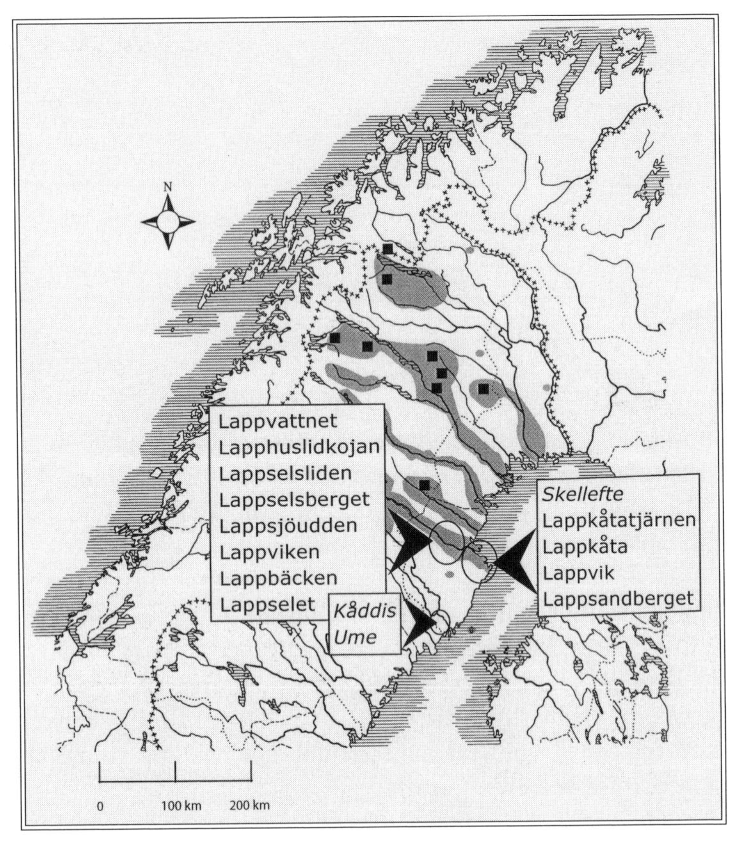


*Figure 192. Map of some Saami place-names and characteristic Lapp place-names near Skelletfteå and Umeå in coastal Västerbotten.*

Two of the most significant names in Västerbotten that are considered by Nordic linguists as being of Saami origin are the two largest river names, the *Ume* and *Skellefte* (*Svensk Etymologisk Ordbok* 1948: 931, 1276). The Skellefte River runs from Arjeplog in the mountain foothills through Lapland and down to the northern coast of Västerbotten. Its upper course is named *Seldutiedno* and its lower course is named *Syöldateiednuo* in Ume Saami. The suffix *-iedno, -iednuo* means "river." Ume can derive from the Ume Saami name *Ubmejeiednu*, meaning "large roaring river" (Wahlberg 2003:277, 337; *Svensk Etymologisk Ordbok* 1948:931, 1276). This is the largest river in the region and it joins with the Vindel River about 50 km upstream before flowing into the Bay of Bothnia. Even other major river names such as the Lule and Pite Rivers are also probably of Saami origin. The "å" at the end of these Saami names refers to Swedish settlements and towns that were founded near the river estuaries where there was also the most arable land (Fries 1970). With state formation and the taxation of salmon, these rivers and their harbors became the regional hubs of Crown administration and commerce. Umeå and Skellefteå are still the largest cities in the county.

Another name that is probably of Saami origin is *Kåddis*. This place is located about 10 km upstream from Umeå on the north side of the Ume River. The high elevation (40 m above sea level) finds

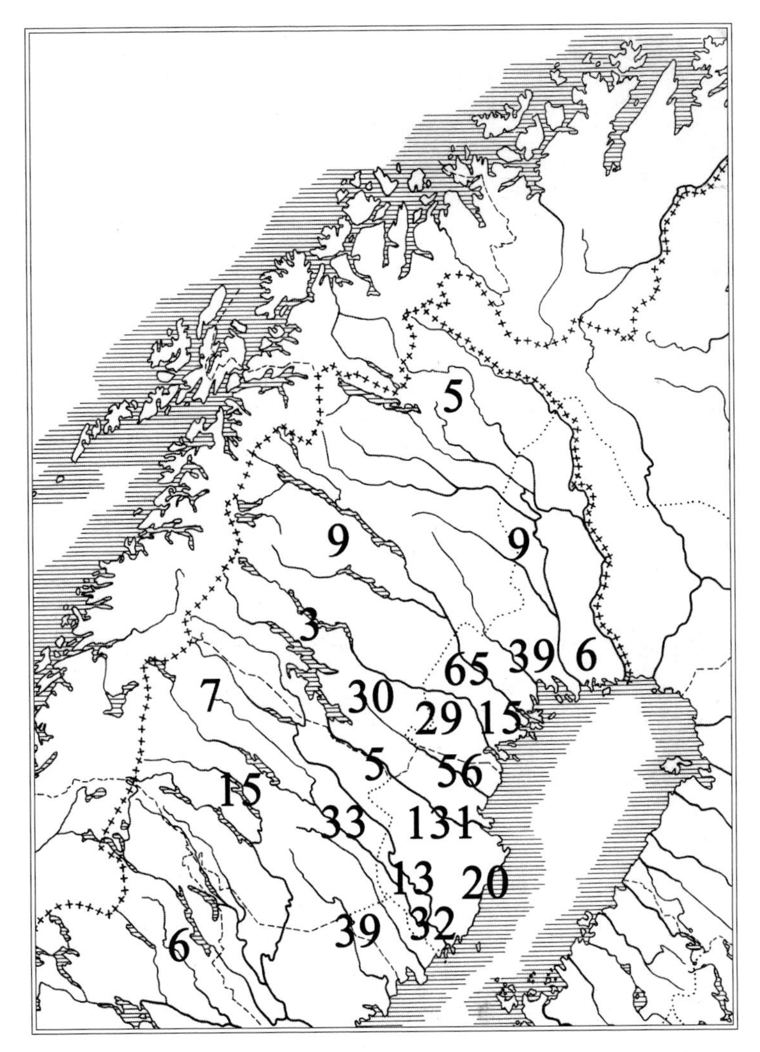


*Figure 193. Numbers of place-names with the prefix "Lapp" in Upper Norrland. The major river names Ume, Skellefte, Pite and Lule are all Saami names.*

of Stone Age settlements and the aforementioned characteristic stone tools (a bifacial projectile, a slate point, a grooved stone club) indicate that the area was first settled in the Late Neolithic, ca. 1800 B.C. (Broadbent 1984). The Nordic linguist Holm (1973) interpreted the place-name *Kåddis* as non-Nordic in origin and as deriving from *kadde,* meaning "shore or beach" in Saami. He suggested this site on the Ume River had been a Saami fishing place of some antiquity. In Ume Saami, *gáddie* means shore (Wahlberg 2003:180). The name *kodde* also means "wild reindeer" (Collinder 1964). Gunnar Pellijeff (1982) prefers to associate the name with that of medieval settlements, and to the Finnish word *kodis,* which means "farmyard."

From the archaeological perspective and the Ume River location, a Saami origin seems most convincing. The archaeological contexts of many northern sites are often unknown to linguists whose frame of reference is that of historic maps and written sources. Kåddis is located downstream from the waterfall and rapids of Stornorrfors, where there are more prehistoric settlement remains and rock art. This is one of the richest salmon fishing places on the Ume River, so much so that Uppsala Cathedral claimed ownership of it in 1316. Continuity in place-naming was undoubtedly founded on the same principles as hunting and fishing itself, the richness, reliability, access to natural resources and the physical appearances of these places (Figure 192).

The same principles of shore-level association used for sites can be applied to the Nordic names Lövånger, Kräkånger and Hertsånger, which are found in Lövånger parish. These names derive from the Nordic word *angr,* which means "fjord" or "narrow inlet" (Holm 1949, 1991). The name is common in West Norway where it dates to the period A.D. 500–800. While the name *angr* can theoretically date to as early as A.D. 500, the elevation for the shoreline below the settlement and church village at Lövånger aligns with the 10 m elevation, which dates to A.D. 950. Lövånger parish (*Lavanger*) was first established under the Archbishop in Uppsala, Jakob Ulfsson, in 1340. The inlet leading up to this trading site is named *avan*. Holm (1949:92) believes that the *angr* name was the original name of the inlet Avafjärden. Hertsånger and Kräkånger can be associated with the 15 m levels and the period A.D. 500, but do not conform as well to the *angr* topography as Lövånger. These names refer to coastal waterways, not settlements, and are probably connected to the heyday of the Germanic fur trade that was based in the Mid-Nordic region. Even names like Tarv, Täfteå, Obbola and Hiske have this maritime connection (Rathje 2001:177–182).

Lövånger is paralleled by archaeological sites at Broänge and Mångbyn, located 3 km upstream (Broadbent and Rathje 2001). The oldest reference to a church in the area is from nearby Kyrksjön (church lake) and could date to the thirteenth century. But the *angr* names and the archaeological data show that trading had been underway before then. This makes perfect sense as trade was of interest to both the Saami and Germanic groups, who could have met there a thousand or more years ago, and hundreds of years before the area became settled by Swedish farmers.

Table 56. Low-lying Lapp place-names in Lövånger parish.

| SITE | ELEVATION | DATE |
| --- | --- | --- |
| *Lappkåtatjärnen (Storön)* | 8–10 m | A.D. 950–1150 |
| *Lappkåtatjärnen (V.Uttersjön)* | 10–15 m | A.D. 600–950 |
| *Lappvik* | 8–10 m | A.D. 950–1150 |

There are, as noted by Holm and others, no Nordic Iron Age settlement names in this region, but there are many landscape and land-use associations with Lapp names. *Lappkåtamyren* (Lapp Hut Bog), for example, is near Broänge and Mångbyn. The small mountain named *Lappsandberget* (Lapp Sand Mountain) on Bjurön Island has a Saami circular sacrificial feature just below its highest point. A second mountain in the parish, near Blacke on the former fjord Högfjärden, is named *Lappmyrberget* (Lapp Bog Mountain) (Holm 1949:143–145). Adjacent to it is *Lappmyren* (Lapp Bog). The ritual significance of islands and mountains is well attested in the literature on the Saami (cf. Manker 1957). *Lappkåtatjärn* (Lapp Hut Lake) is near Västra Uttersjön. A second place with the same name *Lappkåtatjärnen* (Lapp Hut Lake) is situated on Storön Island at 8 to 10 m above sea level, which would date to A.D. 950–1150. This site is one of the lowest-lying Lapp place-names in Lövånger and coincides with the radiocarbon date from Broänge (Figure 194).

Ulf Lundström of Skellefteå Museum has documented the cultural and place-name associations of eskers in Skellefteå Municipality (Lundström n.d.). Eskers are sinuous ridges of glacial drift that had formed from river tunnels in glaciers. There are many smaller and several larger eskers in Västerbotten and some that extend for up to 100 km in a southeast to northwest direction. They not only lead down to the coasts, but they continue into the Gulf of Bothnia and form offshore islands. These islands were major seal hunting sites and extensions of the land-based hunting systems. The eskers form natural dry-land highways for both humans and animals. The Bure esker (*Bureåsen*) runs from Uttersjön in Lövånger parish to the Skellefte River and from there proceeds toward Lapland. The important archaeological sites of Harrsjöbacken, Nedre Bäck, Fahlmark and Lundfors are found along this natural line. It meets up with an even longer esker that runs through Burträsk. It starts in Ånäset near the coast and continues by Hertsånger, Vebomark,

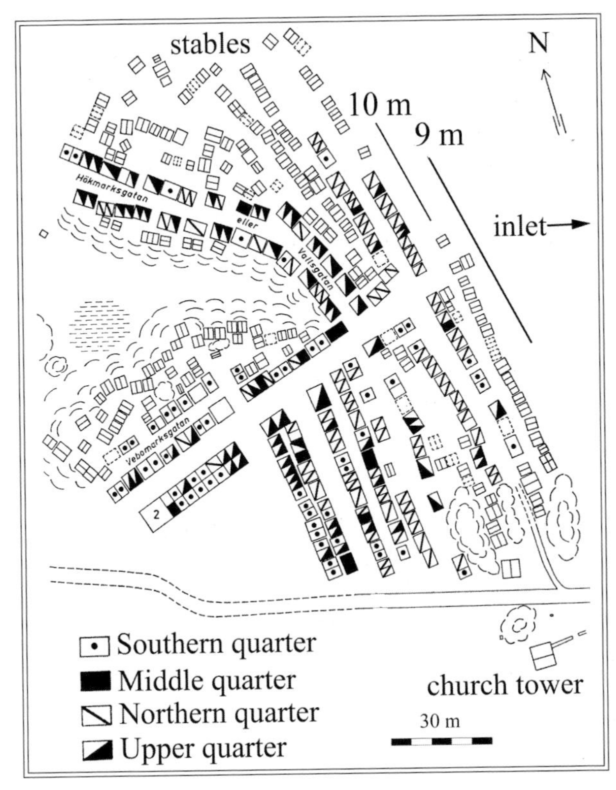


*Figure 194. Map of Lövånger church town from 1936 (Based on Bergling 1964:95). A distinctive beach ridge can still be seen just below town at the 10 m elevation. This elevation dates to ca. A.D. 950.*

Lappvattnet and up to where the Malå waterway meets the Skellefte River. Burvik Bay was the richest fishing bay on this northern coast and many people were attracted to the area, including the Saami. A Franciscan monastery (*Bure kloster*) was established there in the fifteenth century for the express purpose of Christianizing them. One archaeological complex near Bureå that relates directly to the seal hunting sites of Lövånger is Harrsjöbacken and Hamptjärn. Iron slag was found in a forging pit, and an oval cooking pit at the settlement was radiocarbon-dated to 1845±70 B.P. (A.D.79–245) (Sundqvist et al. 1992). Seal oil was identified in one pit, and what is even more revealing than the iron working and sealing at these sites is that textile-impressed and asbestos-tempered ceramics were found there. This early form of asbestos ceramics is considered to be one of the most distinctive traits of Saami culture.

The Bure esker was an important migration route for reindeer and the location of the Fahlmark hunting site, with numerous bifacial arrowheads, makes sense in this context. A Saami place-name is likewise found near Fahlmark, *Koppisbacken*, which derives from the Saami word *gåbba*, meaning "a small hill." There are a number of other place-names and references to Saami sites along the Bure and Burträsk esker routes including *beditje* [Petikån]; *leaggie* [Eggliden], which means "mire"; *jaldda* [Gilta], which means "an even rolling landscape"; *gåbba* [Kopisbacken]; and three other names of probable Saami origin: *Iltoberget, Situträsk* and *Kinnilia* (Lundström n.d.). This landscape of Saami names, encompassing both sacred and profane features, offers numerous archaeological opportunities for investigating Saami land uses in the coastal zone.

### The Geography of "Lapp" Place-Names

It is possible to gain an overview of the locations and associations of "Lapp" place-names in Västerbotten using the National Land Survey place-name database. These place-names were broken down into two major categories: settlements and natural landscape features. These are shown by municipality in Table 57. The overwhelming majority of these names are found in Skellefteå Municipality, which includes Lövånger parish, with some 6 settlement names and 125 environmental names. Altogether, there are 390 of these place-names in the county, which is by far the greatest concentration in the whole country. This is an astonishing number of places ascribed to the Saami. While

Table. 57. Lapp place-names in Västerbotten County.

| MUNICIPALITY | SETTLEMENTS | NATURAL FEATURES | TOTALS | PERCENTAGES |
|---|---|---|---|---|
| Bjurholm | 0 | 39 | 39 | 10 |
| Dorotea | 0 | 6 | 6 | 1.5 |
| Lycksele | 1 | 32 | 33 | 8.5 |
| Malå | 0 | 5 | 5 | 1.3 |
| Nordmaling | 0 | 0 | 0 | 0 |
| Robertsfors | 1 | 19 | 20 | 5.0 |
| Skellefteå | 6 | 125 | 131 | 34.0 |
| Sorsele | 0 | 7 | 7 | 1.8 |
| Storuman | 1 | 10 | 11 | 2.8 |
| Umeå | 0 | 32 | 32 | 8.0 |
| Vilhelmina | 1 | 14 | 13 | 3.8 |
| Vindeln | 1 | 77 | 28 | 20.0 |
| Vännäs | 0 | 13 | 13 | 3.3 |
| Åsele | 0 | 0 | 0 | 0 |
| Total | 11 | 379 | 390 | 100 |

Table 58. Place-name associations by county (%).

| | NORRBOTTEN | VÄSTERBOTTEN | VÄSTERNORRLAND | GÄVLEBORG | JÄMTLAND | DALARNA |
|---|---|---|---|---|---|---|
| Group 1 (water). | 28 | 28 | 13 | 23 | 31 | 18 |
| Group 2 (land). | 33 | 33 | 47 | 38 | 44 | 53 |
| Group 3 (bogs). | 22 | 28 | 34 | 38 | 17 | 26 |
| Group 4 (other). | 17 | 7 | 6 | 7 | 8 | 3 |

there are 11 settlement names in the county, 28 of the environmental names in Skellefteå include the word *kåta,* which is the Swedish version of the Saami name *goahte,* for "hut" or "dwelling." The most common of these names is *Lappkåtamyren* (Lapp Hut Bog) with eight examples, followed by *Lappkåtakläppen* (Lapp Hut Knoll) with six examples. The names often cluster, for example *Lappmyren* and *Lappmyrberget* near Blackehamn in Lövånger parish.

In order to see how these Lapp-prefixed names were associated with landscape features, they were further divided into four categories: 1) references to water – streams, rapids, waterfalls, lakes, bays and beaches; 2) references to land – mountains, hills, points or peninsulas, islands, cliffs and caves; 3) references to meadows, mires, bogs or pastures and 4) other, such as brush. Of the first group, the most prevalent names are for streams and lakes (17 places). Of the second group, the most common names are for mountains (9 places) and hills (20 places). Of the third group, meadows number 17 places, and mires 10 places. The last group has four place-names referring to brush (*sly*). This breakdown has roughly equal proportions of land, water, meadows and mires and thus a relationship to the whole landscape, not just historically known settlements or nomadic herding routes. The presence of so many Swedish place-names referring to Lapps implies that the Saami and Scandinavians had been in direct contact for a considerable period of time. If this region had been solely occupied by Swedish speakers, there should be no Saami names or references to Lapps at all. Instead, the maps are awash in them.

There are obviously different chronological horizons embodied in this material and many of the place-names can be relatively recent and connected with nomadic herding. But the numbers of places referring to reindeer corrals (*rengårdar*) are evidence of intensive (settled) reindeer husbandry. The archaeological finds of reindeer and sheep/goat and cattle bones dating to the Iron Age, together with pollen-analytical evidence of grazing, show that these activities pre-dated the Swedish settlers and nomadic reindeer herders in the region by centuries.

These north Swedish coastal place-names can be compared with a place-name analysis in Utsjoki Finland, where Saami is still spoken and there is continuity of Saami settlement (Rankama 1993). Saami place-names generally consist of two parts, a root such as a topographic feature (mountains, mires, etc.) and a determinative that can describe this feature, make reference to man-made structures – such as a hut (*goahti*) or corral (*gárdi*) – or refer to a personal name, resources, vegetation or ground-cover (Rankama 1993:55–56). These place-names tend to cluster and can overlap in various ways. Some are nested, which is a convenient way for indicating proximity, while others can be linear and form chains of descriptions along rivers and eskers. Associations with prominent landmarks, such as mountains and waterways, were also the basis of way-finding. Technically, the ethnonym *Lapp* is just an additional determinative, but one that also connects physical geography to landscape knowledge. In other words, in coastal Västerbotten we have a Saami landscape that follows Saami place-naming practices and way-finding, but somehow translated into Swedish. The logical source of this knowledge would have had to be people who were familiar with the landscape and, above all, had an interest in attaching Saami/Lapp identities to these places. If the settlers were not solely responsible for this, another explanation is that they were identified by the Saami themselves, possibly by people who were becoming or had already become Swedish speakers.

There are a number of indications that some Saami had settled down and had accepted title to the land by converting to Christianity. The first three settlers of Holmön Island are just such a group (Sandström 1988). King Magnus Eriksson's government offered free land in northern Västerbotten, without taxes until 1323, to "all who believed in Christ or will convert to Christianity" (Huss 1942:356). mtDNA evidence from the Christian cemetery at Björned in Ångermanland indicates that conversions had already taken place (Göterström 2001). Obviously many women could have simply intermarried and brought their landscape knowledge with them. The Scandinavian settlers soon became the majority population, however, and language replacement was surely rapid, with the blessing of the Swedish state and church authorities.

### Lapp Place-Names in Sweden

Seen on a larger scale, the *Lapp* place-name distributions in Sweden concentrate along the whole Bothnian coast down to the Mälar Valley (Mälardalen) in Uppsala County. They are even found scattered in southern Sweden (Figure 195). The trend in pure numbers shows an increase from south to north (Uppsala to Norrbotten), which probably reflects the relative presence of Saami in the coastland and the renaming process associated with colonization or later contacts (cf. Zachrisson 1997a:185–188).

A number of these place-names contain the determinative nouns *kåta, koja* and *stuga* (Saami hut, hut and cottage). In addition, there are references to *gärde* (corrals). In Norrbotten, there are 26 sites with the name *kåta* and nine with the nouns *torp, stuga* and *bod* (croft, cottage and shed). Fifty-eight percent of them are in the coastal parishes. In Västerbotten, there are 39 Lapp place-names that refer to a *kåta*, seven with a *hus* (house) and two with a *gärde*. In Västernorrland there are only four sites with references to a *kåta*, but 24 with a *koja*, two with a *stuga* (cabin) and six with a *källa* (spring). In Jämtland, there are two *kåta* place-names, seventeen with a *koja* and one with a *torp*.

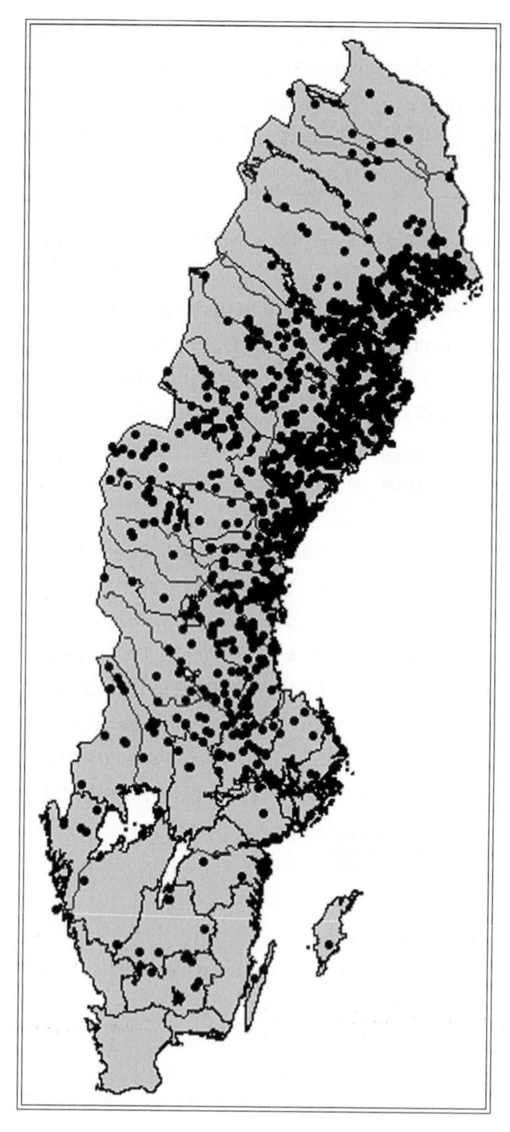

*Figure 195. Distribution of 1,147 Lapp place-names in Sweden.*

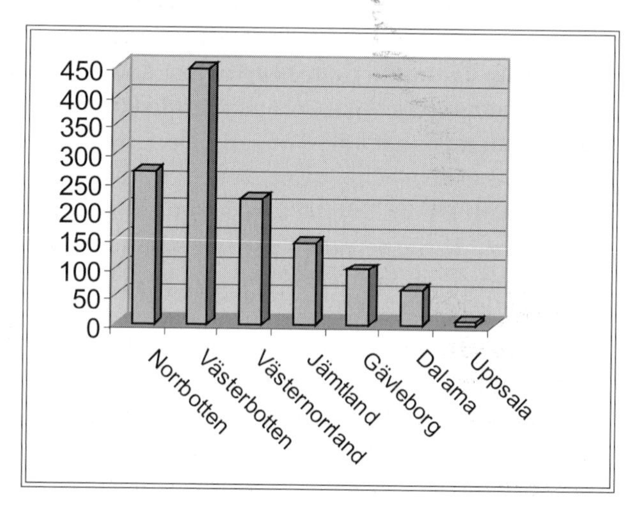


*Figure 196. Numbers of place-names with the prefix "Lapp" by county, north to south.*

Comparisons by county from south to north show varying percentages with regard to water, land and mires. The two northernmost counties show identical percentages with reference to land and water, although there are more references to mires in Västerbotten than Norrbotten. As compared to Västernorrland there are far fewer places with references to water. The same is true of Gävleborg County. The counties of Jämtland and Dalarna have more references to land than water and fewer references to mires and bogs.

### Conclusions about Place-Names

Linguistically, there are two trends marked by the effects of colonization in Västerbotten. The first is the relative lack of place-names in the Saami language. This is due in large part to a lack of research, as shown by the work by Steckzén (1964) and Lundström (n.d.). But there are names, and they are very old. These names refer to mountains, rivers and, in one case, a shore. They are landscape names, not anecdotal personal names.

The Saami inevitably had to choose between settled lives on the coast as Christianized non-Saami, or leaving. There is, not unexpectedly, little evidence of coastal Saami names in the cameral records from the 1500s. Northern farmsteads are nevertheless often located on old Saami sites, made especially attractive by the richness of the soils due to fertilization through animal husbandry and the by-products of hunting and fishing. There is thus even a close physical association between these older sites and "Swedish" farmsteads. Perhaps a majority of them are not Swedish at all, but shadows of an almost forgotten past.

The river valleys and the eskers still functioned as Saami roadways, but as was the case in many regions, the rich fishing waters and arable terraces along the rivers drew Swedish and Finnish settlers inland and increased competition there as well. These conflicts were a major motivation for what became the Agricultural Limit in 1865. This border, designed to keep the settlers and Saami from interfering with each other, was an effort by the Swedish state to protect these Saami from extinction.

Rankama (1993:62) commented on the potential archaeological value of the place-names she had documented in northern Finland. These names have much to tell us about the environment of shared landscapes and the processes of cultural integration throughout northern Sweden. I have only scratched the surface of the place-name evidence, but the results give a good sketch of an ancient Saami landscape in the coastal region that complements the archaeological evidence we have thus far.

## A Model for Coastal Settlement in Lövånger

A reconstruction of the 10 m shoreline in Lövånger provides a picture of the coastal landscape that was contemporary with the main period of the Iron Age sealers. Place-names of likely antiquity add to this picture, and historical tax records provide a framework for envisioning how this local region could have been organized (Figure 191). This model offers a means for re-creating the "missing" parts of a regional settlement system that would have supported the sealers (cf. Broadbent 1991). There are few settlement remains preserved in this region except for those built of stone on the outermost coast. It is not known what their other dwellings looked like although it can be assumed there is some similarity to historically known Saami structures. These were undoubtedly made of wood, sod and bark and probably were of the same sizes and shapes as the sealers' huts.

Looking more closely at Lövånger parish, there are three place-names of particular interest in this context: *Rengårdstjärn* (Lapp Corral Lake) near *Lappkåtatjärnen* (Lapp Hut Lake), and to the east, *Lappvik* (Lapp Bay) (Wennstedt 1988:12). The place-name *Lappvik* is the earliest known in the parish and is recorded from 1539 as *Lapuiken* (Holm 1949:144). The location and elevation of this place today (10 m = A.D. 950) is on what was once a major fjord and potential grazing area during the Iron Age. Twelve percent of the Lapp place-names in Skellefteå Municipality are between the 50 and 10 m curves. None are lower. *Lappvik* was strategically located near the sealing sites on Bjurön. This locale was on a south-facing slope and bay located in the center of an open passage when the shore level was at the 15 m level. Bjuröklubb, Jungfruhamn and Grundskatan are located only 5 km away and were in use when the shoreline was 10 to 15 m higher than today.

Both Bygdeå and Lövånger were connected to the sea by coastal waterways and Lövånger, in particular, was characterized by long fjord-like passages that made communication along the coast very effective. This system existed from at least the Early Metal Age (Bronze Age) and numerous large grave cairns are found at the 35 m level. The Lövånger inlet landscape was even more effective during the Iron Age as waterways connected productive fishing and sealing areas with bottom lands for livestock and farming. This maritime network could be efficiently combined with lake fishing, the hunting of moose, beaver and fur-bearing animals, and livestock raising. Fishing and fowling is evidenced by a group of two to three small foundations located by Fågelvattnet, a small lake in Bureå Parish that has produced a radiocarbon date of 1115±65 B.P. (Viklund 2000).

This water network continued into the Medieval Period, but the region lost much of its connectivity after A.D. 1500 because of land uplift. From this point on, Lövånger became part of a mercantile-religious state system with a higher dependence on fishing and agriculture. The possibility of a church at Kyrksjön in Lövånger (Hedqvist 1949: 276–277) is paralleled by the possibility of an even earlier trading center at Mångbyn and Broänge, about three kilometers to the northwest of Lövånger. Mångbyn has rendered remains of houses, pottery and even boat rivets, and is mentioned in local folklore as a trading center. Hallström (1949:81) described foundations at elevations of 7 to 8 m above sea level.

I led some limited student excavations at Broänge in the late 1980s. This site had been identified by Seth Jansson, a marine archaeologist, who believed there could even be remains of boats in the mire at the bottom of the inlet (Jansson 1981). The name *Broänge* refers to the fact that there had been some sort of wooden constructions, pilings or a causeway, in this inlet. The site at Broänge is situated on a point at the mouth of Åviken and the Gärdefjärden, which once connected to the Gulf of Bothnia. The point rises just above the 9 m level, which in terms of shoreline displacement calculates to A.D. 900–1000. The most notable aspect of the site is a 30–50 cm high and 4 m wide, symmetrical U-shaped earthwork. The modern farmstead has caused some disturbance of this feature, but it can still be seen from a distance looking both north and east. Toward the northwest, however, the construction of the road and barns has more or less demolished whatever structures might have been there (Figure 197).

Five trenches were dug into this earthwork. In one trench, a layer of stones had been found capping the wall. In others, stones seemed to have been incorporated in the structure. In a deeper trench, deposits of rust-colored soil mixed with carbon were found buried beneath an older soil cover. Under the mixed material at a depth of 50 cm and beneath several larger stones, a thicker carbon level was found. This deposit was radiocarbon dated to 1025±70 B.P and calibrated to between A.D. cal. 890 and 1160, which coincides well with the calculated contemporary shoreline just below the site. A second distinctive shoreline terrace below the site lies at 8.5 m, which would date to around A.D. 1100. It is not likely that the site would have been usable as a harbor after this date. The Broänge site is intriguing and could very well represent a trading place predating Lövånger (Broadbent and Rathje 2001). The low wall could have been the footing for a wooden palisade that would have offered shelter and security. The thick carbon layer suggests it had burned. The ground within the ca. 40 m × 20 m enclosure is remarkably level and almost stone free, with most of the surface

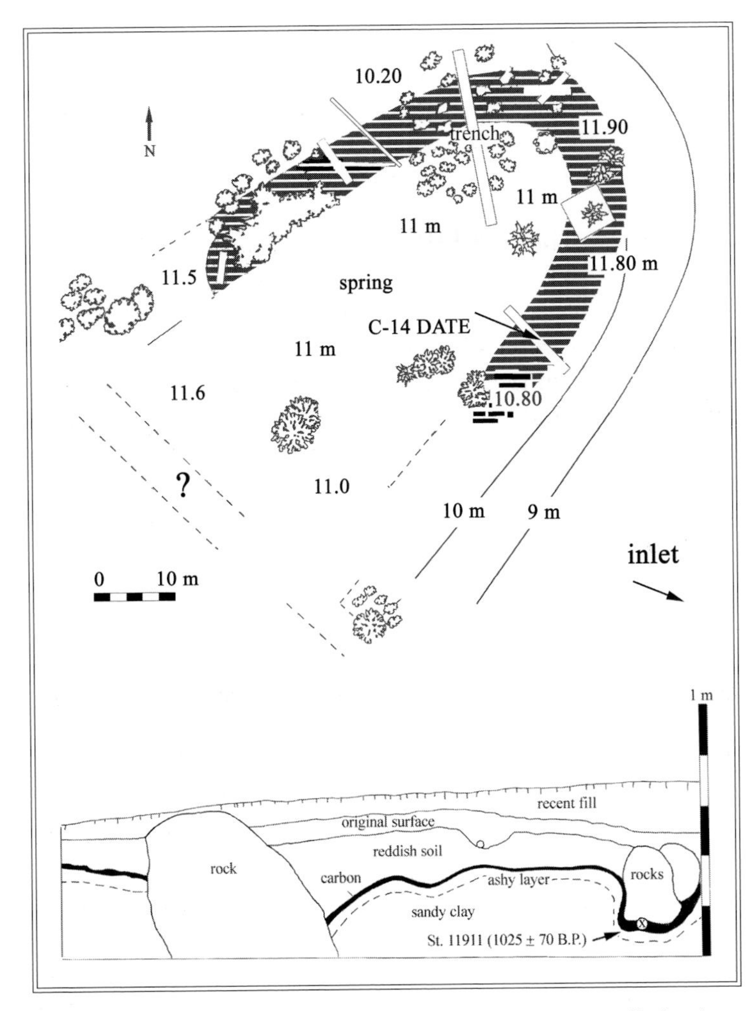


*Figure 197. (top) Map of the low earth wall at Broänge. (bottom) Profile drawing through the wall and the carbon layer that radiocarbon-dated to the Viking Period.*

about 11 m above sea level. There is also a fresh water source within the enclosure. This was not a large area for a settlement but could have housed some storage buildings for seasonal use. In line with this idea, the church town at Lövånger was also a temporary market site, used only on church "weekends" and also situated right on the water for easy access.

The radiocarbon date and shoreline elevation at Broänge coincide with the dates of the seal hunting sites farther out on the coast, and it is feasible that there was not only a regional settlement system, but a system involving organized mercantile activities. Seal oil and skins, furs and fish were commodities the region could produce beyond subsistence needs and were undoubtedly important means for obtaining grain, salt and other goods. Another important aspect of this particular area, as pointed out by the geologist Erik Granlund (1943), is the availability of bog iron, which is especially prevalent in the Mångbyn-Nolbyn area. Iron was of the utmost importance and the iron on the sealing sites could very well derive from these local sources. Assuming that Broänge was no longer usable as the water retreated from the point, the next site to take on the role of market center was Lövånger. This site was excellently served by the Avafjärden inlet. Significantly, and unlike other church towns in northern Sweden, the church town at Lövånger was not organized around the church, but lies right on the inlet. The main street leads straight down to the shore and there are distinctive shorelines immediately below the town between 9 and 10 m above present sea level. At Böle, a farm and field site opposite Lövånger, and 1.5 km across the Gärdefjärden, radiocarbon dates fell into the period A.D. 1200–1300 (Rathje 2005) and mark the appearance of Swedish colonists. From this point on, Lövånger became the center of local medieval trade and religious and state influence.

## The Church Town

Beyond the question of the ages of the respective sites at Broänge and Lövånger is the nature of the church town itself. These "towns" are unique manifestations in northern Sweden, for example at Arvidsjaur, some 100 km inland, and at the famous Saami winter market town of Jokkmokk. A detailed analysis of church towns was published in 1964 by the geographer Ragnar Bergling. From an archaeological perspective these towns, which are really temporary villages, provide some wonderful perspectives about land use in the region. They were built by villagers from the surrounding countryside and were used by households from each respective village during Sundays and especially during important religious holidays such as Easter and Christmas. They were important centers for social intercourse, trade and even legal proceedings. Bergling describes how the villagers built their cabins along small streets that pointed in the directions from which they had come (Figures 47, 194). He determined that each street contained a number of dwellings equal to the number of households in each respective rural community and also correlated with how far away these communities were from the church towns. In other words, the church towns accurately depict regional demography. Bergling calculated the distances peasants traveled from the village areas to their churches for the years 1543, 1601 and 1618 (Bergling 1964:52–60).

The Lövånger figures are, by comparison with Norrbotten and Västerbotten as a whole, close to half the distance traveled, reflecting the nature of the more compact coastal landscape and coastal waterways. To explore the meaning of these distances in terms of economic activity in the Lövånger landscape, I was fortunate to have access to data collected by a colleague of mine, historian Dr. Roger Kvist, who examined the tax records of peasants in Lövånger for the year 1560. Following Bergling's example, I calculated the distances of villages from the coastline on the basis of Kvist's three economic categories: Type 1 (coastal economy), Type 2 (mixed coastal and inland economy) and Type 3 (inland economy). These results are given in table form (Table 60). The Type 1 villages (coastal) averaged 5.25 households and ranged in size from two to 11 households. The mean distance of these villages from the coast was only 3.1 km and none were more than 7.5 km from the shore. Type 2 villages averaged 5.7 households, with a range of three to nine households. They were on average 8.7 km from the coast (Figures 198, 199). The Type 3 villages (inland settlers) averaged 8.7 households, with ranges of three to 17 households. They averaged 20.5 km from the coast.

Table 59. Distances traveled between farmsteads and church towns.

| LÖVÅNGER: | | |
|---|---|---|
| YEARS | MEDIAN | MIDDLE QUARTILE |
| 1543 | 8 km | 4–13 km |
| 1601 | 8 km | 4–15 km |
| 1618 | 8 km | 4–15 km |
| VÄSTERBOTTEN: | | |
| YEARS | MEDIAN | MIDDLE QUARTILE |
| 1543 | 14 km | 7–23 km |
| 1601 | 15 km | 7–25 km |
| 1618 | 13 km | 6–21 km |
| NORRBOTTEN: | | |
| YEARS | MEDIAN | MIDDLE QUARTILE |
| 1543 | 17 km | 8–32 km |
| 1601 | 16 km | 10–34 km |
| 1618 | 14 km | 8–24 km |

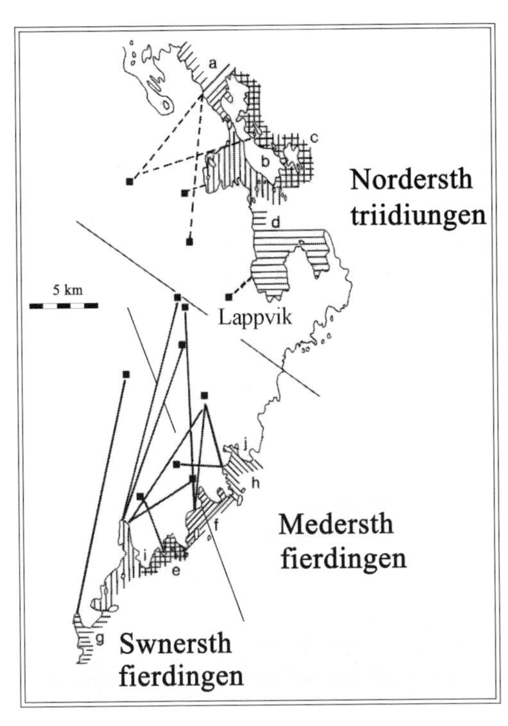


Figure 198. Sixteenth-century seal-netting areas of Lövånger parish.

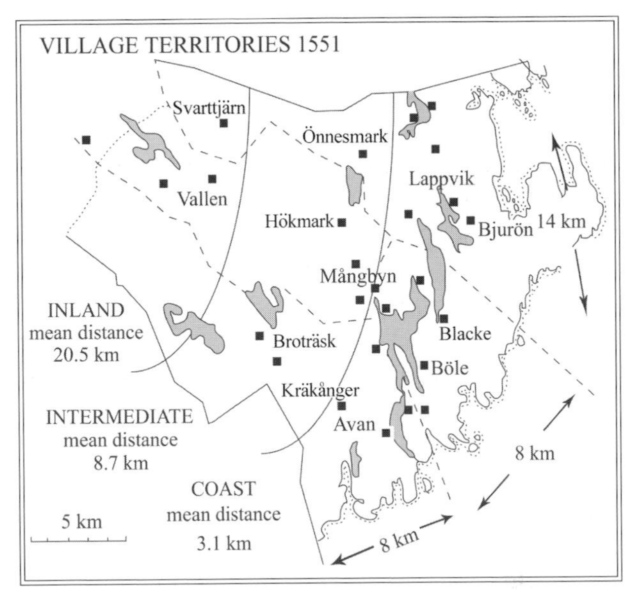


Figure 199. Map of villages and economic zones in terms of distances from the coast. The coastal villagers aligned their sealing and fishing areas with the fjords and inlets, and divided up their coastlines into 8–14 km wide segments. This pattern is comparable to typical hunter-gatherer territories and also corresponds to the clustering of Bronze Age grave cairns along these northern coasts.

The distances traveled and exploited are remarkably similar to hunter-gatherer carrying capacity models. These Bothnian coastal people appear to have resided within approximately 8 to 10 km wide economic zones. In addition to this zonation, the Lövånger coastline had been segmented into three territories called *Swnersth fierdingen* (Southern quarter), *Medersth fierdingen* (Middle Quarter) and *Nordersth triidiungen* (Northern third). These were, from south to north, 8 km to 14 km in extent. The boundary between the *Nordersth triidiungen* and the *Medersth fierdingen* corresponds to the natural waterway leading past Lövånger and out the Avafjärden. The villagers within each of these zones exploited the bays, harbors and islands within their respective working territories, although could have joined forces when necessary. They practiced a mixed economic strategy in which hunting, fishing and herding were still dominant in the economy. By the 1500s agriculture and fishing had nevertheless become the mainstay of the economy (Huss 1949).

Based on this model, and using the combinations of Lapp place-names with the Viking Period shoreline and grazing lands, a model can be projected for a regional settlement system during the Iron Age. The clustering of the sealers' huts into groups of three to five, sometimes up to nine huts, reflects the settlement communities behind these activities. These units are directly comparable to what is known about Saami *sijdda* settlement organization in northern coastal Norway (cf. Bjørklund 1985:39; Grydeland 2001:18). Like the coastal Saami settlements at Kvænangen, these Lövånger *sijddas* circle the points, fjords and islands into village territories that could be exploited

Table 60. The villages of Lövånger parish.

| COASTAL | HOUSEHOLDS | DISTANCE FROM SHORE (KM) |
|---|---|---|
| Fjälbyn | 9 | 7.5 |
| Blacke | 8 | 3.0 |
| Fällan | 2 | 1.5 |
| Bjurön | 4 | 1.0 |
| Sunnanå | 2 | 3.0 |
| Nolbyn | 6 | 5.5 |
| Kräkånger | 11 | 1.0 |
| Kåsböle | 5 | 1.0 |
| Västanå | 4 | 1.5 |
| Selet | 9 | 1.0 |
| Uttersjön | 6 | 4.0 |
| Risböle | 3 | 1.0 |
| Böle | 3 | 1.0 |
| Lappvik | 2 | 2.0 |
| Avan | 5 | 1.0 |
| Gammalbyn | 5 | 1.0 |
| | **Mean 5.2** | **Mean 3.1 km** |
| | **Range 2–11** | **Range 1.0–7.5 km** |

| INTERMEDIATE | HOUSEHOLDS | DISTANCE FROM SHORE (KM) |
|---|---|---|
| Broträsk | 3 | 8.0 |
| Önnesmark | 7 | 7.0 |
| Bissjön | 8 | 5.0 |
| Svedjan | 6 | 11.0 |
| Bodan | 5 | 11.0 |
| Mångbyn | 3 | 10.0 |
| Gärde | 8 | 9.0 |
| | **Mean 5.7** | **Mean 8.7** |
| | **Range 3–9** | **Range 5–11 km** |

| INLAND | HOUSEHOLDS | DISTANCE FROM SHORE (KM) |
|---|---|---|
| Hötjärn | 3 | 8.0 |
| Bjursiljum | 7 | 26.0 |
| Svarttjärn | 7 | 16.0 |
| Vallen | 5 | 30.0 |
| Hökmark | 17 | 13.0 |
| Vebomark | 17 | 16.0 |
| Tjärn | 5 | 26.0 |
| | **Mean 8.7** | **Mean 20.5 km** |
| | **Range 3–17** | **Range 8–30 km** |

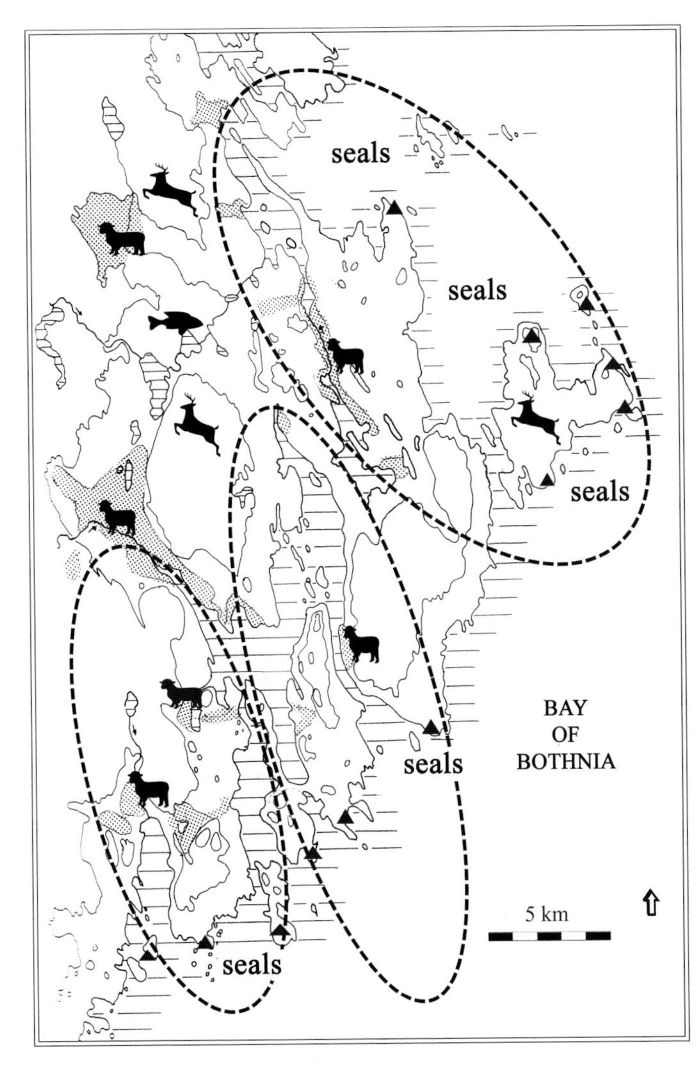


*Figure 200. Reconstructed territories encompassing sealing sites, grazing lands and waterways in Lövånger during the Late Iron Age. These territories bear a striking resemblance to the coastal Saami siidas of North Norway.*

by groups of seal hunters from five to nine families (Figure 200). The seal hunters' dwellings clustered in groups of three to five dwellings, sometimes nine dwellings when greater efforts were called for, and like the church town, mirror local demography during the Iron Age.

## Assimilation and Change

Lars Beckman had, for four decades, looked into the genetics of populations living in Norrbotten and Västerbotten. This body of work was presented in a collection of articles published in 1996. The Saami, as defined by various blood-group markers and mtDNA and Y chromosomes, were found to be a unique European population that separated from other Europeans, including the Finns, thousands of years ago (Tambets et al. 2004). In this regard they are like the Basques (Sajantila et al. 1995). This said, they display a high degree of admixture with Swedes and the Finns, especially the latter (15–20%). Beckman (1996) has mapped these admixtures and found that, as expected, these are greatest near the Finnish border (60–80%). Even in Swedish Lapland the Finnish influence can be 30–40%. Swedish genetic dominance is greatest on the Västerbotten coast, although in Bureå, Lövånger and Skellefteå, Finnish influence is still 5%, and Saami influence 2%. Although these studies were based on living populations, and must be viewed with caution regarding prehistory, Beckman and his colleagues' results on the Västerbotten coast coincide with what we know about colonization history. It is possible that the percentages of Swedes in the region before A.D. 1300 were quite the reverse: 2% Swedish, 4% Finnish and 94% Saami. The abandonment of the sealing sites, and the rapid colonization of this region, speaks of a major, but not total, population replacement. As noted earlier, there is mtDNA evidence of admixture at the Late Iron Age and Early Medieval Christian cemetery at Björned in the lower Ångermanland River valley (Götherström 2001).

Even the ultimate artifact of the Bothnian sealing tradition, the *fälbåt* [seal boat] is believed by one of its foremost experts, Bertil Bonns (1988:56), to be derived from Saami boat-building traditions. Bonns, following Tegengren's lead regarding the Kemi region in Finland, comments that even though the Saami seemingly disappeared in many church records in the sixteenth century, they had undoubtedly only been assimilated (1988:56). The archaeological evidence pinpoints when this happened in Västerbotten: A.D. 1279–1300. From this point on there are almost no coastal Saami in the census and tax records, only Christian souls with Swedish surnames.

## Summary and Discussion

This material gives us a testable model for culturally contextualizing the Iron Age seal hunting societies of Västerbotten. Another perspective, but regarding the issue of Saami settlement continuity, is provided by a study regarding farmstead organization in Västerbotten and Norrbotten (Roeck-Hansen 2002). This study encompassed the coastal region between the Ume River in the south of Västerbotten and the Torne River valley on the Finnish border. The goal was to distinguish between Finnish and Swedish farmsteads on the basis of organization, including consolidated plots of land containing farm buildings and scattered arable lands. The sources go back to the sixteenth century. Based on these comparisons, it can be stated that there was indeed a clear difference between the Swedish coastlands and Finland, and also regarding what was normal for contemporary Swedish farms in the south. The Swedish Bothnian farmsteads were dispersed into smaller units and, while every farm had its own fields and pastures, hunting and fishing were of far greater importance and carried out collectively (Roeck-Hansen 2002:74). In this regard they are much more like the Iron Age people of Västerbotten, as I have characterized them, than the agrarians of the Mid-Nordic region or of South Sweden.

Rathje (2001) has approached these differences from a gender-archaeological and cognitive-folklore perspective. Her main thesis is that this region was permanently occupied during the Late Iron Age and was not a seasonal hunting ground for sealers from Middle Norrland or Finland. She detailed the nature of such a system and the use of shielings (seasonal pastures and huts) that emphasized the importance of women in north Swedish pastoralist society (Rathje 2001:68–82). She found no evidence for a Germanic hierarchy as seen in three-aisled houses, grave mounds and chiefdoms. Village society in Västerbotten was basically unstratified and egalitarian, and this social system had deep local roots. Women, the so-called Amazons mentioned by Adam of Bremen in A.D. 1081, controlled and seasonally lived at these shielings. Equally intriguing is that these peasants had an altogether different relationship to the environment than southern Swedish peasants. Illnesses and other fears were ascribed to supernatural beings called *vittra,* who also lived in family units and engaged in livestock husbandry and reindeer herding (Rathje 2001:170–174). A corresponding belief system in the region was that of the many hunting taboos connected with sealing (cf. Edlund 2000).

Rathje has seen this coast as a unique and multicultural region, but while true, there was little that separated this region from the interior before A.D. 1300. The long-term continuities in the Skellefteå region not only go back to Lundfors 6,000 years earlier, but align with the interior through eskers and river valleys in an east–west system of social and economic dependencies and networks. These contacts reached across the Bay of Bothnia to Finland, and to the Baltic and beyond, judging by the artifact material. This system first came to a halt in A.D. 1323 with the Treaty of Nöteborg and the interests of the Swedish state to control trade and territory. Long-term change also came with the Christian church, which not only tried to assert its power over people's hearts and minds, but also appropriated the land and its resources. This took on its full impact on merging with the state under Gustav Vasa in 1523. Vasa clearly recognized the power of religion and, after throwing out the Danes, established one of the greatest administrative and religious bureaucracies in Europe.

To summarize, coastal Västerbotten is indeed a unique cultural region. There were Swedish and Finnish influences, but the source of this uniqueness is the fact that these were embedded into an indigenous matrix that can only have been Saami in origin.

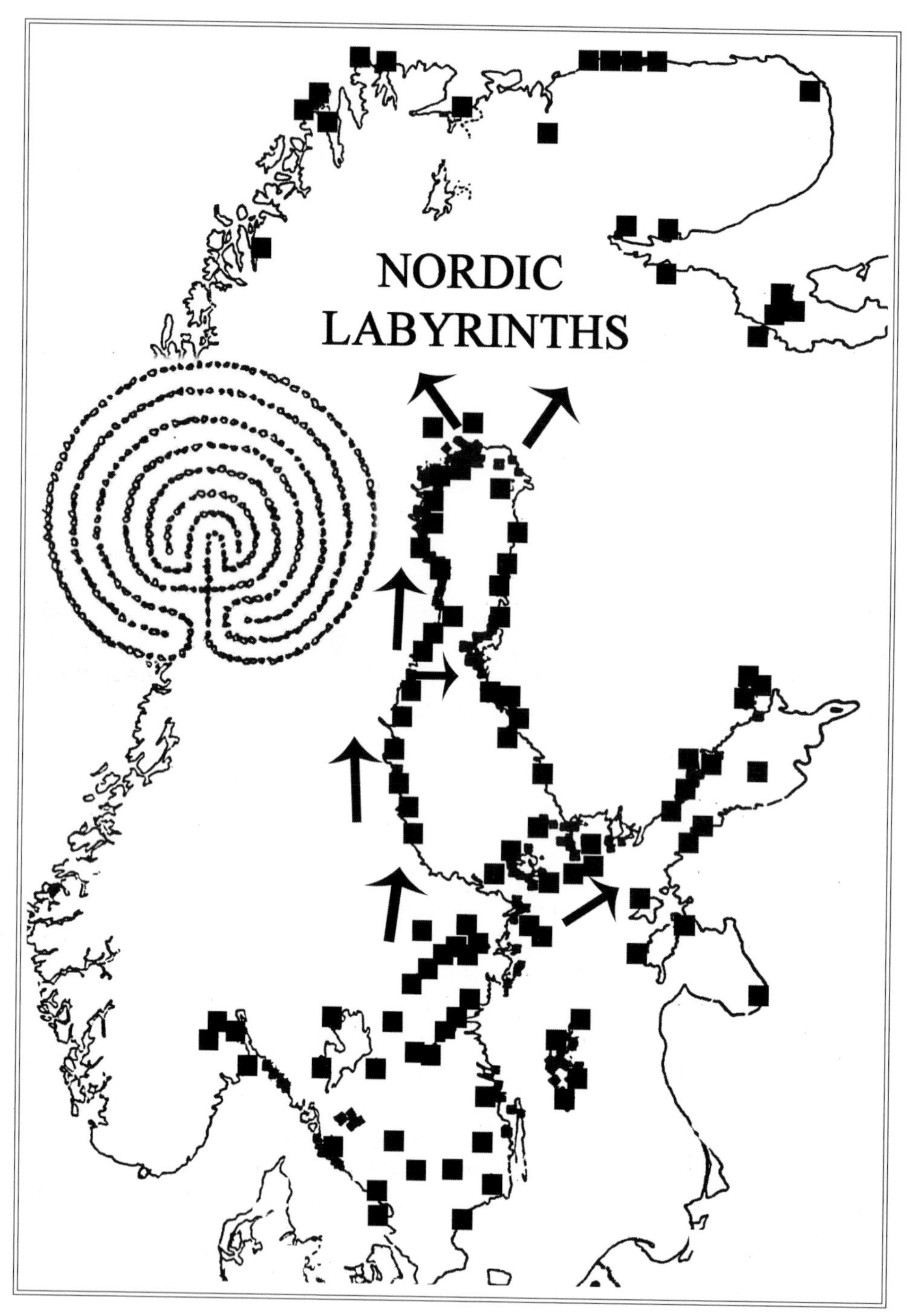


*Figure 201. Map of Nordic labyrinths. The Bothnian labyrinths date to A.D. 1300–1850. They mark the appropriation of the northern coastlands and the assertion of Christian hegemony, even over the past.*

# 10

# The Labyrinth and the Bear

The stone labyrinth is the consummate symbol of Swedish colonization of the Bothnian coasts. There are more than three hundred known in Sweden, of which more than 156 are found between Söderhamn, south of Hornslandet, and the Finnish border. John Kraft, Sweden's foremost expert on labyrinths, calculated that of these, 128 are found on islands, 70 are within 200 m of herring fishing sites and an additional 19 are within 500 m of fishing sites (Kraft 1977, 1982). Their association with medieval fisheries and old sailing routes is indisputable (Westerdahl 1995b), even those found upstream on rivers (Kraft 1977). The distribution of labyrinths on the Finnish and Baltic coasts coincides with Swedish settlements or seasonal fisheries as well. Kraft (1977) has also noted that most are found less than 5 m above sea level and a dozen between 10 and 15 m. Only 15 are found higher than this. The majority are less than 1,000 years old. Rabbe Sjöberg and I have confirmed this using lichenometry and rock weathering and determined that the Bothnian labyrinths date to the period A.D. 1300–1850, with a majority from the sixteenth century (Broadbent and Sjöberg 1990).

The purpose of this analysis is to discuss the labyrinths found on or near Stor-Rebben, Grundskatan, Stora Fjäderägg, Snoän and Hornslandet. The main question is why these medieval labyrinths were built on or near these sites, and how could this relate to the labyrinth builders' perceptions about these places?

Kraft (1977, 1982) has painstakingly gone through the historical materials, interviewed locals, mapped many sites himself and evaluated all the evidence regarding their functions. Ideas about them vary from pastimes by shipwrecked sailors to the Russian invasions of the 1700s and 1809, or children's games and dances. In fact, there is a scarcity of oral histories about them and informants tended to profess ignorance or speak of strangers, implying a much more serious and an even ominous context. Fishing was a risky undertaking in the North and is still one of the most dangerous jobs in the world. The labyrinths were physically associated with this working environment and were logically related to protection at sea and good luck in fishing. "Walking the labyrinth" was a way of magically entering dangerous waters, real or imagined, and then returning safely. Kraft has even documented this rite as having been performed as late as the 1950s (Kraft 1981:13).

The labyrinth is an ancient symbol of death and dangerous journeys that harkens back to Crete and Greece and the stories of the Minoan labyrinth and *The Odyssey*. Their forms vary but the classic "Cretan" labyrinth consists of a single entrance and an endpoint. The Nordic labyrinths are overwhelmingly of Cretan type and have no dead-ends. There is one way in and one way out. The Bothnian labyrinths were constructed using cobbles on beaches or on bedrock and can have six, eight or even twelve walls. With few exceptions they start with a cross and the walls' lines are then added from this center and to additional corner points (Figure 203). These two aspects, the cross and the single pathway, are the labyrinth's most important symbolic attributes.

The labyrinth is one of the most magical and universal of symbols and has been likened to the brain, the bowels and womb of Mother Earth, a city (Troy) and the cosmos. As a pathway, it relates to an individual's journey through life, a pilgrimage and The Way (Purce 1974). It was readily adopted as a Christian symbol and is found in medieval European churches, especially in Italy and France (Bord 1976). In Sweden, labyrinths are found in Hablingbo church and by Fröjel church on Gotland, in churches at Mörklinta, Enköping, Viby and Horn, as well as in Linköping's cathedral in southern Sweden. There are also labyrinths at Sibbo church in Finland, Telemark church in Norway, and Gerninge and Skive Old Church in Denmark (Kraft 1977:74). While magic and superstition were closely connected to both hunting and fishing, as already noted regarding taboo words, the cross was the literal center of the meaning of the labyrinth. This is where one must begin when building one, and this is no less than the early Christian symbol and monogram Chi-Rho, the two Greek letters $\chi$ and $\rho$ – the name of Christ. The symbol originated with the Roman Emperor Constantine, who ordered his

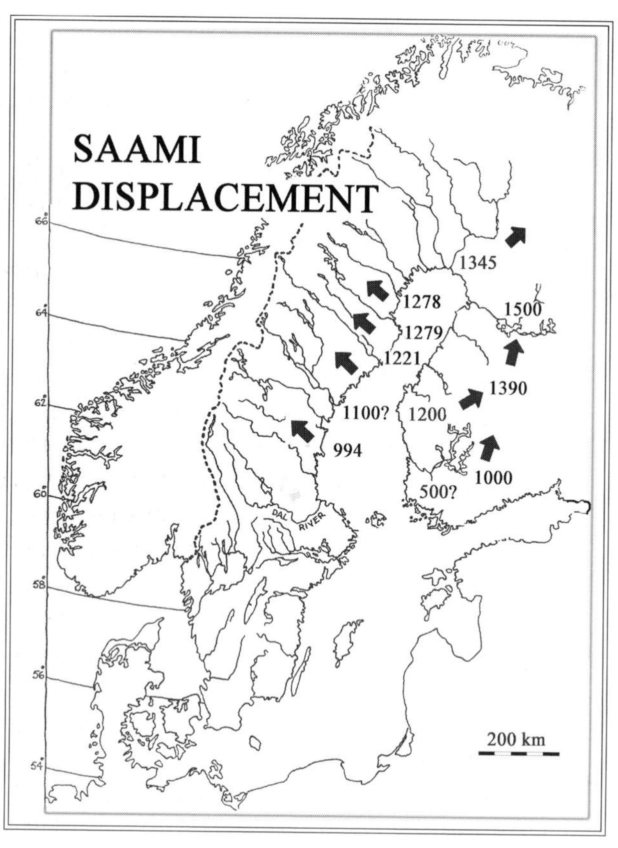


*Figure 202. Displacement of the Saami from the Bothnian coastland based on calibrated radiocarbon dates. Finnish dates from Itkonen 1947.*

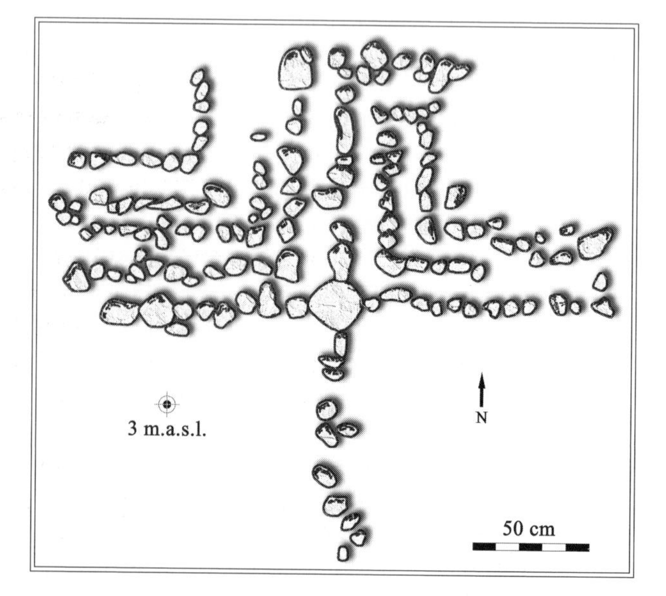


*Figure 203. Half-built labyrinth at Svarthällviken on Bjurön. This feature lies at 3 m above sea level and cannot be older than the seventeenth century. It illustrates the construction of the labyrinth around the central cross and the curve at the top of the cross that can be interpreted at the Good Shepherd's crook.*

soldiers to place the cross on their shields with one extremity of the cross bent around to form the Good Shepherd's crook (Russel 1969; Bord 1976:19). This is exactly how a labyrinth is constructed. By form and chronology the Bothnian labyrinths, as Christian symbols, were built near places where there was a need for protection – be it from the sea or from heathenism.

Christian churches were frequently built directly on top of heathen shrines in Scandinavia, the most prominent example of which is Gamla Uppsala, the site of the last heathen temple and human sacrificial site in Sweden, as described by Adam of Bremen in A.D. 1081. The principle of super-position was formalized through statues of Saint Olav Haraldsson of Norway, who was martyred on July 29, 1030, and subsequently became a popular cult figure in the Catholic Church. Olav is depicted holding an axe and trampling a troll beneath his feet. These pathetic figures are being humiliated, have gaping mouths and can even have their pants drawn down. The Norwegian coat of arms shows the royal lion holding Olav's axe. The "troll" is heathenism and witchcraft personified, and in a drawing of a now-lost Saint Olav statue from Jämtland in northern Sweden, the troll is clearly a Saami *noaidi* (Lidén 1999:346). Many of the Saint Olav statues were put into church towers, mutilated and destroyed during the Reformation. One statue, now kept in the tower of Enånger church in Hälsingland, was found to have both his hands chopped off and axe cuts to his groin (Figure 204). The Lutheran church did not look kindly on these Catholic saints, nor on Saami *noaidis* for that matter!

If the bear burial at the Grundskatan site is one of its most remarkable finds and expressions of cultural identity in the circumpolar world of animism, polytheism and shamanism, then the stone labyrinth that was deliberately built on top of a sealer's hut at this site is equally significant. The hut radiocarbon-dated to the eleventh century and the labyrinth dated by lichenometry to the sixteenth century, like the majority of labyrinths, and at the height of the Reformation. Their stratigraphic relationship is unequivocal. This is a classic expression of super-positioning as power and is an archetypal Christian response to the perceived dangers of the place. Grundskatan was not a herring-fishing site, but the largest visible pre-Christian dwelling complex in the region.

In a similar Christian response to the past, a labyrinth had been built using stones taken from a Bronze Age grave cairn that overlooks the sea at Jävre near Piteå, not too far from the Stor-Rebben site (Kraft 1982). Rock-weathering differences were used to establish that the labyrinth stones had indeed come from the cairn, and lichens growing on the overturned stones were used to date the labyrinth. These results indicated that the labyrinth dated to A.D. 1299±31 (Broadbent 1987a). Jävre is among the oldest Bothnian labyrinths we know of, and coincides with the first medieval colonization of the Piteå region (cf. Axelson 1989).

Against this background, the labyrinths found by huts on Stor-Rebben Island were probably not made by Iron Age sealers, but by the medieval fishermen who had used their readily accessible stones to build them. The Stor-Rebben labyrinths, the labyrinth near the circular sacrificial feature at Yttre Bergön on Hornslandet, and a labyrinth near the complex of Saami circles on Stora Fjäderägg Island can all be interpreted in this light. They are related by the need of later settlers and fishermen to explain these older constructions, and to either build on their power, or diminish it.

Kraft (1977:71–73) has documented 15 labyrinth locales in southern Sweden that are near to Bronze Age or Iron Age cairns or cemeteries, but one can suspect that a number of these sites were appropriated during later periods, especially since many of the locales were still meeting places. Two coastal labyrinths built by Bronze or Iron Age cairns described by Kraft, at Gaddenäset in Småland and Risön in Halland (Kraft 1977:71), appear to be add-ons, very much like the Jävre labyrinth.

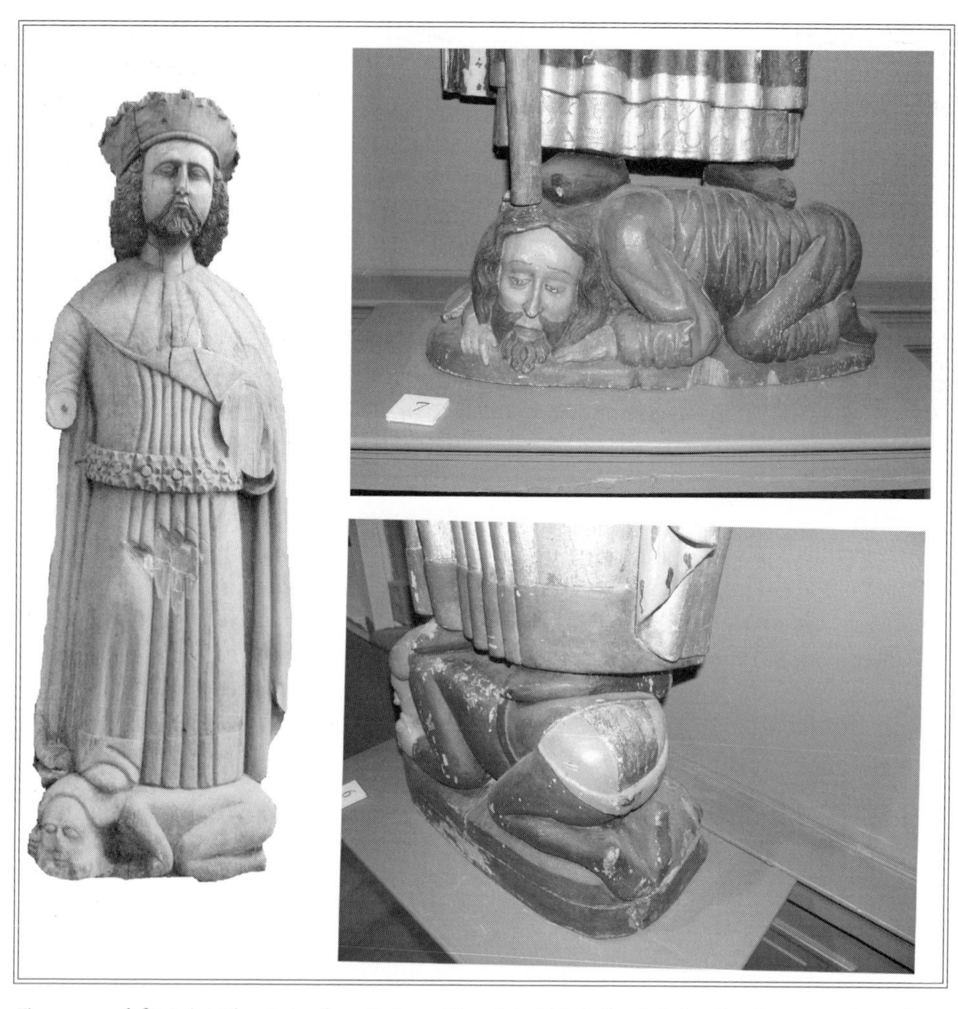

*Figure 204. (left) Saint Olav statue from Enånger Church in Hälsingland. Saint Olav is portrayed standing on a troll representing the victory of Christianity over heathenism. This statue shows signs of desecration, presumably during the Reformation. The hands have been chopped off and axe cuts were delivered to the groin. (right, top and bottom) Two additional wretches being trod on by Saint Olav. These figures are at the Hälsingland Museum in Hudiksvall.*

Gaddenäset has two labyrinths that were awkwardly squeezed in between graves, which means that they were not only built later, but that they ran out of room in the process of doing so.

There is some evidence in the White Sea region that the Saami may have themselves used labyrinths (Manyukhin and Lobanova 2002; Olsen 2002; Hansen and Olsen 2004:227), but this conclusion is based on their proximity to circular sacrificial sites with concentric rings and *seites*. Some Christianized Saami may have nevertheless taken up labyrinth building, a syncretistic act already observed regarding their readiness to take up Norse religious practices. As another form of religious re-alliance, this is no different than placing bear bones in anatomical order to enable resurrection.

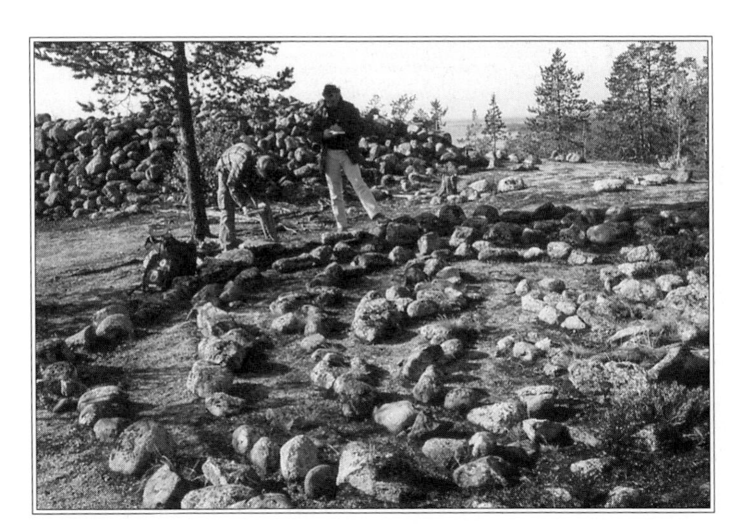

*Figure 205. The labyrinth at Jävre, which dates to A.D. 1299±31, and the Bronze Age cairn from which the stones had been taken. The Bay of Bothnia is visible in the background. Rabbe Sjöberg and Atholl Anderson are measuring rock weathering using the Schmidt Test Hammer.*

The Grundskatan labyrinth may even have been built by a zealous Saami convert. But the builder of the labyrinth at Grundskatan could hardly have had any idea that there was a bear burial some 100 m away, although the memory of the place as spiritually powerful may have been retained in local folklore. The Grundskatan bear burial and labyrinth are explicit assertions of the identities of these people and their different relationships to the coastal landscape. These two symbols are at the core of this narrative, expressing two worldviews, and the religious and cultural struggles that played out here more than 500 years ago.

# 11

# Synthesis

This analysis of the Bothnian Saami has been structured around three perspectives: the long-term perspective, the maritime perspective and the regional cultural-ecological perspective.
Five overarching hypotheses were posed.

1) The Saami are an indigenous people with roots going back at least 7,000 years in northern coastal Västerbotten.
2) There are two major cultural-ecological regions in Sweden, the Circumpolar and the European. During the Iron Age the Germanic settlement boundary coincided with the 63rd parallel on the Bothnian coast.
3) Proto-Saami, Proto-Finnish and Proto-Germanic societies had been in close contact for thousands of years and were heterogeneous and overlapping.
4) Coastal and interior settlement in northern Sweden occurred in semi-sedentary cycles relating to peaks and declines in terrestrial and marine resources. Animal husbandry changed this pattern and contributed to sedentism as well as nomadism.
5) Northern Sweden was part of a World System of trade and information exchange that had roots going back to the Stone Age.

The methodological approach has been interdisciplinary and has included, in addition to archaeological techniques, geology, cultural and physical geography, osteology, botany, ethnology, history, linguistics and anthropology. Site analysis and sampling has been based on a 400–800 km long north-to-south transect of the Bothnian coast (including sites and place-names), and shoreline displacement studies at sites between 3 m and 20 m above sea level.

The theoretical orientation has been that of resiliencies and the adaptive strategies of Saami societies, as opposed to continual crises and conflicts in their interactions with majority societies. This approach shifts attention to the strategies of successful adaptation and Saami societies as flexible, heterogeneous, syncretistic and heterarchical. Their successful interactions with other societies hold the key to understanding Saami identities.

The maritime perspective is central to this analysis. The coastlands provided the economic foundations for settlement stability and complexity. The maritime climate zone has also been the "environmental corridor" that introduced animal husbandry, metallurgy and many other cultural elements into northern Sweden from the south. These two elements, which have been viewed as part of the process of Saami ethnogenesis in Norway and Finland, thus represent the southern stimulus package that helped to form Saami society in Sweden. This material is of equal antiquity to that long proposed by Nordic linguists for North Norway.

The long-term perspective has been used to establish arguments for continuities and cultural trajectories as opposed to successive immigrations. This coastland had been a virtual mixing bowl of southern, northern and eastern influences within a region that had been intimately connected with the interior since the Early Stone Age, and probably even more so during the Late Metal Age/ Saami Iron Age. The Ume Saami and Pite Saami speakers had lived on these coasts until "the Lapps were driven away from there." It was easy to pinpoint when the modern state had transformed these regions into Swedish territory, the late thirteenth century (A.D. 1279).

There may never be complete agreement among archaeologists about what is Saami or not Saami, and even what the state calls Saami and Swedish today. As noted in the introduction, this inevitably becomes a question of majority and minority power relations.

In order to deal with these realities using archaeological data, I have used the concept of cultural clines (Caulkins 2001). My analytical strategy has involved:

1) Viewing cultures as seamless cultural topographies.
2) Mapping differences across landscapes as clines of continuous variations.
3) Emphasizing commonalities.

Resilience theory (Holling and Gunderson 2002; Holling et al. 2002; Redman and Kinzig 2003) has provided an excellent model for interpreting this material. This theory builds on four central ideas:

1) Flexibility and heterogeneity.
2) Change as episodic and punctuated in time and space.
3) Change in adaptive cycles.
4) Resiliency as maintained by communication and reinforced through symbols, ceremonies, reciprocity, trade and "traditional" culture.

Resilience theory applies well to the older prehistoric material summarized in Chapter 3, as well as to the period A.D. 1–1500. The episodic or punctuated nature of this coastal system is one of its most interesting characteristics. Resilience theory defines the "ecosystem functions" of adaptive cycles as occurring in four stages: growth, conservation, release and reorganization.

Growth and conservation periods are marked by stability and increasing "capital" in the form of population and resource growth, social connectedness, increased specialization, trade and so forth. Social cohesion is reinforced through symbols, ceremonies and trade. The release stage is marked by reorganization into new settlement and regional exploitation patterns, new economic strategies, new technologies and new religious practices. Using these definitions, modern Saami ethnogenesis as seen on the Bothnian coast can be broken down in the following periods:

600 B.C.–A.D. 700 Growth: systematic and increasing interactions with Germanic and Finnish societies (early modern ethnogenesis).

| | |
|---|---|
| A.D. 700–1200 | Conservation: strong internal cohesion; social stratification; expanded exploitation of coastal, forest and alpine resources; extensive trade; intensified rituals. |
| A.D. 1200–1300 | Release: Swedish colonization, the Christian mission, European mercantilism, Saami assimilation and the abandonment of the Swedish coastland. |
| A.D. 1300–1500 | Reorganization: Swedish state control, the Reformation, Lapland created, the development of reindeer nomadism and new polities in Saami society (modern ethnogenesis). |

The elements that contributed to the growth period are well known: metallurgy, animal husbandry, cultivation, greater mobility, economic diversification as a response to environmental changes, and a greater dependence on reindeer. The conservation stage is the best known period of Saami prehistory in Sweden as seen through the specialized exploitation of the alpine, forest and coastal regions, widespread trade, metal offer sites, bear rites, social stratification and the growth of individual ownership of animals and goods. The release stage is seen all over the Nordic North. This was a major period of Swedish colonization. The reorganization process took form through the implementation of state power, religious control, the creation of a nomadic herding system and cultural and linguistic assimilation.

Colonialism derives from the Latin *colonia* referring to a settlement in hostile or conquered territory. The term has reference to *colere* (to cultivate) and this in turn has been the basis of land ownership and tenure as recognized by the state. Chris Gosden (2004) has formulated three types of colonial encounters: the shared cultural milieu, the middle ground and *terra nullius*. These are readily applicable to the prehistory of the Bothnian coast, and especially the changing forms of cultural contact that characterized Saami interactions during the Iron Age and Medieval Period.

The shared cultural milieu of the period 5000 B.C.–A.D. 1 is a history of interactions with the outside world within a World System that introduced ideas, technologies and economies, and new forms of cultural capital at the regional and local level. There is little evidence of actual colonization by outsiders.

The Iron Age corresponds to the idea of a middle ground, which is analogous to the interactions between the Algonquian Indians and the French fur traders in the Great Lakes region of North America during the seventeenth century (cf. White 1991). The middle ground created a working relationship appealing to the values of both groups (Gosden 2004:31). This is precisely what occurred during the period of the Roman Iron Age fur trade, and especially during the Viking Period. This led, among other things, to the growth of wealth, social stratification and adoption of Germanic religious practices among the Saami. Objects, especially valuable metal items, became embedded in local cosmologies and social relations.

*Terra nullius* coincides with colonization starting in the late thirteenth century and efforts by the Swedish state and church to assert control through land and resource ownership. The full impacts occurred with the merging of the church and state under King Gustav Vasa in the sixteenth century. Culture contact changed into confrontation, suppression and obligatory acculturation.

The issue of Saami cultural identity, as discussed in the introduction, relates directly to these colonial processes. Strathern (1988) has coined the term "dividuals" as opposed to "individuals."

Dividuals are made up of the social relations and attributes of societies as a whole; identity is relational and relative. Individualism is more related to quantifiable values, ownership, title, prestige tied to individual power and to currency (Gosden 2004:37). The transformation of Saami society from the fourteenth century was the change from diverse and variable forms of circumpolar adaptive communities, to narrower, constrained and legally prescribed identities. This was a formalization of "The Other" in north Swedish society. This also led to internal dissension among the Saami, principally the reindeer owners versus non-owners and between reindeer herders and settlers over grazing lands.

## Summary of Results

1) Seen in terms of economy, settlement, technology, ideology and religion, all the components associated with the processes of Saami ethnogenesis have been identified in northern coastal Västerbotten, and there is little difference in these respects from Northern Norway, interior Sweden or Finland.
2) There is a long-term historical trajectory in coastal Västerbotten from the deep past and into late prehistory defined by circumpolar adaptive strategies at the local, regional and World System levels. This is seen through settlement organization and cultural landscapes, as well as networks of travel, trade and resource exploitation.
3) Coastal settlements were highly dependent on sealing and occurred in cycles coinciding with peaks in regional productivity. These periods also led to the expansion of European and Eurasian technologies, ideologies and economies into the North, and these were readily adopted by northern societies.
4) Coastal societies during the Metal Ages (Bronze Age and Iron Age) manifested their territories along the Bothnian coast through cairn graves that segmented the shores and bays into units 5–15 km in length, depending on topography. These hunting and pastoralist systems continued into historic times, even after Christianity had taken possession of the dead.
5) The coast and interior were intimately connected through natural east–west networks, economic routes and interdependencies. As seen by artifact distributions, these connections were intensified during the Early and Late Metal Ages, but were also in evidence during the Mesolithic/Early Stone Age. These social connections enabled reciprocal utilizations of interior and coastal resources, both of which were subject to major population cycles. Peaks in resources facilitated periods of semi-sedentism, as well as periodic depopulations and re-settlements of both regions, referred to as "punctuated sedentism." This was most likely the basis of pre-agrarian sustainability.
6) From at least the first centuries A.D. there was a well-organized coastal settlement system incorporating hunting, animal husbandry and, with certainty from A.D. 500, intermittent cultivation on the North Bothnian coast. Iron working was practiced during the whole period and had both practical functions (tools, ornaments and boat rivets) and symbolic meanings.
7) Bothnian coastal societies were organized in bands analogous to Saami *sijddas/siidas*, flexible groups of three to five, but sometimes up to nine households. These groups were involved in collective hunting and herding strategies. The largest aggregations occurred

during the Viking Period during which there was an intensification of husbandry, seal hunting, fur trapping and trade.

8) Settlements in the coastland were based on the seasonal exploitation of seals on the outer coast and animal husbandry within 8–10 km of the coast. These were analogous to shielings (cf. Rathje 2001). Seasonal indicators show that the sealing sites were occupied during late winter, spring, summer and fall. There also is evidence that domestic animals were kept on sealing sites, some of which were year-round. Storage caches indicate economic planning beyond subsistence needs. There is evidence that sealers were part of an organized trading network with local trading sites. Boat building was part of the local system and may have been one incentive for operating forges on or near beaches.
9) The ritual bear burial at Grundskatan, iron slag placed in hearths in dwellings, and circular sacrificial features of Saami type are *longue durée* expressions of Saami identity. Saami religion was syncretistic and incorporated Germanic/Norse grave forms, including cremations, and thereafter shifted to Christian practices.
10) The north to south transect between Stor-Rebben Island and Hornslandsudde shows that there were coastal Saami settlements between latitudes 61° and 65°N. The hut forms, consisting of contemporary oval, round and rectilinear forms, suggest that there were interactions at the settlement level with Germanic and Finnish groups, particularly during the Viking Age. These sites were located in regions well north of contemporary Germanic Iron Age settlement territories and deep within such regions. The northern region was predominantly Saami, and hut-based sealing was probably a Saami specialty. It is probable that there was a high degree of mutually beneficial economic interaction, as well as in iron technology and religion.
11) Linear alignments of huts relate to aggregations of hunters and herders involved in larger-scale activities. These arrangements reflect intensified production of surpluses for trade.
12) The chronology of the sealing sites spans from A.D. 1 to 1279. There were three periods of expansion: ca. A.D. 100–400, A.D. 400–600 and A.D. 800–1100. There was a regression during the seventh century, which was a regional-wide period of decline. By A.D. 1279 all the coastal sealing sites along the Bothnian coast had been abandoned.
13) The abandonment of the sealing sites coincides with other major changes throughout northern Europe, including the beginnings of the Little Ice Age, but, above all, the formation of the Swedish state and the expansion of the Christian Church into the North. Systematic colonization by Swedish settlers and new systems of land tenure resulted in the assimilation of many coastal hunter-gatherers/herders as settled Christians and as land owners. Many Saami, as well as other non-Christians, probably made this change with little difficulty. The remaining populations were displaced inland.
14) Place-names referring to *Lapps* are found along the whole Bothnian coast with the greatest density in Västerbotten. These place-names reflect the interactions of Saami with non-Saami (Finns and Swedes) and coincide with the colonization of the northern coastal Västerbotten, and also with areas with reindeer pastoralism. Seventy-four place-names with reference to reindeer are found in Skellefteå Municipality, 37 of which refer to intensive (non-nomadic) reindeer husbandry.

15) Herring fisheries rapidly expanded northward starting in the thirteenth century, and small harbors and chapels soon dotted the Bothnian coasts. The stone labyrinth is interpreted as an iconic Christian symbol that marked the Swedish appropriation of coastal territory and religious hegemony throughout the Bothnian region.
16) In the fourteenth century the state began to systematically tax resources, regulate trade and cut off the east–west networks that had been operating for thousands of years. This also led to an artificial border with the interior and the creation of increasingly reindeer-dependent societies. According to historical accounts in Sweden, small herds became large herds with fewer owners starting in the sixteenth century, requiring greater pasturing, leading to nomadic herding in many regions.
17) In Västerbotten, Norrbotten and northern Ångermanland, the Forest Saami lived on into the nineteenth century in the same ways the coastal Saami had before them. The coastal settlers of Swedish Västerbotten still lived in coastal territories analogous to those who came before them, hunted seals and fished in household- and village teams, made boats and nets using Saami methods, used Saami taboo words, and still believed in reindeer herding forest spirits.

## Final Thoughts

This study has focused on evidence that illuminates multiple aspects of Saami prehistory. It is far from complete, but serves to shift the narratives of both Swedish and Saami prehistory in northern Sweden. There can be little doubt that Saami culture has left few physical remains in the northern landscape as compared with Nordic society, and it is paradoxical that Saami culture is often first recognizable in the archaeological record through non-Saami trade goods and adopted ritual practices. One need not look far, however, to see beyond this veil. The postcolonial discourse is a global phenomenon within archaeology and it is now widely acknowledged that colonial societies are themselves "ambiguous hybrids" that are full of divergent lines of interest and evidence of interactions (Murray 2004:7). Saami culture has left an indelible mark on north Swedish society and culture.

The biogeography of the Nordic region has been a key factor in the development of Saami identities. Strong eastern (Uralic) influences have, since early post-glacial times, extended into Sweden from the Finnish and Norwegian land bridge to the north. The maritime effects on the Bothnian and Norwegian coasts have at the same time enabled southern influences to reach northward in pulses of expansions and regressions. This dynamic combination of biological, cultural, technological and ideological forces characterizes both the process and substance of what we know as Saami and north Swedish culture today.

Archaeology is a tool for filling in the gaps of history, especially for those who have been relegated to sidebars in our own narratives. From once being a means for creating national myths, archaeology has evolved into a tool for average men and women who were left out of history, and for minorities and colonized peoples who have been denied their histories.

The Saami are among the best-known indigenous peoples in the world and yet, like most cultural minorities, are still struggling for recognition and cultural survival. These indigenous Saami societies, while capable of maintaining their unique ethnic identities, have also been increasingly marginalized through the creation of the narrow territorial and economic constraints that define their rights differently across four nations today.

The 4th International Polar Year (2007–2008) has just been completed, and this era of rapid global change reminds us of the challenges and promises facing all Arctic residents (Krupnik et al. 2005). In the larger scheme of things, these challenges are like those of many other peoples. There are lessons to be learned from this 7,000-year narrative: the strengths of diversity – socially, culturally, linguistically and spiritually; using natural ecological variability in order to achieve sustainability and, above all else, the value of multiculturalism. The resiliencies of the Saami and other northern peoples are testimonies to the strengths of their spirits and examples of how meaningful futures can derive from the many threads that have woven the fabric of all nations.

APPENDIX 1

# Osteological Material

Includes burned, charred and unburned bone fragments.

A) Identified species at site locales, numbers of identified specimens, NISP.

| SPECIES | BJURÖKLUBB | GRUNDSKATAN | HORNSLANDET | JUNGFRUHAMN | SNÖAN | STOR-REBBEN | STORA FJÄDERÄGG | TOTAL |
|---|---|---|---|---|---|---|---|---|
| Ringed seal | | 8 | | 1 | | | 7 | 16 |
| Harp seal | | | 1 (?) | | | | 17 | 18 |
| Indeterminate Seal | 1 | 180 | 1 | 4 | 2 | | 4213 | 4401 |
| Bear | | 66 | | | | | | 66 |
| Cattle | | | | | | | 1 | 1 |
| Sheep/goat | | | 1 | 1 | | 2 | 1 | 5 |
| Reindeer | | | | | | 1 | | 1 |
| Large ungulate | | 2 | | 2 | 1 | | 3 | 8 |
| Ungulate | | | | | | 2 | | 2 |
| Ungulate? | | | | | | 1 | | 1 |
| Hare | | 1 | | | 1 | | | 2 |
| Indeterminate duck | | | | | | | 1 | 1 |
| Indeterminate bird | | 5 | | 9 | | | 1 | 15 |
| Indeterminate bird? | | | | | | | 2 | 2 |
| Total | 1 | 262 | 3 | 17 | 4 | 6 | 4246 | 4539 |

B) Identified species in huts (referred to by numbers or letters) at all locales, NISP.

| SPECIES | BJURÖKLUBB | GRUNDSKATAN | | | | HORNSLANDET | | JUNGFRUHAMN | | SNÖAN | | STOR-REBBEN | | STORA FJÄDERÄGG | | | | TOTAL |
|---|---|---|---|---|---|---|---|---|---|---|---|---|---|---|---|---|---|---|
| | 67 | 1 | 3 | 4 | 14 | 13 | 132B | A | B | A | B | C | D | A | B | D | G.HAMNEN | |
| Ringed seal | | | 5 | 3 | | | | | 1 | | | | | | 7 | | | 16 |
| Harp seal | | | | | | | 1 (?) | | | | | | | | 17 | | | 18 |
| Indeterminate Seal | 1 | 8 | 129 | 42 | 1 | | 1 | 3 | 1 | | 2 | | | 2 | 4112 | 98 | 1 | 4401 |
| Bear | | | | 66 | | | | | | | | | | | | | | 66 |
| Cattle | | | | | | | | | | | | | | | 1 | | | 1 |
| Sheep/goat | | | | | | 1 | | 1 | | | | | 2 | | 1 | | | 5 |
| Reindeer | | | | | | | | | | | | | 1 | | | | | 1 |
| Large ungulate | | 2 | | | | | | | 2 | 1 | | | | | 1 | | 2 | 8 |
| Ungulate | | | | | | | | | | | | 1 | 1 | | | | | 2 |
| Ungulate? | | | | | | | | | | | | 1 | | | | | | 1 |
| Hare | | | 1 | | | | | | | | 1 | | | | | | | 2 |
| Indeterminate duck | | | | | | | | | | | | | | | 1 | | | 1 |
| Indeterminate bird | | 2 | 1 | 2 | | | | | 9 | | | | | | 1 | | | 15 |
| Indeterminate bird? | | | | | | | | | | | | | | | 2 | | | 2 |
| Total | 1 | 12 | 136 | 113 | 1 | 1 | 2 | 4 | 13 | 1 | 3 | 2 | 4 | 2 | 4143 | 98 | 3 | 4539 |

C) Anatomical representation for seals at all locales (including ringed seal, harp seal and indeterminate seal), NISP.

| SPECIES | BJURÖKLUBB | GRUNDSKATAN | | | | HORNSLANDET | | JUNGFRUHAMN | | SNÖAN | STORA FJÄDERÄGG | | | | TOTAL |
|---|---|---|---|---|---|---|---|---|---|---|---|---|---|---|---|
| | 67 | 1 | 14 | 3 | 4 | 119 | 132B | A | B | B | A | B | D | GAMLA HAMNEN | |
| Cranium | | | | 30 | 9 | | | 1 | | | | 168 | 3 | | 211 |
| Vertebral column | | 2 | | 2 | | | | | | | | 1251 | 6 | | 1261 |
| Rib cage | | | | 3 | | | | | | | | 10 | | | 13 |
| Front extremity | 1 | | | 1 | | | | 1 | | | | 15 | | | 18 |
| Front flipper | | 1 | | 44 | 13 | | | | | | | 65 | 1 | | 124 |
| Rear extremity | | 3 | | 1 | | | | 1 | 1 | | | 125 | 1 | | 132 |
| Rear flipper | | 2 | 1 | 50 | 20 | | 1 | | 1 | 2 | 2 | 1898 | 63 | 1 | 2040 |
| Front/rear flipper | | | | 2 | | | | | | | | 127 | | | 129 |
| Long bone fragment | | | | | | | 1 | | | | | 2 | | | 2 |
| Sesamoids, baculum | | | | 1 | 3 | | | | | | | 475 | 24 | | 503 |
| Total | 1 | 8 | 1 | 134 | 45 | 0 | 2 | 3 | 2 | 2 | 2 | 4136 | 98 | 1 | 4435 |

D) Anatomical representation for ungulates by site and hut (Cattle, Sheep/goat, Reindeer, Large ungulate, Ungulate, Ungulate?), NISP.

| SPECIES | GRUNDSKATAN | HORNSLANDET 119 | JUNGFRUHAMN | | SNÖAN | STOR-REBBEN | | STORA FJÄDERÄGG | | TOTAL |
|---|---|---|---|---|---|---|---|---|---|---|
| | 1 | 13 | A | B | A | C | D | B | GAMLA HAMNEN | |
| Tooth | | 1 | | | | | | | | 1 |
| Rib cage | | | | | | | 1 | | | 1 |
| Front extremity | | | | 2 | | 1 | | 1 | | 4 |
| Rear extremity | | | 1 | | | | 3 | 1 | | 5 |
| Foot | 2 | | | | | | | | 1 | 3 |
| Hand/foot | | | | | | 1 | | 1 | | 2 |
| Long bone | | | | | 1 | | | | 1 | 2 |
| Total | 2 | 1 | 1 | 2 | 1 | 2 | 4 | 3 | 2 | 18 |

APPENDIX 2

# Radiocarbon and AMS Dates

| SITE | FEATURE | ELEVATION (M) | SAMPLE | B.P. | RATIO ¹³C‰ | MEDIAN A.D. | A.D. (±1 S.D.) | A.D. (± 2 S.D.) | COMMENTS |
|---|---|---|---|---|---|---|---|---|---|
| ***Stor-Rebben*** | | | | | | | | | |
| A1 | Hut | 16m | St.11910 | 1845±135 | –25.5 | 172 | 23–340 | 171(BC)–532 | |
| A2 | Hut | 16m | St.11178 | 1495 ± 70 | –26.6 | 558 | 443–643 | 423–656 | |
| B | Hut | 13m | St.11179 | 1045 ±110 | –25.7 | 985 | 880–1155 | 716–1217 | |
| C | Hut | 13m | St.11180 | 945 ± 110 | –26.3 | 1092 | 999–1212 | 880–1280 | |
| ***Stora Fjäderägg*** | | | | | | | | | |
| A | Hut | 20m | St.11181 | 1015±100 | –27.5 | 1021 | 898–1155 | 779–1219 | |
| B1 | Hut | 19m | St.11900 | 1660±70 | –24.9 | 386 | 259–529 | 230–559 | |
| B2 | Hut | 19m | St.11182 | 1235±315 | –24.5 | 779 | 465–1154 | 90–1385 | |
| C | Hut | 15m | St.11183 | 955±75 | –26.3 | 1093 | 1018–1163 | 900–1251 | |
| D | Hut | 13m | St.11184 | 1110±145 | –26.8 | 913 | 714–1036 | 656–1208 | |
| Gamla Hamnen | Hut | 8 m | St.11901 | 310±70 | –26.7 | 1572 | 1490–1650 | 1441–1953 | |
| ***Grundskatan (Site 78)*** | | | | | | | | | |
| 1 | Hut | 13m | St.10787 | 1160±70 | –25.8 | 866 | 779–968 | 690–1014 | |
| 3a | Hut | 16m | St.11907 | 1500±100 | –25.6 | 542 | 435–643 | 263–762 | |
| 3b | Hut | 16m | St. 11906 | 1205±70 | –25.4 | 819 | 695–894 | 673–972 | |
| 4a | Hut | 15m | Beta-196486 | 190±40 | –26.7 | 1773 | 1662–1952 | — | contaminated |
| 4b | Hut | 15m | St.10785 | 1110±110 | –25.3 | 912 | 780–1020 | 674–1155 | |
| 4c | Bear bone | 15m | Ua-19830 | 1080±45 | –21 | 958 | 898–1014 | 830–1030 | bone |
| 4d | Hut | 15m | Beta-196487 | 420±40 | –26.1 | 1470 | 1433–1611 | — | contaminated |
| 4e | Hut | 15m | Beta- 210236 | 1500±40 | –21.6 | 568 | 536–621 | 434–644 | bone |
| 10 | Oven | 10m | St.10784 | <250 | –25.5 | 1750 | — | — | Russian Oven |
| 11 | Hut | 13m | St.11170 | 1175±100 | –25.8 | 848 | 723–972 | 663–1021 | |
| 12 | Hut | 13m | St.11171 | 1430±110 | –26.1 | 605 | 437–760 | 390–867 | |
| 13a | Hut | 13m | St.11908 | 1045±110 | –25.3 | 985 | 880–1155 | 716–1217 | |
| 13b | Hut | 12m | St.11172 | 880±80 | –25.8 | 1144 | 1044–1220 | 1020–1272 | |
| 13c | Hut | 12m | Beta-196488 | 1200±40 | –25.3 | 825 | 777–884 | 690–946 | |
| 14a | Hut/laby | 13m | St.11173 | 1145±100 | –25.4 | 878 | 776–990 | 661–1118 | |
| 14b | Hut/laby | 13m | St.11174 | 1000±185 | –25.3 | 1017 | 870–1231 | 659–1296 | |
| 15a | Pit | 17m | Beta-196489 | 320±40 | –25.7 | 1562 | 1515–1641 | — | contaminated? |
| 15b | Pit | 17m | St. 11175 | 670±245 | –26.1 | 1295 | 1033–1467 | 779–1952 | old surface layer |

*(continued)*

| SITE | FEATURE | ELEVATION (M) | SAMPLE | B.P. | RATIO $^{13}C‰$ | MEDIAN A.D. | A.D. (±1 S.D.) | A.D. (± 2 S.D.) | COMMENTS |
|---|---|---|---|---|---|---|---|---|---|
| ***Jungfruhamn (Sites 138–139)*** | | | | | | | | | |
| A1 | Hut | 15m | St.11176 | 985±70 | –25.8 | 1066 | 990–1155 | 898–1211 | |
| A2 | Hut | 15m | Beta-196490 | 1210±50 | –26.3 | 813 | 722–887 | 678–950 | |
| B | Hut | 15m | St.11177 | 1300±130 | –27.2 | 745 | 636–886 | 443–1015 | |
| C | Hut | 17m | St.11909 | 1710±125 | –25 | 323 | 139–526 | 58–597 | |
| ***Site 70*** | Hut | 12m | Beta -196485 | 1020±60 | –25.8 | 1015 | 902–1149 | 893–1157 | |
| ***Site 67*** | Hut | 17m | St.10786 | 1485±70 | –25.3 | 567 | 467–648 | 425–660 | |
| ***Oval hearth*** | Hearth | 5m | Beta-191232 | 230±40 | –25 | 1742 | 1641–1953 | — | Saami hearth |
| ***Broänge*** | Wall | 11m | Beta-196484 | 550±50 | –25.2 | 1378 | 1319–1428 | — | contaminated? |
| ***Broänge*** | Wall | 11m | St. 11911 | 1025±70 | –24.3 | 1011 | 899–1149 | 831–1185 | |
| ***Snöan*** | | | | | | | | | |
| *49A* | Hut | 15m | Ua-1322 | 1150±100 | –25 | 872 | 775–988 | 660–1115 | |
| *49B* | Hut | 15m | Ua-1323 | 255±100 | –25 | 1658 | 1491–1952 | — | contaminated? |
| 53A | Hut | 5m | St.11904 | 735±120 | –26.5 | 1258 | 1167–1392 | 1039–1416 | |
| *53B* | Hut | 3m | St.11905 | 445±105 | –27 | 1481 | 1401–1631 | 1296–1481 | |
| 92A | Oven | 5m | St.11902 | 430±95 | –24.7 | 1494 | 1413–1630 | | |
| *92B* | Oven | 5m | St.11903 | 470±95 | –24.8 | 1450 | 1320–1618 | | |
| ***Hornslandsudde (Sites 119,132)*** | | | | | | | | | |
| 5 | Hut | 18m | Ua-32857 | 1390±30 | –27.6 | 646 | 632–664 | 602–674 | bone |
| 12a | Hut | 16m | Beta-207939 | 1820±40 | –23.3 | 191 | 136–236 | 85–323 | |
| 12b | Hut | 16m | Beta-209908 | 1570±40 | –27.2 | 488 | 434–537 | 409–575 | |
| 132b | Hut | 20m | Beta-210238 | 1130±40 | –24.8 | 920 | 881–980 | 780–991 | |
| 5 | Hut | 18m | Beta-217790 | 140±40 | –28.5 | | | | contaminated |
| 15 | Hut | 12m | Beta-210237 | 260±70 | –23.5 | | | | contaminated |
| 132a | Hut | 20m | Beta-217789 | 210±40 | –26.9 | | | | contaminated |

# References


Aikio, A. 2004. *"Palaeo-Laplandic" Substrate Words in (North) Saami*. Brochure, Nordic Archaeological Conference. University of Oulu, Oulu.

Akino, S. 1999. Sending-Spirit Ceremonies. In *Ainu, Spirit of Northern People*, edited by W. W. Fitzhugh, C. O. Dubreuil, pp. 288–255. Arctic Studies Center, National Museum of Natural History, Smithsonian Institution, Washington, D.C.

Alexandersen, V. 1997. Hvad viser tænderne? In *Möten i gränsland. Samer och germaner i Mellanskandinavien*, edited by I. Zachrisson, pp. 99–116. Statens historiska museum monographs 4, Stockholm.

Ambrosiani, B. 1971. *Arkeologisk undersökning 1966. Hornslandsudde, Rogsta sn, Hälsingland*. B2. Riksantkvarieämbetet rapport 1971, Stockholm.

Ambrosiani, B., E. Iregren and P. Lahtiperä. 1984. *Gravfält i fångstmarken. Undersökningar av gravfälten på Smalnäset, Krankmårtenhögen, Härjedalen*. Riksantikvarieämbetet och Statens historiska museer 1984 (6), Stockholm.

Andersen, O. 1992. *Ofuohtagat: samer och nordmenn i Ofoten*. Hovedfagsoppgave i arkeologi, University of Bergen, Bergen.

———. 2004. Hva kan teltplassene fortelle om rendriftenss oppkomst? In *Samisk forhistorie*, edited by M. Krogh, K. Schanche, pp. 135–149. Varanger Samiske Museum, Indre Sandvik, Porsanger.

Andersson, D. 2007. *Iron Working at Hornslandsudde. Archaeometallurgic analyses*. Geoarkeologiskt Laboratoriet, Analysrapport nr 7, Uppsala.

Aronsson, K.-Å. 1991. *Forest Reindeer Herding AD 1–1800*. Archaeology and Environment 10. Umeå University, Umeå.

———. 2005. Arkeologiska och paleoekologiska undersökningar av renskötarboplatser. In *Fra villrenjakt til rendrift 1*, edited by O. Andersson, pp. 109–123.

Arwill, E. 1975. *Preliminär rapport över undersökning av boplats vid Östra Falmark, Bureå sn, Västerbotten*. Skellefteå Museum, Skellefteå.

Atterman, I. 1977. Fiskelägen på blekingekusten. *Blekingeboken* 55:73–116.

Axelson, A. W. 1989. *Pitebygdens historia. En kort historik till omkring 1900*. Eget förlag. Accidenstryckeriet, Piteå.

Baeksted, A. 1970. *Gudar och Hjältar i Norden*. Bokförlaget Forum AB, Uddevala.

Bakka, E. 1976. *Arktisk og Nordisk i Bronsealdern i Nordskandinavia*. Det Kunglige Norske Videnskapers Selskab Museet, Miscellanea 25, Trondheim.

Banton, M. 1981. The Direction and Speed of Ethnic Change. In *Ethnic Change*, edited by C. F. Keyes, pp. 31–52. University of Washington Press, Seattle.

Barth, F. 1969. *Ethnic Groups and Boundaries*. Little, Brown and Company, Boston.

———. 1994. *Manifestasjon och process*. Det Blå Bibliotek, Oslo.

Baudou, E. 1968. *Forntida bebyggelse i Ångermanlands kustland. Arkeologiska undersökningar an ångermanländska kuströsen*. Arkiv för norrländsk hembyggdsforskning XVII, Härnosand.

———. 1974. Samernas invandring till Sverige ur arkeologisk synpunkt. In *Sameforskning idag och imorgon. Rapport från symposium rörande den samiska kulturen. Nordiska Museum jubileumssymposier*, pp. 27–51. Stockholm.

———. 1977. Den förhistoria fångstkulturen i Västernorrland. In *Västernorrlands förhistoria*, pp. 11–152. Västernorrlands läns landsting, Motala.

———. 1987. Samer och germaner i det förhistoriska Norrland. En kritisk översikt över tio års forskning. *Samer och germaner. Bebyggelsehistorisk tidskrift* 14:9–23.

———. 1992. *Norrlands forntid – ett historiskt perspektiv*, Höganäs.

———. 2004. *Den nordiska arkeologin*. Kungliga Vitterhets Historiska och Antikvitets Akademien, Stockholm.

Beckman, L. 1996. *Samerna – en genetiskt unik urbefolkning*. Institutionen för medicinsk genetik, Umeå universitet, Umeå.

Benedict, J. B. 1967. Recent glacial history of an alpine area in the Colorado Front Range, USA. Establishing a lichen growth curve. *Journal of Glaciology* 6(48):817–832.

———. 1985. *Arapaho Pass. Glacial Geology and Archaeology at the Crest of the Colorado Front Range*. Research Report 3. Center for Mountain Archaeology, Ward, Colorado.

Bergling, R. 1964. *Kyrkstaden i Övre Norrland*. Skytteanska Samfundets Handlingar 3, Umeå.

Berglund, B. 1964. Littorina Transgressions in Blekinge, South Sweden. *Geologiska Föreningens i Stockholm Förhandlingar* 94:625–652.

Berglund, B., S. Helmfrid and Å. Hyenstrand. 1994. Ten Thousand Years in Sweden. In *Landscape and Settlements*, edited by S. Helmfrid, pp. 12–17. National Atlas of Sweden, Stockholm.

Bergman, I. 1991. Spatial Structures in Saami Landscapes. In *Readings in Saami History Culture and Language II*, edited by R. Kvist, pp. 59–68. Umeå University, Umeå.

———. 1998. Visar keramiken att de var samer? *Populär arkeologi* nr 4:26–28.

Bergman, I., L. Liedgren, L. Östlund and O. Zachrisson. 2008. Kinship and Settlements: Sami Residence Patterns in the Fennoscandian Alpine Areas around A.D. 1000. *Arctic Anthropology* 45(1):97–110.

Bergman, I., A. Olofsson, G. Hornberg, O. Zachrisson and E. Hellberg. 2004. Deglaciation and Colonization: Pioneer Settlements in Northern Fennoscandia. *World Prehistory* 18(2):155–177.

Bergman, I., L. Östlund, O. Zachrisson and L. Liedgren. 2008. Värro Muorra: The Landscape Significance of Sami Sacred Wooden Objects and Sacrificial Altars. *Ethnohistory* 55(1):1–28.

Bergqvist, E. 1977. Postglacial Land Uplift in Northern Sweden. Some remarks on its relation to the present uplift and the uncompensated depression. *Geologiska Föreningens i Stockholm Förhandlingnar* 99:347–357.

Bergström, R. 1968. *Stratigrafi och isrecession i Södra Västerbotten*. Serie C Nr 634, Årsbok 63 nr 5. Sveriges Geologiska Undersökning, Stockholm.

Bergstøl, J. 2004. Fangstfolk eller samer i Østerdalen? In *Samisk forhistorie*, edited by M. Krogh and K. Schanche, pp. 62–80. Varanger Samiske Museum, Varanger.

———. 2008. *Samer i Østerdalen? En studie av etnisitet i jernaldernen og middelalderen i det nordøstre Hedmark*. Det humanistiske fakultet, Oslo.

Bergstøl, J. and G. Reitan. 2008. Samer på Dovrefjell i vikingtiden. *Norsk Historisk Tidsskrift* 87:9–27.

Bergvall, M. and P. Persson (eds.). 2004. *Västernorrland – Sameland: Om samisk närvaro i Ångermanland och Medelpad*. Länsmuseet Västernorrland, Härnösand.

Bergvall, A. and J. Salander. 1996. *Rösen i mellersta Västerbotten. Dateringar och discussion utifran nivåavvägningar*. Institutionen för arkeologi, Umeå University, Umeå.

Berkes, F. and C. Folke. 1998. *Linking social and ecological systems: management practices and social mechanism for building resilience.* Cambridge University Press, Cambridge.

Berkes, F. 1999. *Sacred Ecology: Traditional Ecological Knowledge and Resource Management.* Taylor and Francis, Philadelphia.

Beschel, R. E. 1950. Flechten als Altersmasstab rezenter Moränen. *Zeitschrift für Gletscherkunde und Glacialgeologie* 1:152–161.

Björk, S. 1995. Late Weichselian to Early Holocene Development of the Baltic Sea, with Implications for Coastal Settlements in the Southern Baltic Region. In *Man and Sea in the Mesolithic. Coastal Settlement above and below the Present Sea Level,* edited by A. Fisher, pp. 23–34. Oxbow Monograph 53. Oxbow Books, Oxford.

Björk, S., B. Kromer, S. Johnson, O. Bennike. D. Hammarlund, D. Lerndahl, G. Possnert, T. L. Rasmussen, B. Wohlfarth, C. U. Hammer and M. Spurk. 1996. Synchronized terrestrial-atmospheric deglacial records around the North Atlantic. *Science* 274:1155–1160.

Bjørklund, I. 1985. *Fjordfolket i Kvaenangen. Fra samisk samfunn till norsk utkant 1550–1980.* Universitetsforlaget, Oslo.

Bjørklund, I. and S. E. Grydeland. 2001. *Spildra – med fortida inn i framtida.* Spildra Grendeutvalg i samarbeid med Tromsø Museum, Tromsø.

Black, D. 2007. *Wood Charcoal Remains from Several Saami Sites along the Northeastern Coast of Northern Sweden.* University of Western Michigan, Kalamazoo.

Bogoras, W. 1909. *The Chukchee.* Memoirs of the American Museum of Natural History XI. American Museum of Natural History, New York.

Bolin, H. 1999. *Kulturlandskapets korsvägar. Mellersta Norrland under de två sista årtusendena f. Kr.* Stockholm Studies in Archaeology 19. Stockholm University, Stockholm.

Bonns, B. 1988. Fälbåtar och fälmän. In *Bottnisk Kontakt IV,* pp. 47–57. Skellefteå Museum, Skellefteå.

Bord, J. 1976. *Mazes and Labyrinths of the World.* The Anchor Press Ltd., London.

Bosworth, J. (ed.). 1885. *Alfred the Great. A Description of Europe and the Voyages of Othere and Wulfstan.* Oxford University Press, Oxford.

Bourdieu, P. 1977. *Outline of a Theory of Practice.* Cambridge Studies of Social and Cultural Anthropology 16. Cambridge University Press, Cambridge.

Braudel, F. 1949. *Les mémoires de la Méditerranée: préhistoire et antiquité.* Editions de Fallois, Paris.

Brightman, R. 1993. *Grateful Prey: Rock Cree Human-Animal Relationships.* University of California Press, Berkeley.

Brink, S., O. Korhonen and M. Wahlberg. 1994. Place Names. In *Cultural Heritage and Preservation,* edited by K.-L. Selinge, pp. 134–145. National Atlas of Sweden, Stockholm.

Broadbent, N. D. 1979. *Coastal Resources and Settlement Stability. A case study of a Mesolithic site complex in northern Sweden,* AUN 3. Uppsala University, Uppsala.

———. 1982. *Den förhistoriska utvecklingen under 7000 år.* Skelleftebygdens historia 3. Skellefteå kommun, Skellefteå.

———. 1983. Too Many Chiefs and Not Enough Indians. A Peripheral View of Nordic Bronze Age Society. In *Struktur och förändring i bronsålderns samhälle,* pp. 7–22. Report Series 17. Institute of Archaeology, Lund University, Lund.

———. 1984. A Late Neolithic Site at Kåddis, Umeå Parish, Västerbotten. In *Papers in Northern Archaeology,* edited by E. Baudou pp. 45–56. Archaeology and Environment 2. Umeå University, Umeå.

———. 1985. New Knowledge of Early Iron Age Settlement in Northern Sweden. Cooperation between the University of Umeå and Västernorrland County Museum. In *In Honorem Evert Baudou,* pp. 387–393. Archaeology and Environment 4 Umeå University, Umeå.

———. 1986. Perforated Stones, Antlers and Stone Picks: Evidence for the Use of Digging Sticks in Scandinavia and Finland. *Tor* XVII: 63–106.

———. 1987a. Datering av labyrinter genom lavtillväxt. *Norrbottens museums årsbok 1987*, 83–97.

———. 1987b. *Iron Age and Medieval Seal Hunting Sites*. Research Reports 5. Center for Arctic Cultural Research, Umeå University, Umeå.

———. 1987c. Chronological Analysis of Lichen Growth on Headstones in Northern Sweden. In *Theoretical Approaches to Artifacts, Settlement and Society*, ed. G. Burenhult, A. Carlsson, Å. Hyenstrand and T. Sjøvold, pp. 76–82. BAR International Series 366, London.

———. 1987d. *Lichenometry and Archaeology. Testing of Lichen Chronology on the Swedish North Bothnian Coast*. Research Reports 2. Center for Arctic Cultural Research, Umeå University, Umeå.

———. 1989a. En kort redogörelse för nyligen erhållna C14-dateringar från Bjuröklubb, Grundskatan, Stora Fjäderägg och Stor-Rebben i Västerbotten och Norrbotten. *Bottnisk kontakt* 4:21–23.

———. 1989b. Bjuröklubbs arkeologi. *Oknytt* 1–2:15–23.

———. 1991. Järnålderns sälfångst i bottniska viken. Om ett nordligt socioekonomiskt och kognitivt system. *Gunneri* 64:223–231.

———. 1997. Towards an Integration of the Human and Natural Sciences in Arctic Research. In *Climate and Man in the Arctic*, pp. 12–17. Danish Polar Center, Copenhagen.

———. 2000. Seal Hunters, Labyrinth Builders and Church Villagers: The Seal Hunting Cultures Project. *Tidsperspektiv* 1:7–21.

———. 2001a. Fulfilling the Promise. On Swedish Archaeology and Archaeology in Sweden. *Current Swedish Archaeology* 9:25–38.

———. 2001b. Northern Pasts. Northern Futures. *Scandinavian-Canadian Studies* 13:6–21.

———. 2003. *Flurkmark, RÄA 510. Umeå socken, Västerbotten. Excavation Report: 1996–2001*. Möten i Norr, Umeå.

———. 2004a. Global Climate Change, Settlement and Sedentism: North Swedish Prehistory from 7000 BC to the Present. Integrated Regional Impact Studies in the European North. In *Basic Issues, Methodologies and Regional Climate Modelling II*, edited by M. A. Lange and D. Poszig, pp. 95–106. Zufo Berichte 2. Westfälische Wilhelms-Universitet, Münster.

———. 2004b. *Saami Prehistory, Identity and Rights in Sweden*. Paper given at the Northern Research Forum, Yellowknife. http://www.nrf.is/Publications/The%20Resilient%20North/Plenary%203/3rd%20NRF_plenary%203_Broadbent_final.pdf.

———. 2006. The Search for a Past. The Prehistory of the Indigenous Saami in Northern Coastal Sweden. In *People, Material Culture and Environment in the North. Proceedings of the 22nd Nordic Archaeological Conference, University of Oulu, 18–23 August 2004*, edited by V. P. Herva, pp. 13–25. Humanistinen tiedekunta, Oulun yliopisto, Oulu.

Broadbent, N. D. and K. I. Bergqvist. 1986. Lichenometric Chronology and Archaeological Features on Raised Beaches: Preliminary Results from the Swedish North Bothnian Coastal Region. *Arctic and Alpine Research* 18(3):297–306.

Broadbent, N. D. and J. Graham. 2006. *Excavation Report. Hornslandsudde, Hälsingland, Sweden*. Arctic Studies Center. National Museum of Natural History. Smithsonian Institution, Washington D.C.

Broadbent, N. D. and L. Rathje. 2001. Vikingatiden fanns även i norr. *Populär arkeologi* 2:17–18.

Broadbent, N. D. and R. Sjöberg. 1990. Så gamla är labyrinterna. *Västerbotten* 1:292–297.

Broadbent, N. D. and J. Storå. 2003. En björngrav i Grundskatan. *Populär arkeologi* 1:3–6.

Broadbent, N. D. and P. Lantto. 2008. Terms of Engagement: An Arctic Perspective on the Narratives and Politics of Global Climate Change. In *Anthropology and Climate Change: From Encounters to Actions*, edited by Susan A. Crate and Mark Nuttall, pp. 341–355. Left Coast Press, Walnut Creek.

Broadbent, N. D. and B. Wennstedt Edvinger. n.d. Sacred Sites, Settlements and Place-Names: Ancient Saami Landscapes in Northern Coastal Sweden. In *Landscape and Culture in the Siberian North*, edited by P. Jordan. University London College Press, London.

Broberg, G. and N. Roll-Hansen (eds.). 2005. *Eugenics and the Welfare State*. Michigan State University Press, East Lansing.

Broberg, G. and M. Tydén. 2005. Eugenics in Sweden: Efficient Care. In *Eugenics and the Welfare State. Norway, Sweden, Denmark and Finland*, edited by G. Broberg, H. Roll-Hansen, pp. 77–149. Michigan State University Press, East Lansing.

Buggey, S. 2004. An Approach to Aboriginal Cultural Landscapes in Canada. In *Northern Ethnographic Landscapes: Perspectives from Circumpolar Nations*, edited by I. Krupnik, R. Mason and T. Horton. National Museum of Natural History. Smithsonian Institution, Washington, D.C.

Burenhult, G. (ed.). 1999. *Arkeologi i Norden*. Natur & kultur, Stockholm.

Bursche, A. 1996. Archaeological Sources as Ethnical Evidence: The Case of the Eastern Vistua Mouth. In *Cultural Identity and Archaeology: The Construction of European Communities*, edited by P. Graves-Brown and C. Gamble, pp. 228–234. Routledge, London and New York.

Burström, M. 1990. Järnframställning och gravritual. En strukturalisk tolkning av järnslag i gravar i Gästrikland. *Fornvännen* 85:261–272.

Bäckman, L. 1975. *Sájva: föreställningar om hjälp- och skyddsväsen i heliga fjäll bland samerna*. Stockholm Studies in Comparative Religion 13. Acta Universitatis Stockholmiensis. Stockholm University, Stockholm.

Bäckman, L. and Å. Hultkrantz. 1978. *Studies in Lapp Shamanism*. Stockholm Studies in Comparative Religion 16, Acta Universitatis Stockholmiensis. Almqvist and Wiksell International, Stockholm.

Campbell, Å. 1948. *Från vildmark till bygd*. Två Förläggare Bokförlag, Umeå.

Carlsson, A. 1998. *Tolkande arkeologi och svensk forntidshistoria*. Stockholm Studies in Archaeology 17. Acta Universitatis Stockholmiensis. Stockholm University. Almqvist and Wiksell International, Stockholm.

Carlsson, D. 1979. *Kulturlandskapets utveckling på Gotland. En studie av jordbruks- och bebyggelseförändringar under järnåldern*. Kulturgeografiska Institutionen, Stockholms Universitet Meddelande B49. Pressförlag, Visby.

Carlsson, M. 2002. *Norrbotten under yngre metallålder. Sammanställning över lösfynd i Norrbottens län 200 f.Kr.-300 e. Kr.* Institutionen för arkeologi och samiska studier. Umeå universitet, Umeå.

Carpelan, C. 1975a. Om samerna och samekulturens ursprung. In *Kemijoki 8000-Laxälv i norr*, edited by A. Erä-Esko, pp. 38–41. Statens historiska museum, Stockholm.

———. 1975b. En översikt över den forhistoriska tiden i området kring Kemi älv. In *Kemijoki 8000 – Laxälv i norr*, edited by A. Erä-Esko, pp. 16–37. Statens historiska museum, Stockholm.

———. 1977. *Älg- och björnhuvudföremål från Europas nordliga delar*. Finska fornminnesföreningen. Finsk Museum, Helsinki.

———. 1993. Problems of Archaeological Research in the Arctic Areas of Fennoscandia. In *Cultural Heritage of the Finno-Ugrians and Slavs*, edited by V. Lang and J. Selirand, pp. 180–189. Varrak, Tallinn.

———. 2001. Late Paleolithic and Mesolithic Settlement of the European North. In *Early Contacts Between Uralic and Indo-European: Linguistic and Archaeological Considerations*, edited by C. Carpelan, A. Parpola and P. Koskikallio, pp. 37–53. Mémoire de la Société Finno-Ougrienne 242. Suomalais-Ugrilainen Seura, Helsinki.

Carr, D. D. 1986. Narrative and the Real World. An Argument for Continuity. *History and Theory* 15:117–131.

Caulkins, D. D. 2001. Consensus, Clines and Edges in Celtic Cultures. *Cross-Cultural Research* 35(2):109–126.

Chappell, J. M. 2009. Sea Level Change, Quaternary. In *Encyclopedia of Paleoclimatology and Ancient Environments*, edited by V. Gornitz, pp. 893–989. Springer, Dordrecht.

Chase-Dunn, C. and T. D. Hall. 1997. *Rise and Demise. Comparing World Systems*. Westview Press, Boulder.

Chernykh, E. N. 1992. *Ancient Metallurgy in the USSR. The Early Metal Age*. Cambridge University Press, Cambridge.
Christiansen, C. 1995. The Littorina Transgressions in Denmark. In *Man and Sea in the Mesolithic. Coastal Settlement above and below the Present Sea Level*, edited by A. Fischer, pp. 15–22. Oxbow Monograph 53. Oxbow Books, Oxford.
Christiansson, H. 1969. Obbolagraven och des runda spännen. In *Nordsvensk forntid*, edited by H. Christiansen and Å. Hyenstrand. Skytteanska Samfundets Handlingar 6, Umeå.
Christiansson, H. and K. Knutsson. 1989. *The Bjurselet Settlement III*. Occasional Papers in Archaeology 1. Societas Archaeologica Upsaliensis, Uppsala.
Clark, G. 1946. Seal-hunting in the Stone Age of North-Western Europe: A Study in Economic Prehistory. *Proceedings of the Prehistoric Society* XII:12–48.
Cnieff, J. D. 1757. *Berättelse om själ-fångst i Österbotten*. Kungliga Vitterhets, Historie och Antikvitets Akademiens Handlingar XVIII:177–197.
Collinder, B. 1953. *Lapparna. En bok om samefolkets forntid och nutid*. Forum, Stockholm.
———. 1964. *Ordbok till Sveriges Lapska Ortnamn*. Kungliga Ortnamnskomissionen. Almqvist & Wiksell, Uppsala.
Cribb, R. 1991. *Nomads in Archaeology*. New Studies in Archaeology. Cambridge University Press, Cambridge.
Crosby, A. W. 1986. *Ecological Imperialism. The Biological Expansion of Europe, 900–1900*. Cambridge University Press, Cambridge.
Crowell, A. L. 1997. *Archaeology and the Capitalist World System. A Study from Russian America*. Plenum Press, New York and London.
Crumley, C. L. (ed.). 1994. *Historical Ecology: Cultural Knowledge and Changing Landscapes*. School of American Research Press, Santa Fe, N.M.
Dahlstedt, K.-H. 1965. Place-Names, Linguistic Contact and Prehistory. In *Hunting and Fishing*, pp. 135–158. Norrbottens Museum, Luleå.
D'Andrade, R. 1995. *The Development of Cognitive Anthropology*. Cambridge University Press, Cambridge.
Davidson, H. R. E. 1964. *Gods and Myths of Northern Europe*. Penguin Books Ltd., Baltimore.
Denton, G. H. and W. Karlén. 1973. Holocene Climate Variations. Their Patterns and Possible Causes. *Quaternary Research* 3:155–205.
Digerfeldt, G. 1975. A Standard Profile for Litorina Transgressions in Skåne, Southern Sweden. *Boreas* 4:125–142.
Drake, S.1918 (1979). *Västerbottenslapparna under förra hälften av 1800-talet*. Två Förläggare Bokförlag, Umeå.
Dubois, T. A. 1999. *Nordic Religions of the Viking Age*. University of Pennsylvania Press, Philadelphia.
Dunbar, M. J. 1954. Arctic and Subarctic Marine Ecology: Immediate Problems. *Arctic* 7:3–4.
———. 1968. *Ecological Development in Polar Regions*. Prentice Hall, New York.
Dunfjeld-Aagård, L. 2005. *Sörsamiske kystområder – Tolkning av fortidig samisk tilstedevaerelse i Ytre Namdal*. University of Tromsø, Tromsø.
Düben, G. v. 1977 (1873). *Om Lappland och Lapparne, Förträdesvis de Svenske*. Gidlunds, Östervåla.
Edlund, A.-C. 1989. *Sjökatt och Svarttjäder. Studier över säljaktens noaord inom det bottniska området och östersjöområdet*. Umeå universitet, Umeå.
———. 2000. *Sälen och jägaren. De bottniska jägarnas begreppssystem för säl ur ett kognitivt perspektiv*. Norrlands Universitetsförlag, Umeå.
Edlund, L.-E. 1988. Några maritima perspectiv på det bottniska ortnamnsförrådet samt aspekter på kulturgränser inom det nordnorrländska området. In *Det maritima kulturlandskapet kring bottenviken*, pp. 91–150. Bottenvisprojektet, Umeå.

Edsman, C.-M. 1994. *Jägaren och makterna. Samiska och finska björnceremonier* Ser. C:6. Publications of the Institute of Dialect and Folklore Research, Uppsala.

Ehrenreich, R. M., C. Crumley and J. Levy (eds.). 1995. *Heterarchy and the Analysis of Complex Societies*. Archaeological Papers of the American Anthropological Association 6, Arlington.

Eidtlitz Kuoljok, K. 1991. *På jakt efter Norrbottens medeltid. Om nordösteuropas historia och etnologi*. Miscellaneous Publication 10. Center for Arctic Cultural Research, Umeå University, Umeå.

Ekman, J. and E. Iregren. 1984. *Osteologiska studier över material från norrländska boplatser*. Early Norrland 8. Kungliga Vitterhets Historie och Antikvitets Akademien, Stockholm.

Ekman, S. 1982 (1910). *Norrlands jakt och fiske*. Två Förläggare Bokfölag, Umeå.

Eldjarn, G. and J. Godal. 1988. *Nordlandsbåten og Åfjordsbåten*. Båten i bruk. Bind 1. A. Kjellands forlag, Lesja.

Engelmark, R. 1976. The Vegetational History of the Umeå Region During the Past 4000 Years. In *Paleo-Ecological Investigations in Coastal Västerbotten, N. Sweden*, pp. 75–111. Early Norrland 9. Kungliga Vitterhets Historie och Antikvitets Akademien, Stockholm.

Englund, L.-E., E. Hjärthner-Holdar and E. Larsson. 1996. *Järnhanteringen på boplatsen vis Lappnäset- analys av slaggar och järn. Ångermanland, Nora sn*. Riksantikvarieämbetet Rapport 5. Geoarkeologiskt Laboratorium Analysrapport 15, Uppsala.

Englund, L.-E. 2000. *Arkeometallurgiskt material från Lill-Mosjön. Grundsunda sn RAÄ 356, Ångermanland, Nora sn*. Geoarkeologiskt Laboratorium Analysrapport 1, Uppsala.

Ericson, P. 2004. Samer från fjäll, skog, bygd och kust. In *Tidsspår – Västernorrland – Sameland. Om samisk närvaro i Ångermanland och Medelpad*, edited by M. Bergvall and P. Persson, pp. 150–186. Härnosand Museum, Härnosand.

Eriksen, T. H. 1993. *Etnicitet och nationalism*. Bokbolaget Nya Doxa AB, Nora.

Eriksson, L. 1975. *Kartering av fornlämningsområde 1966, 1973. Hornlandsudde, Rogsts sn, Hälsingland*. Riksantikvairieämbetet Rapport B11, Stockholm.

Fagen, B. 2001. *The Little Ice Age: How Climate Made History, 1300–1850*. Perseus Book Group, New York.

Fahlgren, K. 1953. Bygden organiseras In *Skellefte Sockens historia 1*, pp. 224–308. Almqvist and Wiksells boktryckeri AB, Uppsala.

Fairbridge, R. 1963. Mean Sea Level Related to Solar Radiation During the Last 20,000 Years. *Symposium of the Rome Symposium Organized by UNESCO, Liege, 229–242*.

Fairbridge, R. W. 2009. History of Paleoclimatology. In *Encyclopedia of Paleoclimatology and Ancient Environments*, edited by V. Gornitz, pp. 414–428. Springer, Dordrecht.

———. 2009. Medieval Warm Period. In *Encyclopedia of Paleoclimatology and Ancient Environments*, edited by V. Gornitz, pp. 551–554. Springer, Dordrecht.

Fandén, A. 2002. *Schamanens berghällar. Nya tolkningsperspektiv på den norrländska hällristnings- och hällmålningstraditionen*. Lofterud Produktion HB, Nälden.

Federova, N. V. 2002. West Siberia and the World of Medieval Civilizations: History of Interactions on the Trade Routes. *Archaeology, Ethnology and Anthropology of Eurasia* 4(12):91–101.

Fellman, I. 1906. *Handlingar och uppsatser angående finska lappmarken och Lapparne* IV, Helsinki.

Fischer, A. (ed.). 1995. *Man and Sea in the Mesolithic. Coastal Settlement above and below the Present Sea Level*. Oxbow Monograph 53. Oxbow Books, Oxford.

Fjellström, P. 1985. *Samernas samhälle i tradition och nutid*. Kungliga Skytteanska Samfundets Handlingar 27, Umeå.

———. 1987. Den nordsvenska kulturbäraren – en symbol för den mångkulturella Norrland. *Bebyggelsehistorisk tidskrift* 14:42–56.

Fjellström, P. 1755 (1981). *Kort berättelse, om lapparnas björna-fänge, samt deras der wid brukade widskeppelser*, Stockholm (Umeå).

Forsberg, L. 1985. *Site Variability and Settlement Patterns. An Analysis of the Hunter-Gatherer Settlement Systems in the Lule River Valley 1500 B.C.–B.C./A.D.* Archaeology and Environment 5. Umeå University, Umeå.

———. 1992. Proto-Saami Bronze Age in Northern Scandinavia: A Provocative View. In *Readings in Saami History, Culture and Language III*, edited by R. Kvist, pp. 1–8. Miscellaneous Publications 14. Center for Arctic Cultural Research, Umeå University, Umeå.

———. 1999. The Bronze Age Site at Mårtensfäboda in Nysätra and the Settlement Context of the Cairns of the Coast of North Sweden. In *Dig It All. Papers Dedicated to Ari Siiriäinen*, pp. 251–285. The Finnish Antiquarian Society, Helsinki.

———. 2001. Keramiken från Råingetlokalerna. Mångfald och formspråk. In *Tidsspår -forntidsvärld och gränslöst kulturarv*, edited by M. Bergvall and O. George, pp. 129–150. Länsmuseet Västernorrland, Härnosand.

Forstén, A. 1972. The Refuse Fauna of the Suomusjärvi Period in Finland. *Finskt Museum* 79:74–84.

Fossum, B. 2006. *Förfädernas land. En arkeologisk studie av rituella lämningar i Sápmi.* Studie Arkeologica Universitatis Umensis 22. Umeå universitet, Umeå.

Frachetti, M. 2008. *Pastoralist Landscapes and Social Interactions in Bronze Age Eurasia.* University of California Press, Berkeley.

Franzén, G. 1939. Ortnamn. In *Nordisk kultur* 5, pp. 124–171. Albert Bonniers Förlag, Stockholm.

Friis, J. A. 1871. *Lappisk mytologi, eventyr og folkesagn*, Christiania.

Giddens, A. 1977. *Studies in social and political theory.* Basic Books, New York.

Gimbutas, M. 1965. *The Bronze Age Cultures in Central and Eastern Europe.* Mouton and Company, The Hague.

Gjessing, G. 1944. *The Circumpolar Stone Age.* Acta Arctica II, Copenhagen.

———. 1942. *Yngre Stenalder i Nord-Norge.* Oslo.

———. 1955. Prehistoric Social Groups in North Norway. *Proceedings of the Prehistoric Society* 21:1–10.

Goodnow, K. and H. Akman (eds.). 2008. *Scandinavian Museums and Cultural Diversity.* Berghahn Books, Oxford.

Gollwitzer, M. 1997. Yngre Järnålder i fjälltrakterna. In *Möten i gränsland. Samer och germaner i Mellanskandinavien*, edited by I. Zachrisson, pp. 27–33. Statens historiska museum monographs 4, Stockholm.

Goody, J. 1977. *The Domestication of the Savage Mind.* Cambridge University Press, Cambridge.

Gornitz, V. 2009a. Ancient Cultures and Climates. In *Encyclopedia of Paleoclimatology and Ancient Environments*, edited by V. Gornitz, pp. 6–10. Springer, Dordrecht.

———. 2009b. Sea Level Change, Post-Glacial. In *Encyclopedia of Paleoclimatology and Ancient Environments*, edited by V. Gornitz, pp. 887–893. Springer, Dordrecht.

Gosden, C. 2004. *Archaeology and Colonialism. Cultural Contact from 5000 BC to the Present.* Cambridge University Press, Cambridge.

Graan, O. 1672 (1983). *Relation, Eller En Fullkomblig Beskrivning on Lapparnas ursprung, så wäl som om heela dheras Lefwernes Förhållande. Berättelser om samerna i 1600-talets Sverige.* Skytteanska Samfundets Handlingar, Umeå.

Graburn, N. H. H. and B. S. Strong. 1973. *Circumpolar Peoples: An Anthropological Perspective.* Goodyear Publishing, Pacific Palisades, CA.

Grandin, L., E. Hjärthnar-Holdar and E. Grönberg. 2005. *Järnhantering vid Bjuröklubb och Grundskatan: Analysrapport* Arkeometalurgiska analyser 13. Geoarkeologiskt Laboratorium, Uppsala.

Granlund, E. 1932. *De svenska högmossornas geologi.* Sveriges Geologiska Undersökning. Avhandlingar. Årsbok 26(C), Stockholm.

———. 1943. *Beskrivning till jordsartskarta över Västerbottens län nedanför odlingsgränsen*, Serie Ca. 26. Sveriges Geologiska Undersökning, Stockholm.

Green, A. M. 2002. Any Old Iron! Symbolism and Ironworking in Iron Age Europe. In *Artifacts and Archaeology: Aspects of the Celtic and Roman World*, edited by A. M. Green and P. Webster, pp. 8–19. University of Cardiff Press, Cardiff.

Grove, J. M. 1988. *The Little Ice Age*. Methuen, London and New York.

Grundberg, L. 2001. Där som inga lagliga köpstäder äro. Medeltida urbaniseringstendenser i ett norrländskt perspektiv. *Bebyggelsehistorisk tidskrift* 42:75–102.

———. 2006. *Medeltid i centrum: europeisering, historieskrivning och kulturarvsbruk i norrländska kulturmiljöer*. Studia archaeologica Universitatis Umensis, Kungliga Skytteanska Samfundets Handlingar, Umeå.

Grydeland, S. E. 2001. *De Sjøsamiske siida-samfunn*. Nord-Troms Museums Skrifter I/2001, Sørkjosen.

Gräslund, B. 1980. Climate Fluctuations in the Early Subboreal Period. A Preliminary Discussion. *Florilegium Florinis Dedicatum, Striae* 14:13–22.

Gullberg, K. (ed.). 1994. *Järnåldern i MittNorden*. Förlagsaktiebolaget Scriptum 3, Vasa.

Gunderson, L. H. and C. S. Holling (eds.). 2002. *Panarchy: Understanding Transformations in Human and Natural Systems*. Island Press, Washington, D.C.

Gustafsson, P. 1971. Om Västerbottnisk säljakt. *Västerbotten*, 65–105.

———. 1988. Sälisen och fälbåten. *Bottnisk kontakt* IV: 28–47.

———. 1990. Du skall inte söka sälen – du skall söka isen. *Västerbotten*, 243–291.

Götherström, A. 2001. *Acquired or Inherited Prestige? Molecular Studies of Family Structures and Local Horses in Central Svealand during the Early Medieval Period*. Theses and Papers in Scientific Archaeology 4. Archaeological Research Laboratory. Stockholm University, Stockholm.

Haaland, G., R. Haaland and D. Dea. 2004. Furnace and Pot: Why the Iron Smelter Is a Big Pot Maker. A Case Study from South-Western Ethiopia. *Azania* XXXIX:146–165.

Haaland, R. 2004. Technology, Transformation and Symbolism: Ethnographic Perspectives on European Iron Working. *Norwegian Archaeological Review* 37(1):1–19.

Haavio, M. 1952. Finsk-ugriska religioner. In *Nordisk Teologisk Uppslagsbok 1–3*, edited by R. Askmark. Gleerups Förlag, Malmö.

Haetta, O. M. 2002. *Samene. Nordkalottens urfolk*. Høyskole Forlaget, Kristiansand.

Halén, O. 1994. *Sedentariness during the Stone Age of Northern Sweden in the light of the Alträsket site, c. 5000 B.C., and the Comb Ware site Lillberget, c. 3900 BC*. Acta Archaeologica Lundensia Ser 4 (20). Lund University, Lund.

Hall, T. D. 1999. World-Systems and Evolution: An Appraisal. In *World-Systems Theory in Practice: Leadership, Practice and Exchange*, edited by N. P. Kardulias, pp. 1–23. Rowman & Littlefield, New York.

Hallowell, A. I. 1926. Bear Ceremonialism in the Northern Hemisphere. *American Anthropologist* 28:1–175.

Hallström, G. 1929. Kan lapparnas invandringstid fixeras? En arkeologisk studie. *Norrlands försvar*:39–42.

———. 1932. Lapska offerplatser. In *Arkeologiska studier tillägnade H. K. H. Kronprins Gustaf Adolf*, pp. 111–131. P. A. Norstedt, Stockholm.

———. 1942. Lövånger sockens forntid belyst av fynd och fornlämningar. In *Lövånger. En sockenbeskrivning I*, edited by C. Holm, pp. 228–352. Aktiebolaget Nyheternas tryckeri, Umeå.

———. 1949. Lövånger sockens forntid. In *Lövånger. En sockenbeskrivning II*, edited by G. Holm, pp. 13–89. Aktiebolaget Nyheternas tryckeri Umeå.

———. 1960. *Monumental Art of Northern Sweden from the Stone Age*. Almqvist and Wiksell, Stockholm.

Hamayon, R. N. 1996. Shamanism in Siberia: From Partnership in Supernature to Counter-power in Society. In *Shamanism, History and the State*, edited by N. Thomas and C. Humphrey, pp. 76–89. University of Michigan Press, Ann Arbor.

Hansen, L.-I. 1990. *Handel i Nord, samiske samfundsendringer ca. 1500–ca.1700*. Universitetet i Tromsø, Tromsø.

Hansen, L.-I and B. Olsen. 2004. *Samenes historie fram till 1750*. Cappelen Akademisk Forlag, Oslo.

Hasselbrink, G. 1981, 1983. *Sudlappisches Wörterbuch. Band I, II.* Schriften des Instituts fur Dialektforschung und Volkskunde in Uppsala Serie C:4, Uppsala.

Hedeager, L. 2001. Asgard Reconstructed? Gudme, A Central Place in the North. In *Topographies of Power in the Early Middle Ages*, edited by F. T. de Jong and C. van Rhijn, pp. 476–508. Brill, Leiden.

Hedman, S.-D. 2003. *Boplatser och offerplatser. Ekonomisk strategi och boplatsmönster bland skogssamer 700–1600 AD.* Studie Archaeologica Universitatis Umensis 17. Umeå University, Umeå.

Hedqvist, J. 1949. Lövångers kyrka och dess inventarier. In *Lövånger. En sockenbeskrivning 2*, edited by G. Holm, pp. 276–366. Aktiebolagets nyheternas tryckeri, Umeå.

Helle, E. 1974. On the Biology of the Ringed Seal in the Bothnian Bay. In *Proceedings of the Symposium on the Seal in the Baltic*, pp. 38–42. Statens Naturvårdsverk, Solna.

Helmfrid, S. (ed.). 1994. *Landscape and Settlements.* National Atlas of Sweden, Stockholm.

Helskog, K. 1988. *Helleristingene i Alta. Spor etter ritualer og dagligliv i Finnmarks forhistorie.* Alta Museum, Alta.

Helskog Thrash, E. 1983. *The Iversfjord Locality. A Study of Behavioral Patterning During the Stone Age of Finnmark, North Norway.* Tromsø Museums Skrifter XIX, Tromsø.

Herbert, E. 1993. *Iron, Gender and Power: Rituals and Transformations in African Societies.* Indiana University Press, Bloomington.

Hicks, S. 1988. The Representation of Different Farming Practices in Pollen Diagrams from Northern Finland. In *The Cultural Landscape: Past, Present and Future*, edited by H. J. B. Birks, P. E. Kaland and D. Moe, pp. 189–207. Cambridge University Press, Cambridge.

———. 1994. Present and Past Pollen Records of Lapland Forests. *Review of Paleobotany and Paynology* 83:17–35.

Hjärne, E. 1917. Bronsfyndet från Storkåge. Ett vittnerbörd om handelsförbindelser mellan Västerbotten och Östersjöprovinserna under äldre järnåldern. *Fornvännen* 12:147–172, 203–225.

Hjärthner-Holdar, E. 1993. *Järnets och järnmetallurgins introduktion i Sverige.* AUN 16, Societas Archaeologica Upsaliensis, Uppsala University, Uppsala.

Hjärthner-Holdar, E. and C. Risberg. 2001. The Innovation of Iron, from Bronze Age to Iron Age Societies in Sweden and Greece. In *Sixth Annual Meeting European Association of Archaeologists, 2000*, edited by B. Werbart, pp. 29–45. BAR International Series 985, Lisbon.

Hodder, I. 1991. Archaeological Theory in Contemporary European Societies: The Emergence of Competing Traditions. In *Archaeological Theory in Europe*, edited by I. Hodder, pp. 1–24. Routledge, London.

Hodges, H. 1970. *Technology in the Ancient World.* Penguin Books, Middlesex.

Holling, C. S. and L. H. Gunderson. 2002. Resilience and Adaptive Cycles. In *Panarchy: Understanding Transformations in Human and Natural Systems*, edited by L. H. Gunderson and C. S. Holling, pp. 25–62. Island Press, Washington, D.C.

Holling, C. S., L. H. Gunderson and D. Ludwig. 2002. A Quest of a Theory of Adaptive Change. In *Panarchy: Understanding Transformations in Human and Natural Systems*, edited by L. H. Gunderson and C. S. Holling, pp. 3–24. Island Press, Washington, D.C.

Holm, B. 1921. De bottniska själarnas levnadsvanor. *Fauna och flora*, 241–261.

Holm, G. 1949. Ortnamnen i Lövånger. In *Lövånger. En sockenbeskrivning II*, edited by G. Holm, pp. 90–157. Aktiebolaget Nyheternas tryckeri, Umeå.

———. 1973. Bynnamnet Kåddis. In *Studier från runtid till nutid tillägnade Carl Ivar Ståhle*, pp. 53–58, Malmö.

———. 1991. *De nordiska anger-namnen.* Lund University Press, Lund.

Holm, L. 2006. *Stenålderskust i norr. Bosättning, försörjning och kontakter i södra Norrland.* Studia Archaeologica Universitatus Umensis 19, Umeå University, Umeå.

Holmqvist, V. 1936. On the Origin of the Lapp Ribben Ornament. *Acta Archaeologica* 5:265–282.

Hornborg, A. and C. Crumley (ed.). 2007. *The World System and the Earth System. Global Socioenvironmental Change and Sustainability since the Neolithic.* Left Coast Press, Walnut Creek, CA.

Huggert, A. 1984. Flint Also Came from the East. A Contribution to the Knowledge of Upper Norrland. In *Papers in Northern Archaeology*, edited by E. Baudou, pp. 57–74. Archaeology and Environment 2. Umeå University, Umeå.

———. 1996. Early Copper in Northern Fennoscandia. *Current Swedish Archaeology* 4:69–82.

———. 2000. A Church at Lycksele and a Sacrificial Site on Altarberget — The Two Worlds of the Saami. *Acta Borealia* 1:51–75.

———. 2001. Praktfull flintyxa låg i ett stenkummel. *Västerbotten*, 56–61.

Hult, I. 1943. Sälen och säljakten i Östersjön under sennaste decennierna. *Svenskt Jakt* 81:365–372.

Hultblad, F. 1968. *Övergång från nomadism till agrar bosättning i Jokkmokks socken*. Meddelande från Uppsala universitets Geografiska Institutioner A 230. Lund.

Hulthén, B. 1991. *On Ceramic Ware in Northern Scandinavia During the Neolithic, Bronze and Early Iron Age*. Archaeology and Environment 8. Umeå University, Umeå.

Hultkrantz, Å. 1964. Type of Religion in the Arctic Hunting Cultures. In *Hunting and Fishing*, pp. 265–318. Norrbottens Museum, Luleå.

Hurrell, J. W. 1995. Decadal Trends in the North Atlantic Oscillation. Regional Temperatures and Precipitation. *Science* 269:676–679.

Huss, G. 1942. Lövångers äldre bebyggelse. In *Lövånger. En sockenbeskrivning I*, edited by C. Holm, pp. 353–407. Aktiebolaget Nyheternas tryckeri, Umeå.

Huttunen, P. and K. Tolonen. 1972. *Pollen-Anaytical Studies of Prehistoric Agriculture in Northern Ångermanland*. Early Norrland 1. Kungliga Vitterhets Historie och Antikvitets Akademien, Stockholm.

Hülphers, A. A. 1789. *Samlingar till en beskrivning över Norrland* 3 (Lappland). P. A. Norrstedt and Sons, Stockholm.

Hvarfner, H. 1957. *Fångstmän och nybyggare i Ångermanlands källområden under järnålder*. Arkiv för Norrländsk Hembyggsforskning 15, Härnosand.

Hyenstrand, Å. 1974. *Järn och bebyggelse. Studier I Dalarnas äldre kolonisationshistoria*. Falu Nya Boktrykeri AB, Falun.

Hämäläinen, A. 1930. Hylkeenpyynti keskisen Pohjanlahaden suomenpuoleisella nannalla. *Finska Fornminnesföreningens Tidskrift* XXXVII:1–162.

Högström, P. 1747 (1980). *Beskrifning öfwer de til Sweriges Krone lydnande Lappmarker*. Norrländska skrifter 3, Umeå.

Indreko, R. 1956. *Steingeräte mit rille*. Handlingar, Antikvariska Serien 4. Kungliga Vitterhets Historia och Antikvitets Akademien, Stockholm.

Ingold, T. 1978. The transformation of the siida. *Ethnos 1978* 43:146–162.

———. 1980. *Hunters, Pastoralists and Ranchers. Reindeer Economies and Their Transformations*. Cambridge Studies in Social Anthropology 28. Cambridge University Press, Cambridge.

———. 1983. The Significance of Storage in Hunting Societies. *Man* 18:553–571.

———. 1986. *The Appropriation of Nature: Essays on Human Ecology and Social Relations*. Manchester University Press, Manchester.

———. 2000. *The Perception of the Environment. Essays in Livelihood, Dwelling and Skill*. Routledge, London and New York.

Iregren, E. 1997. Människoskeletten. In *Möten i gränsland. Samer och germaner i Mellanskandinavien*, pp. 84–99. Monographs 4. Statens historiska museum, Stockholm.

———. 1999. *Vi har hittat Yggdrasil – med Ratatosk och Eiktyrnir!* Arkeologiska nyheter and facta Internet, Malmö.

Itkonen, I. T. 1947. Lapparnas förekomst i Finland. *Ymer* 1:42–57.

———. 1951. The Lapps of Finland. *Southwestern Journal of Anthropology* 7(1):32–68.

Jacobsen, H. and J.-R. Follum. 1997. *Kulturminner og skogbruk*. Skogbrukets kursinstitut, Biri.

Jaarola, M., H. Tegelström and K. Fredga. 1999. Colonization History in Fennoscandinavian Rodents. *Biological Journal of the Linnean Society* 68:113–127.
Jansson, S. 1981. *Båtfyndet från Avafjärd*. Arkeologiska institutionen,Umeå universitet, Umeå.
Jirlow, R. 1930. Västerbottnisk säljakt. *Västerbotten*, 77–111.
Johansson, L. 1947. Offerplatser och andra heliga ställen inom Frostvikens lappmark: komplettering av uppsats i Jämten 1946. *Jämten*, 124–126.
Jones, S. 1997. *The Archaeology of Ethnicity*. Routledge, London and New York.
Jordan, P. 2003. *Material Culture and Sacred Landscape: The Anthropology of the Siberian Khanty*. Rowman & Littlefield Publishers, Oxford.
Julku, K. 1986. *Kvenland-Kainuunmaa*. Kustannusosakeyhtio Pohjoinen, Oulu.
Jönsson, S. 1985. *Hälsingland runt på två år. Arkeologi i Sverige 1982–1983*. Riksantikvarieämbetet rapport 1985:5, Stockholm.
Jørgensen, R. 1986. The Early Metal Age in Nordland and Troms. *Acta Borealia* 2:61–86.
Jørgensen, R. and B. Olsen. 1988. *Asbestkeramiske grupper i Nord-Norge 2100 f.Kr.–100 e.Kr.* Tromura, Kulturhistorie 13. Universitetet i Tromsø, Tromsø.
Kardulias, P. N. 1999. *World-Systems Theory in Practice: Leadership, Practice and Exchange*. Rowman and Littlefield, New York.
Karlén, V. 1975. *Lichenometrisk datering i norra Skandinavien-metodens tillförlitlighet och regionala tillämpning*. Naturgeografiska Institutionen, Forskningsrapport 22, Stockholms universitet, Stockholm.
Karlsson, L. 1931. Brännudden, Arvidsjaur. In *Folkminnesuppteckningar från Arvidsjaurs socken, Lappland*, edited by E. Brännström. Språk-och folkminnesinstitutet, Vol. 4373a. Uppsala.
Karlsson, N. 2006. *Bosättning och resursutnyttjande. Miljöarkeologiska studier av boplatser med härdar från perioden 600–1900 e.Kr. inom skogssamiskt område*. Studia archaeologica universitatis umensis 21. Umeå universitet, Umeå.
Kent, S. 2002. *Ethnicity, Hunter-Gatherers and the "Other": Association or Assimilation in Africa*. Smithsonian Institution Press, Washington, D.C.
Keyes, C. F. 1981. The Dialectics of Ethnic Change. In *Ethnic Change*, edited by C. F. Keyes, pp. 3–30. University of Washington Press, Seattle.
Khazanov, A. M. 1984. *Nomads and the Outside World*. Cambridge Studies in Social Anthropology. Cambridge University Press, Cambridge.
Khlobystin, L. P. 2005. *Taymyr. The Archaeology of Northernmost Eurasia*. Contributions to Circumpolar Anthropology 5. Arctic Studies Center, National Museum of Natural History, Smithsonian Institution, Washington, D.C.
Kjellström, R. 1974. *Kulturlämningar kring Altsvattnet. Samiska kulturlämningar* Riksantikvarieämbetet rapport D 10: 4–31. Kulturinventeringarna 1974, Stockholm.
———. 1976. Är traditionerna om Stalo historiskt grundade? *Fataburen*, 155–178.
———. 1995. *Jakt och fångst*. Nordiska museets förlag, Stockholm.
———. 2000. *Samernas liv*. Carlssons Bokförlag, Stockholm.
Kjellström, R. and H. Rydving. 1988. *Den samiska trumman*. Nordiska Museet, Stockholm.
Kleppe, E. J. 1977. Archaeological Material and Ethnic Identification: A Study of Lappish Material from Varanger, Norway. *Norwegian Archaeological Review* 10(1–2):32–46.
Klindt-Jensen, O. 1975. *A History of Scandinavian Archaeology*. Thames and Hudson Ltd., London.
Knutsson, H. (ed.). 2005. *Pioneer Settlements and Colonization Processes in the Barents Region*. Vuollerim Papers on Hunter-Gatherer Archaeology I, Vuollerim.
Koivonen, P. and M. Makkonen. 1998. *Yli-Iin Kierikin Kuuselankankaan kaivauket 1993–94*. Meteli. Oulun yliopiston arkeologian laboratorion tutimusrapportii 16, Oulu.

Korhonen, O. 1982. *Samisk-finska båttermer och ortsnamnselement och deras slaviska bakgrund. En studie i mellanspråklig ordgeografi och mellanfolklig kulturhistoria.* Skrifter utgiven av Dialekt-, ortnamns- och folkminnesarkivet i Umeå, Serie A, dialekter nr. 3, Umeå.

———. 1988. Ålderdomliga drag i sentida sälfångst och några samiska sältermer. In *Bottnisk kontakt 4*, pp. 70–79. Skellefteå Museum, Skellefteå.

Kraft, J. 1977. Labyrint och ryttarlek. *Fornvännen* 72:72–79

———. 1981. Labyrintmagi pa Kuggören? *Hälsingerunor*, 5–15.

———. 1982. Aldrig vilse i en labyrint. Norrbotten. *Norrbottens museums årsbok 1980–1981*, 7–16.

Kramer, L. S. 1997. Historical Narratives and the Meaning of Nationalism. *Journal of the History of Ideas* 58(3):525–545.

Kresten, P. 1999. *Slag och metall från Kyrkesviken, Grundsunda sn, RAÄ 121, Ångermanland.* Geoarkeologiskt Laboratorium Analysrapport 22, Uppsala.

Kristiansen, K. 1994. The Emergence of the European World System in the Bronze Age: Divergence, Convergence and Social Evolution during the First and Second Millennia BC in Europe. In *Europe in the First Millennium B.C.*, edited by K. Kristiansen and J. Jensen, pp. 7–30. J. R. Collins Publications, Copenhagen.

Krupnik, I. 1993. *Arctic Adaptations. Native Whalers and Reindeer Herders of Northern Eurasia.* University Press of New England, Hanover.

Krupnik, I., R. Mason and T. Horten (eds.). 2004. *Northern Ethnographic Landscapes: Perspectives from Circumpolar Nations.* Arctic Studies Center, National Museum of Natural History, Smithsonian Institution. Washington, D.C.

Krupnik, I., M. Bravo, Y. Csonka, G. Hovelsrud-Broda, L. Müller-Wille, B. Poppel, P. Schweitzer and S. Sörlin. 2005. Social Sciences and Humanities in the International Polar Year 2007–2008. An Integrating Mission. *Arctic (InfoNorth)* 58(1):91–101.

Kuoljok, S. 1996. *Sami History*. The Saami Parliament, Kiruna.

Kuz'minykh, S. V. 2006. Final Bronze Age and Early Iron Age in the North of Eastern Europe. In *Lighting the Darkness: The Attraction of Archaeology. Papers in Honour of Christian Carpelan*, edited by M. Suvhonen, pp. 75–84. Arkeologia, Helsingin yliopisto, Helsinki.

Kvist, R. 1987. *Sälfångsten i Österbotten och Västerbotten 1551–1610.* Center for Arctic Cultural Research, Research Report 3. Umeå University, Umeå.

———. 1988. *Klimathistoriska aspekter på sälfångsten i Österbotten 1551–1610.* Center for Arctic Cultural Research, Research Report 12. Umeå University, Umeå.

———. 1990. *Sälfångstens roll i den lokala ekonomin i Österbotten och Västerbotten 1551–1610.* Research Reports 18. Center for Arctic Cultural Research, Umeå University, Umeå.

———. 1991. Sealing and Sealing Methods in the Bay of Bothnia, 1551–70. *Polar Record* 27(163):339–344.

Kvist, R. and R. P. Wheelersburg. 1997. Changes in Saami Socioeconomic Institutions in Jokkmokk Parish 1720–1890. *Arctic Anthropology* 34 (2):1–11.

Käck, B.-O. 2001. Boplatsen vid forsen. In *Tidsspår – forntidsvärld och gränslöst kulturarv*, edited by M. Bergvall and O. George, pp. 25–42. Länsmuseet Västernorrland, Härnosand.

Käck, J. 2009. *Samlingsboplatser?* Studia Archaeologica Universitatis Umensis 24, Umeå universitet, Umeå.

Königsson, L. K. 1968. *Traces of Neolithic Human Influence upon the Landscape Development of the Bjurselet Settlement, Västerbotten.* Kungliga Skytteanska Samfundets Handlingar 1, Umeå.

Laestadius, L. L. 1838–1845 (1997). *Fragments of Mythology.* Edited by Juha Pentikäinen. Aspasia Books, Ontario.

Lamb, H. H. 1977. *Climate, Present, Past and Future.* Climatic History and the Future 2. Methuen & Co Ltd., London.

———. 1995. *Climate, History and the Modern World.* Routledge, London.

Lambeck, K. 2009. Glacial Isostasy. In *Encyclopedia of Paleoclimatology and Ancient Environments*, edited by V. Gornitz, pp. 374–380. Springer, Dordrecht.
Lantto, P. 2005. Raising Their Voices: The Sámi Movement in Sweden and the Swedish Sámi Policy, 1900–1960. In *The Northern Peoples and States: Changing Relationships*, edited by A. Leete, pp. 203–234. Tartu University Press, Tartu.
Larsson, T. B. 1999. Symbols in a European Bronze Age Cosmology. In *Communication in Bronze Age Europe*, edited by C. Orrling, pp. 9–16. Studies 9. Statens historiska museum, Stockholm.
Lavento, M. 2001. *Textile Ceramics in Finland and the Karelian Isthmus*. Finska Fornminnesföreningens Tidskrift 109, Helsinki.
Le Roy Ladurie, E. 2004. *Historie humaine et comparèe du climat. Canicules et glaciers XIIIe–XVIIIe siècle*. Libraire Arthème Fayard, Paris.
Lee, R. B. and R. Daly (eds.). 1999. *The Cambridge Encyclopedia of Hunters and Gatherers*. Cambridge University Press, Cambridge.
Leem, K. 1767 (1975). *Beskrivelse over Finmarkens Lapper, dera Tungemaal, Levemaandeog forrige Afgudsdykelse, oplyst ved mange Kaabersstykker* Copenhagen.
Lehtola, V.-P. 2004. *Sami People: Traditions in Transitions*. University of Alaska Press, Fairbanks.
Lepiksaar, J. 1975. *The Analysis of the Animal Bones from the Bjurselet Settlement, Västerbotten, Northern Sweden*. Kungliga Skytteanska Samfundets Handlingar 8, Umeå.
Levy, J. E. 2006. Prehistory, Identity, and Archaeological Representation in Nordic Museums. *American Anthropologist* 108(1):135–147.
Lidén, A. 1999. *Olav den helige i medletida bildkonst. Legendmotiv och attribut*. Kungliga Vitterhets Historie och Antikvitets Akademien, Stockholm.
Liedgren, L. 1985. Gustaf Hallström's Excavation at Onbacken, Hälsingland, 1923. In *In Honorem Evert Baudou*, pp. 339–352. Archaeology and Environment 4. Umeå University, Umeå.
———. 1992. *Hus och Gård i Hälsingland*. Studia Archaeologica Universitatis Umensis 2, Umeå.
Liedgren, L. and M. Johansson. 2005. An Early Iron Age Stone-Setting from Lake Uddjaur in Arjeplog, Lappland. In *En lång historia..Festskrift till Evert Baudou på 80-årsdagen*, edited by R. Engelmark, T. G. Larsson and L. Rathje, pp. 275–295. Archaeology and Environment 19, Kungliga Skytteanska Samfundets Handlingar 57, Umeå.
Liedgren, L., I. Bergman, G. Hörnberg, O. Zachrisson, E. Hellberg, L. Östlund and T. DeLuca. 2007. Radiocarbon Dating of Prehistoric Hearths in Alpine Northern Sweden: Problems and Possibilities. *Journal of Archaeological Science* 4:1276–1288.
Lindgren, C. 2004. *Människor och kvarts*. Stockholm Studies in Archaeology 29, Riksantikavaieämbetet Arkeologiska Undersökningar, Skrifter 54, Stockholm.
Lindkvist, A.-K. 1994. Förromersk och romersk järnålder i Ångermanlands kustland. En mångkulturell variation inom en region. In *Järnåldern i MittNorden 3*, edited by K. Gullberg, pp. 83–100. Förlagsaktiebolaget Scriptum, Vasa.
Lindow, J. 2002. *Norse Mythology. A Guide to Gods, Heroes, Rituals, and Beliefs*. Oxford University Press, Oxford.
Lindqvist, S.-O. 1968. *Det förhistoriska kulturlandskapet I Östra Östergötland*. Studies in North European Archaeology 2, Acta universitatus stockholmiensis. Stockholm University, Stockholm.
Lindstrom, I. and L. Olofsson. 1993. Maritima fornlämningar i den bottniska skärgården. *Arkeologi i norr* 4–5:55–74.
Lloyd, G. E. R. 1990. *Demystifying mentalities*. Cambridge University Press, Cambridge.
Locke, W. W., J. T. Andrews and P. J. Webber. 1980. *A Manual for Lichenometry*. British Geomorphological Research Group Technical Bulletin 26. Geo Abstracts, Norwich.
Loeffler, D. 2005. *Contested Landscapes/Contested Heritage*. Institutionen för arkeologi och samiska studier, Umeå University, Umeå.

Luho, V. 1954. Porin Tuorsniemen verkkölöytö. *Suomen Museo 61.*
Lund, A. A. 1978. *Adam af Bremen. Beskrivelse af Øerne i Norden.* Wormianum, Højbjerg.
Lundberg, Å. and T. Ylinen. 1997. *Rapport över arkeologisk undersökning av boplats Raä 510, fast. Västerdahl 1:1, Flurkmark, Umeå sn, Västerbotten.* Umark 7, Arkeologsk rapport. Umeå universitet, Umeå.
Lundberg, Å. 1997. *Vinterbyar- ett bandsamhälle i Norrlands inland 4500–2500 f.Kr.* Institutionen för arkeologi, Umeå universitet, Umeå.
———. 2001. Värdefulla gravgåvor eller besvärjande offer? *Västerbotten*:25–28.
Lundgren, P. 2001. *Flurkmarkboplatsens redskap och avlag: horisontell stratigrafi och kronologisk ställning.* Institutionen för arkeologi, Umeå universitet, Umeå.
Lundin, K. 1992. Kokgroparna i Norrbottens kustland. Ett försök till tolkning av kokgroparnas funktion. *Arkeologi i norr* 3:139–174.
Lundius, N. 1675 (1905). Descriptio Lapponiæ. In *Svenska landsmål och svenskt folkliv 17*, edited by K. B. Wiklund, pp. 55–41, Uppsala.
Lundmark, L. 1982. *Uppbörd, utarming, utveckling. Det samiska samhällets övergång till rennomadism i Lule lappmark.* Arkiv avhandlingsserie 14. Norrlands universitetsförlag, Umeå.
———. 1998. *Så länge vi har marker.* Prisma, Stockholm.
———. 2002. *"Lappen är ombytlig, ostadig och obekväm," Svenska statens samepolitik i racismens tidevarv.* Norrlands universitetsförlag, Umeå.
———. 2007. *Myten om kvänernas rike.* Retrieved June 1, 2009, from http://lennartlundmark.se/.
Lundqvist, R. 2002. *Fulufjället: nationalpark i Dalafjällen.* Naturvårdsverket, Stockholm.
Lundström, U. n.d. Åsarnas roll för kommunikationer, handel, kulturmöten och samhällsorganisation i Skelleftebygden. Skellefteå museum, Skellefteå.
Löfgren, K. and A.-L. Olsson. 1983. Snöan – ett fiskeskär från medeltid till nutid. *Västerbotten*, 91–103.
Magnus, B. 1974. Fisker eller bonde? Undersökelser av hustufter på yttrekusten. *Tidskrift för norrön arkeologi* 38:68–108.
Magnus, O. 1555 (1976). *Historia om de nordiska folken 1–4.* Gidlunds förlag, Stockholm.
Magnusson, G. 1986. *Lågteknisk järnhantering i Jämtlands län.* Järnkontorets berghistoriska skriftserie 22, Stockholm.
———. 1987. Järn, kolonisation och landskapsutnyttande i Norrlands inland. *Bebyggelsehistorisk tidskrift* 14:127–136.
Malmer, M. P. 2002. *The Neolithic of South Sweden TRB, GRK and STR.* The Royal Swedish Academy of Letters History and Antiquities, Stockholm.
Manker, E. 1944. *Lapsk kultur vid Stora Luleälvs Källsjöar.* Acta Lapponica IV. Nordiska museet, Stockholm.
———. 1957. *Lapparnas heliga ställen.* Acta Lapponica XIII. Nordiska museet, Stockholm.
———. 1960. *Fångstgropar och stalotomter. Kulturlämningar från lapsk forntid.* Acta Lapponica XV. Nordiska Museet, Gebers, Stockholm.
———. 1968. *Skogslapparna i Sverige.* Acta Lapponica XVIII. Nordiska Museet, Almqvist and Wiksell, Stockholm.
———. 1971. Fennoscandias fornskidor. *Fornvännen* 66:77–91.
Manyukhin, N. L. and M. Lobonova. 2002. Archaeological Past of the Solovetskii Archipelago. In *National and Cultural Heritage of the White Sea Islands*, pp. 31–39. Nordic Council of Ministers, Petrozavodsk.
Markgren, G. 1974. The Moose in Fennoscandia. *Naturaliste Canada* 101:184–194.
Martin, C. 1982. *Keepers of the Game. Indian-Animal Relationships and the Fur Trade.* University of California Press, Berkeley.
Martins, I. 1988. *Jernvinna på Møsstrond i Telemark. En studie i teknikk, bosetning og økonomi.* Norske Oldfunn XIII, Universitets Oldsaksampling, Oslo.

Mattingly, H. 1948. *Tacitus on Britain and Germany*. Penguin Books, Baltimore.
Mayewski, P. A., L. D. Meeker, M. C. Morrison, M. S. Twickler, S. Whitlow, K. K. Ferland, D. A. Meese, M. R. Legrand and J. P. Steffenson. 1993. Greenland Ice Core "Signal" Characteristics Offer Expanded View of Climate Change. *Journal of Geophysical Research* 98(D7):12,839–12,847.
Mayewski, P. and F. White. 2002. *The Ice Chronicles: The Quest for Understanding Global Change*. University Press of New Hampshire, Hanover.
McGovern, T. H. 1988. Cows, Harp Seals, and Church Bells: Adaptation and Extinction in Norse Greenland. *Human Ecology* 8:245–274.
McIntosh, R. J., J. A. Tainter and S. K. McIntosh. 2000. Climate, History, and Human Action. In *The Way the Wind Blows*, edited by R. J. McIntosh, J. A. Tainter and S. K. McIntosh, pp. 1–44. Historical Ecology Series. Columbia University Press, New York.
McLaren, I. A. 1958. *The Biology of the Ringed Seal in the Eastern Canadian Arctic*. Bulletin no. 118. Fisheries Research Board of Canada, Ottawa.
Mebius, H. 1968. *Värro. Studier i samernas förkristna offerriter*. Skrifter utgivna av religionshistoriska institutionen i Uppsala 5. Uppsala University, Uppsala.
———. 2003. *Bissie: studier i samisk religionshistoria*. Östersund Jengel, Östersund.
Miller, U. and A.-M. Robertsson. 1979. *Biostratigraphical Investigations in the Lake Anundsjö Region*. Early Norrland 12. Kungliga Vitterhets, Historie och Antikvitets Akademiens Handlingar, Stockholm.
Miller, U., S. Modig and A.-M. Robertsson. 1979. *Geological Investigations in the Anundsjö Region, Northern Sweden*. Early Norrland 12. Kungliga Vitterhets, Historie och Antikvitets Akademiens Handlingar, Stockholm.
Minc, L. and K. Smith. 1989. The Spirit of Survival: Cultural Responses to Resource Variability in North Alaska. In *Bad Year Economics: Cultural Responses to Risk and Uncertainty*, edited by P. Halstead and J. O'Shea, pp. 1–7. Press Syndicate of the University of Cambridge, Cambridge.
Modelski, G. and W. R. Thompson. 1999. The Evolutionary Pulse of the World System: Hinterlands, Incursions and Migrations 4000 BC to AD 1500. In *World-Systems Theory in Practice: Leadership, Practice and Exchange*, edited by P. N. Kardulias, pp. 241–274. Rowman and Littlefield, New York.
Montelius, O. 1876a. Les Tombeaux et la Topographie De La Suède Pedant L'Age De La Pierre. In *Congrès d'Anthropologie & d'Archaèologie Prèhistoriques 1874, Volume 1*, pp. 153–176. P. A. Nordstedt & Söner, Stockholm.
———. 1876b. Les Souvenirs de L'age de La Pierre des Lapons en Suède. In *Congrès D'Anthropologie & D'Archaèologie Prèhistoriques 1874 (Volume 1)*, pp. 188–203. P. A. Nordstedt & Söner, Stockholm.
———. 1876c. L'Age du Bronze en Suède. In *Congrès D'Anthropologie & D'Archaèologie Prèhistoriques 1874 (Volume 1)*, pp. 488–512. P. A. Nordstedt & Söner, Stockholm.
———. 1919. *Forntiden. Sveriges historia till vara dagar. Stenåldern*, Stockholm.
Mulk, I.-M. 1994. *Sirkas. Ett fångstsamhälle i förändring Kr. f -1600 e.Kr.* Studia Archaeologica Universitatis Umensis 6, Umeå universitet, Umeå.
Mulk, I.-M. and E. Iregren. 1995. *Bjorngraven i Karats*. Duoddaris 9. Ajtte, Jokkmokk.
Mulk, I.-M. and T. Bayliss-Smith. 1999. The representation of Sámi cultural identity in the cultural landscapes of northern Sweden: the use and misuse of archaeological knowledge. In *The Archaeology and Anthropology of Landscape*, edited by P. J. Ucko and R. Layton, pp. 358–396. One World Archaeology. Routledge, London.
———. 2006a. Coins in Sámi Sacrificial Sites: Religious, Ritual, Social Organization and the Fur Trade in Northern Sweden, c. 800–1350 A.D. In *The Furthark and the Fur Trade*, edited by P. Poussa and P. Ambrosiani, pp. 71–99. Umeå University, Umeå.
———. 2006b. *Rock Art and Sami Sacred Geography in Badjelánnda, Laponia, Sweden. Sailing Boats, Anthropomorphs and Reindeer*. Archaeology and Environment 22. Kungl. Skytteanska Samfundets Handlingar, Umeå.

Mundal, E. 1996. Co-Existence of Saami and Norse Culture: Reflected in and Interpreted by Old Norse Myths. In *Shamanism and Northern Ecology*, edited by J. Pentikäinen, pp. 97–116. Walter de Gruyter, Berlin and New York.

Murray, T. 2004. *The Archaeology of Contact in Settler Societies*. Cambridge University Press, Cambridge.

Myhre, B. 1972. *Funn, fornminner og ødegårdar*. Stavanger Museums Skrifter 7, Stavanger.

Myrhaug, M. L. 1997. *I modergudinnens fotspor: samisk religion med vekt på kvinnelige kultutøvere og gudinnekult*. Pax forlag, Oslo.

Myrstad, R. 1996. *Bjørnegraver i Nord-Norge. Spor etter den samiske bjørnekulten*. Institutt for samfunnsvitenskap, Universitetet i Tromsø, Tromsø.

Mäkivuoti, M. 1986. Kempeleen Linnakankaan löydöistä ja ajoituksesta. *Faravid* 9:25–30.

Mörkenstam, U. 1999. *Om "Lapparnas Priviligier": Föreställningar om samiskhet i svensk samepolitik 1883–1997*. Statsvetenskapliga institutionen. Stockholms universitet, Stockholm.

Narmo, L. E. 2000. *Oldtid ved Åmøtet. Østerdalens tidlige historie belyst av arkeologiske utgravninger på Rødsmoen i Åmot*. Åmot Historielag, Rena.

Nesheim, A. 1953. Samisk seljakt och jakttabu. In *Lieber Saecularis in honorum J. Quigstadii*. Studie Septentrionalia 4. University of Oslo, Oslo.

Nesje, A. and M. Kvamme. 1989. Holocene Glacier and Climate Variations in Western Norway. Evidence for Early Holocene Glacier Demise and Multiple Neoglacial Events. *Geology* 19:610–612.

Nickel, K. P. 1990. *Samisk Grammatik*. Universitets forlaget, Oslo.

Nilsson, A. C. 1989. *Tomtningar från yngre järnålder utmed övre Norrlands kust*. Research Report 13. Center for Arctic Cultural Research, Umeå University, Umeå.

Nilsson, S. 1866. *Skandinaviska Nordens Ur-Invånare, ett försök i komparativa Etnografin och ett bidrag till menniskoslägtets utvecklings historia* 1. P. A. Norstedt & Söners Förlag, Stockholm.

Nitzelius, T. and H. Vedel. 1966. *Skogens träd och buskar i färg*. Almqvist & Wiksell, Stockholm.

Niurenius, O. P. 1645 (1905). Lappland, eller beskrivning över den nordiska trakt, som lapparne bebo i de avlägsnaste delarne av Skandien eller Sverige. In *Svenska landsmål och svenskt folkliv 17:4*, pp. 7–23, Uppsala.

Norberg, E. 2000. Björngraven – Mer än riter och kult? *Tidsperspektiv* 2:7–19

Nordlund, C. 2001. *Det Upphöjda landet: Vetenskapen, landhöjningsfrågan och kartläggningen av Sveriges förflutna, 1860–1930*. Kungliga Skytteanska Samfundets Handlingar 53, Umeå.

Norman, P. 1993. *Medeltida utskärs fiske*. Nordiska museets handlingar 116, Stockholm.

Nunez, M. 1997. Finland's Settling Model Revisited. In *Reports of the Early in the North Project. MAA – The Land*, pp. 93–102. Helsinki Papers in Archaeology No. 10. Department of Archaeology, University of Helsinki, Helsinki.

Nylander, P.-O. and L. Beckman. 1991. Population Studies in Northern Sweden XVII. Estimates of Finnish and Saamish Influence. *Human Heredity* 41:157–167.

Nyström, L. 1988. *Bidrag tll finlandssvensk sälfångstterminologi*. Miscellaneous Publications 5. Center for Arctic Cultural Research, Umeå University, Umeå.

———. 2000. *Alg, pytare och skridstång. Sälfångstens och säljaktens terminologi i Finlandssvenska folkmål*. Svenska litteratursälskapet i Finland, Helsinki.

Odner, K. 1983. *Finner och Terfinner. Etniska processer i det nordlige Fenno-Skandinavia*. Oslo Occasional Papers in Social Anthropology 9, Oslo.

———. 1992. *The Varanger Saami*. Habitation and Economy 1200–1900. Scandinavian University Press, Oslo.

———. 2000. *Tradition and Transmission*. Bergen Studies in Social Anthropology. Norse Publications, Bergen.

Ohnuki-Tierny, E. 1999. Ainu Sociality. In *Ainu: Spirit of Northern People*, edited by W. W. Fitzhugh and C. O. Dubreuil, pp. 240–245. Arctic Studies Center, National Museum of Natural History, Smithsonian Institution, Washington, D.C.

Ojala, C.-G. 2006. Saami Archaeology in Sweden and Swedish Archaeology in Sápmi: Boundaries and Networks in Archaeological Research. In *People, Material Culture and Environment in the North. Proceedings of the 22nd Nordic Archaeological Conference*, edited by V. Pekka Herva, pp. 33–41. Humanistinen tiedekunta, Oulun yliopisto, Oulu.

Olofsson, A. 1995. *Kölskrapor, mikrospånkärnor och mikrospån*. Institutionen för arkeologi, Umeå universitet, Umeå.

———. 2003. *Pioneering Settlement in the Mesolithic of Northern Sweden*. Archaeology and Environment 16. Umeå universitet, Umeå.

Olofsson, S. I. 1962. Övre Norrlands historia 1. In *Övre Norrlands historia*, pp. 123–252. Norrbottens och Västerbottens landsting, Umeå.

Olsen, B. 1994. *Bosetning og samfunn i Finnmarks forhistorie*. Universitetsforlaget, Oslo.

———. 1998. Samerna – ett folk utan historia? *Populär arkeologi* 3:3–6.

———. 2000. Belligerent Chieftains and Oppressed Hunters? Changing Conceptions of Inter-Ethnic Relationships in Northern Norway during the Iron Age and Early Medieval Period. In *Identities and Cultural Contacts in the Arctic.*, edited by M. Appelt, J. Berglund and H. C. Gulløv, pp. 28–42. Danish National Museum and Danish Polar Center, Copenhagen.

———. 2002. Labyrinths of the North. In *National and Cultural Heritage of the White Sea Islands*, pp. 40–51. Nordic Council of Ministers, Petrozavodsk.

———. 2004. Hva er samisk forhistorie? In *Samisk forhistorie*, edited by M. Krogh and K. Schanche, pp. 20–30. Varanger Samiske Museum, Varanger.

Olsen, I. 1910. Om lappernes vildfarelser og overtro. In *Kildeskrifter til den lappiske mythologi*, edited by J. K. Qvigstad, pp. 7–101. Det kungl. norske videnskabers selskabs skrifter 4, Trondheim.

———. 1934 (efter 1715) Finnernes afgudssteder i Finnmark omkring 1700. In *Aktstykker og oversikter* pp. 134–140. Nordnorske Samlingar 1. M. B. Utne & O. Solberg, Oslo

Olson, C., H. Runeson, B. Sigvallius and J. Storå. 2008. Bjästamons människor och djur i norrländsk stenålder. In *Stenålderns stationer. Arkeologi i Botniabanans spår*, edited by P. Gustavsson, L.-G. Spång, pp. 51–70. Riksantikvarieämbetet. UV Publikationer, Stockholm.

Olsson, A. 1990. *Sälspjutet. Beteckningar inom det bottniska området och Östersjön*. Center for Arctic Cultural Research, Research Report 17. Umeå University, Umeå.

Paine, R. 1957. *Coast Lapp Society*. Tromsø Museums Skrifter 1. Tromsø Museum, Tromsø.

Paproth, H.-J. 1964. *En gammal jägarrit. Albarksprutnignen vid lapparna björnfest*. Skrifter utgivna av Religionshistoriska institutionen i Uppsala Uppsala universitet, Uppsala.

Paulsson, H. and P. Edwards (trans.). 1976. *Egil's Saga*. Penguin Classics.

Paulson, I. 1963. Zur Aufbewahrung der Tierknochen im Jagdritual der nordeurasischen Völker. *Diószegi 1963*, 483–490.

Pellijeff, G. 1982. Bynamnet Kåddis än en gång. In *Språkhistoria och Språkkontakt i Finland och Nord-Skandinavien*, pp. 229–234. Kungliga Skytteanska Samfundets Handlingar 26, Umeå.

Perkar, S. F. 2009. Glacial Eustasy. In *Encyclopedia of Paleoclimatology and Ancient Environments*, edited by V. Gornitz, pp. 254–361. Springer, Dordrecht.

Peterson, R. O. and R. E. Page. 1982. Wolf-Moose Fluctuations at Isle Royale National Park, Michigan, U.S.A. In *Symposia on Lagomorphs, Beaver, Bear, Wolf and Mustelids, Proceedings of the Third International Theriological Congress*, Helsinki, 15–20 August 1982, pp. 251–253. Acta Zoologica Fennica 174, Helsinki.

Peterson, R. O., J. A. Vucetich, R. E. Page and A. Chouinard. 2003. Temporal and Spatial Aspects of Predator–Prey Dynamics. *Alces* 39:215–232.

Petré, B. 1980. Björnfällen i begravningsritualen – statusobjekt speglande regional skinnhandel? *Fornvännen*, 5–14.

Poole, I. 2005. *Analysis of Charcoal.* 3GEO:Archaeology, Biology, Chemistry, Utrecht.
Price, N. S. 2000. Drum-Time and Viking Age Sámi-Norse Identities in Early Medieval Scandinavia. In *Identities and Cultural Contacts in the Arctic,* edited by M. Appelt, J. Berglund and H.-C. Gulløv, pp. 12–27. Danish National Museum and Danish Polar Center, Copenhagen.
———. 2002. *The Viking Way. Religion and War in Late Iron Age Scandinavia.* AUN 31. Archaeology and Ancient History, Uppsala University, Uppsala.
Pruitt, W. O. 1978. *Boreal Ecology.* Studies in Biology 91. Edward Arnold, London.
Purce, J. 1974. *The Mystic Spiral.* Thames and Hudson, London.
Qvigstad, J. K. 1904. Lapiske Navne paa pattedyr, Kyrbdyr og padder, etc. *Nyt Magazine for Naturvidenskaberne* 4:340–387.
———. 1926. *Lappische Opfersteine und heilige Berge in Norwegen.* Oslo etnografiska museums skrifter 1:5, Oslo.
Ramqvist, P. H. 1983. *Gene: On the Origin, Function and Development of Sedentary Iron Age Settlement in Northern Sweden.* Archaeology and Environment 1. Umeå universitet, Umeå.
Ramqvist, P. H., M. Backe and L. Forsberg. 1985. Hällristningar vid Stornorrfors. *Västerbotten,* 66–75.
Ramqvist, P. H. 1992. Hällbilder som utgångdspunkt vid tolkningar i jägarsamhället. *Arkeologi i norr* 3:31–71.
Rankama, T. 1993. Managing the Landscape: A Study of Sámi Place-Names in Utsjoki, Finnish Lapland. *Etudes/Inuit Studies* 17:49–67.
Ranta, H. 2002. *Huts and Houses. Stone Age and Early Metal Age Buildings in Finland.* National Board of Antiquities, Helsinki.
Rathje, L. 2001. *Amasonen och jägaren. Kön/genderkonstruktioner i norr.* Studia Archaeologica . Universitatis Umensis 14. Umeå universitet,Umeå.
———. 2005. Övergången mellan vikingatiden och medeltid längs västerbottenskusten. In *En lång historia . . . festskrift till Evert Baudou på 80-årsdagen,* edited by R. Engelmark, T. B. Larsson and L. Rathje, pp. 363–375. Archaeology and Environment 19, Kungliga Skytteanska Samfundets Handlingar 57, Umeå.
Redman, C. L. and A. P. Kinzig. 2003. Resilience of Past Landscapes: Resilience Theory, Society, and the Longue Durée. *Conservation Ecology* 7(1):1–14.
Regnard, J. F. 1946 (1681). *Resa i Lappland.* Stockholm.
Reuterskiöld, E. 1910. *Källskrifter till lapparnas mytologi.* Bidrag till vår odlings hävder utgivna av Nordiska museet 10, Stockholm.
———. 1912. *De nordiska lapparnas religion.* Populära etnografiska skrifter 8, Stockholm.
Reymert, P. K. 1980. *Arkeologi og etniscitet.* En studie i etniscitet og gravskikke i Nord-Troms og Finnmark 800–1200. Instituut for samfunnsvitenskap, Tromsø.
Rheen, S. 1983 (1671). *En kort relation om Lapparnes Lefwarne och Sedher, Wijd-Skiepellsser, sampt i många Stycken Grovfe wildfarelsser.* Berättelser om samerna i 1600-talets Sverige. Kungliga Skytteanske Samfundets Handlingar 27, Umeå.
Richards, C. R. J. 1992. The Structure of Narrative Explanation in History and Biology. In *History and Evolution,* edited by M. Nitecki and D. Nitecki, pp. 19–53. State University of New York Press, Albany.
Roberts, N. 2009. Holocene Climates. In *Encyclopedia of Paleoclimatology and Ancient Environments,* edited by V. Gornitz, pp. 438–441. Springer, Dordrecht.
Roeck-Hansen, B. 2002. *Gårdsgärdor och tegesskiftesåker: resursutnyttjande och kulturelltinflyttande i det gamla landskapet Västerbotten.* Meddelanden från kulturgeografiska institution vid Stockholms universitet 11, Stockholm.
Ruong, I. 1969. *Samerna.* Aldus/Bonniers, Stockholm.
Russell, G. 1969. The Secret of the Grail. In *Glastonbury: A Study in Patterns.* Research in Lost Knowledge Organization, London.

Rydving, H. 1995. *The End of Drum-Time*. Historia Religionum 12, Acta Universitatis Upsaliensis, Uppsala University, Uppsala.
Ränk, G. 1948. Grundpinciper för disponeringen av utrymmet i de lapska kåtorna och gammerna. *Folkliv* 4(XII–XIII):87–111.
Røed, K. H., Ø. Flagstad, M. Nieminen, Ø. Holand, M. J. Dwyer, N. Røn and C. Vila. 2008. Genetic Analyses Reveal Independent Domestication Origins of Eurasian Reindeer. *Proceedings of the Royal Society, Series B* (275):1849–1855.
Sajantila, A., P. Lahermo, T. Anttinen, M. Lukka, P. Sistonen, M.-L. Savontaus, P. Aula, L. Beckman, L. Tranebjaerg, T. Gedde-Dahl, L. Issel-Tarver, A. Dirienzo and S. Pääbo. 1995. Genes and Languages in Europe: An Analysis of Mitochondrial Lineages. *Genome Research* 5:42–52.
Sahlins, M. 1972. *The Original Affluent Society*. Aldine-Altherton, New York.
Sandén, E. 1995. An Early Bronze Age Site on the Coast of Västerbotten, Sweden, with Hair-Tempered Textile Pottery. *Fennoscandia archaeologica* XII:173–180.
Sandström, Å. 1988. Ortnamn och tidiga bebyggelse på Holmön. In *Bottnisk kontakt IV*, pp. 136–141. Skellefteå museum, Skellefteå
Saressalo, L. 1987. The Threat from Without. In *Saami Religion. Skripti Donneriana Aboensis XII*, edited by T. Ahlbäck, pp. 251–257. Almqvist and Wiksell International, Stockholm.
Schanche, A. 2000. *Samiske graver i ur og berg. Samiske gravskikk og religion fra forhistorisk tid til nyere tid*. Davvi Girji, Karasjok.
Schefferus, J. 1956 (1673). *Lappland (Lapponia)*. Acta Lapponica 7. Nordiska Museet, Stockholm.
Schönfelder, M. 1994. Bear Claws in Germanic Graves. *Oxford Journal of Archaeology* 13(2):217–227.
Segerstråle, G. 1957. The Baltic Sea: Treatise on Marine Ecology and Paleoecology. *Geological Society of America, Memoir* 67(1):751–799.
Segerström, U. and I. Renberg. 1986. Varviga sjösediment avslöar den forntida landhöjningsförlopp. In *Landet stiger ur havet*, edited by O. Stephansson, pp. 27–30. Centek Förlag, Luleå.
Selinge, K.-G. 1974. Fångstgropar. Jämtlands vanligaste fornlämningar. *Fornvårdar* 12.
———. 1977. Den förhistoriska bonderkulturen i Västernorrland. In *Västernorrlands förhistoriska*, pp. 153–459. Västernorrlands läns landsting, Motala.
———. 1997. *Cultural Heritage and Preservation, National Atlas of Sweden*. Almqvist & Wiksell International, Stockholm.
Serning, I. 1956. *Lapska offerplatsfynd från järnålder och medeltid i de svenska lappmarkarna*. Acta Lapponica XI, Stockholm.
———. 1960. *Övre Norrlands järnålder*. Skrifter utgivna av Vetenskapliga biblioteket i Umeå 4, Umeå.
Sjöberg, R. 1987. *Vittringsstudier med Schmidt Test-hammer. Tillämpningar inom geomorfologi och arkeologi*. Research Reports 1. Center for Arctic Cultural Research, Umeå University, Umeå.
Sjögren, P. 1997. *Boplatsen vid Flurkmark. Forntida miljö och näringsfång*. Institutionen för arkeologi, Umeå universitet, Umeå.
Sjøvold, T. (ed.). 1982. *Introduksjonen av jordbruk i Norden*. De Norske Videnskabs-Akademi, Oslo-Bergen-Tromsø.
Sköld, P. 1993. *Samerna och deras historia. Metodövningar i samisk 1600- och 1700-talshistoria*. Research Reports 29. Center for Arctic Cultural Research, Umeå University, Umeå.
Sköld, T. 1979. The Earliest Linguistic Contact between Lapps and Scandinavians. *Fenno-Ugrica Suecana* 2:105–116.
Solbakk, J. T. (ed.). 2004. *Samene – en handbok*. Davvi Girji, Vasa.
Sommerseth, I. 2004. Fra fangstbaserat reindrift till nomadism i indre Troms. Etnografiske tekster og arkeologiske kontekster. In *Samisk forhistorie*, edited by M. Krogh and K. Schanche, pp. 150–161. Varanger Samiske Museum, Varanger.

Sommerström, B. 1966. Renskötsel. In *Bonniers Lexicon 12*, pp. 416–424. Bonnier, Stockholm.

Spång, L. G. 1997. *Fångstsamhälle i handelssystem. Åsele lappmark neolitikum-bronsålder.* Arkeologiska institutionen. Umeå universitet, Umeå

Steckzén, B. 1964. *Birkarlar och Lappar. Birkarlarväsendets, Lappbefolkningens och skinnhandelns historia.* Kungliga Vitterhets Historie och Antikvitets Akademiens handlingar 9. Historiska serien, Stockholm.

Stenberger, M. 1964. *Det forntida Sverige.* Almqvist and Wiksell, Uppsala.

Stenvik, L. 1988. *En ny fjellgrav fra vikingtiden i Verdal.* Verdal historielags årbok 1988, Verdal.

Stoor, K. 1991. Reindeer Herding and Stock Farming in the Swedish Part of Sapmi. In *Readings in Saami History Culture and Language II,* edited by R. Kvist, pp. 85–92 Miscellaneous Publications 12. Center for Arctic Cultural Research, Umeå University, Umeå.

Storli, I. 1991. *Stallo-boplassene.* Institutt for samfunnsvitenskap, Universitetet i Tromsø, Tromsø.

———. 1993. Sámi Viking Age Pastoralism, or the Fur Trade Paradigm Reconsidered. *Norwegian Archaeological Review* 26(1):1–20.

Storå, J. 2001a. Skeletal Development in the Grey Seal *Halichoerus grypus*, the Ringed Seal *Phoca hispida botnica*, the Harbour Seal *Phoca vitulina vitulina* and the Harp Seal *Phoca groenlandica*: Epiphyseal Fusion and Life History. In *Assessing Season of Capture, Age and Sex of Archaeofaunas,* edited by A. Pike-Tay, pp. 199–222. Bibliotheque d'Archeozoologie XI. La Pensee Sauvage, Paris.

———. 2001b. *Reading Bones. Stone Age Hunters and Seals in the Baltic.* Stockholm Studies in Archaeology 21. Stockholm University, Stockholm.

———. 2002. *Flurkmark, RÄA 510. Umeå socken, Västerbotten. Osteologisk analys av djurbensmaterialet från 1996–2001 års undersökningar.* Möten i Norr, Umeå.

———. 2005. Osteologisk analys av ben från Hornslandsudde, Hälsingland. Department of Anthropology, Smithsonian Institution, Washington, D.C..

———. 2008. *Osteologisk analys av ben från Stora Fjäderägg.* Department of Anthropology, Smithsonian Institution, Washington, D.C.

Storå, J. and N. D. Broadbent. 2002. *Osteologisk analys av ben från tomtningslokaler i Övre Norrlands skärgård: Grundskatan, Bjuröklubb, Jungfruhamn, Stor-Rebben.* Department of Anthropology, Smithsonian Institution, Washington, D.C.

Storå, J. and P. G. P. Ericson. 2004. A Prehistoric Breeding Population of Harp Seals (*Phoca groenlandica*) in the Baltic Sea. *Marine Mammal Science* 20(1):115–133.

Storå, J. and L. Lõugas. 2005. Human Exploitation and History of Seals in the Baltic during Late Holocene. In *The Exploitation and Cultural Importance of Sea Mammals, Proceedings of the 9th Conference of the International Council of Archaeozoology,* Durham, August 2002, edited by G. G. Monks, pp. 95–106. Oxbow Books, Oxford.

Storå, N. 1971. *Burial Customs of the Skolt Lapps.* Communications No. 210. Suomolainen Tiedeakatemia. FF, Helsinki.

Strade, N. 1997. Det sydsamiske sprog. In *Möten i gränsland. Samer och germaner i Mellanskandinavien,* edited by I. Zachrisson, pp. 175–184. Stockholm Monographs 4. Statens historiska museum, Stockholm.

Strathern, M. 1988. *The gender of the gift: problems with women and problems with society in Melanesia.* University of California Press, Berkeley.

Stuiver, M. and R. S. Kra (eds.). 1986. Calibration Issue Proceedings of the Twelfth International Radiocarbon Conference. *Radiocarbon* 28(2B):805–1030.

Ståhl, H. 1976. *Ortnamn och ortnamnsforskning.* Almqvist & Wiksell, Stockholm.

Sugden, D. 1982. *Arctic and Antarctic: A Modern Geographical Synthesis.* Basil Blackwell, Oxford.

Sundqvist, L., A.-K. Lindqvist, R. Engelmark, J. Linderholm and K. Viklund. 1992. *Preliminär rapport över arkeologiska undersökningar vid Harrsjöbacken och Hamptjärn, Bureå sn, Västerbotten 1991–1992*. Skellefteå museum, Skellefteå.

Sundström, H. 1984. *Bönder Bryter Bygd.* Bothnica 4. Norrbottens museum, Luleå.

Sundström, J. 1997. Järnålder i fångstlandet. In *Möten i gränsland. Samer och germaner i Mellanskandinavien*, edited by I. Zachrisson, pp. 21–27. Statens historiska museum monographs 4, Stockholm.

*Svensk Etymologisk Ordbok.* 1948 (1922). Edited by E. Hellqvist. C. W. K. Gleerups förlag Berlingska boktryckeriet, Lund.

Svensson, P. 1904. Om säljakten i Bottniska viken. *Svenska Jägarförbundets Nya Tidskrift* 42(I, II), pp. 149–161, 260–273.

Söderberg, S. 1974a. Feeding Habits and Commercial Damage of Seals in the Baltic. In *Proceedings of the Symposium on the Seal in the Baltic*, pp. 66–78. Naturvårdsverket, Solna.

———. 1974b. Seal Hunting in the Baltic. In *Proceedings on the Symposium on the Seal in the Baltic*, pp. 104–116. Naturvårdsverket, Solna.

Tallgren, A. M. 1949. *The Arctic Bronze Age in Europe*. Eurasia Septentrionailes Antigua, Helsinki.

Tambets, K., S. Rootsi, T. Kivisild, H. Help, P. Serk, E.-L. Loogväli, H.-V. Tolk, M. Reidla, E. Metspalu, L. Pliss, O. Balanovsky, A. Pshenichnov, E. Balanovska, M. Gubina, S. Zhadanov, L. Osipova, L. Damba, M. Voevoda, I. Kutuev, M. Bermisheva, E. Khusnutdinova, V. Gusar, E. Grechanina, J. Parik, E. Pennarun, C. Richard, A. Chaventre, J.-P. Moisan, L. Barać, M. Peričić, P. Rudan, R. Terzić, I. Mikerezi, A. Krumina, V. Baumanis, S. Koziel, O. Rickards, G. F. De Stefano, N. Anagnou, K. I. Pappa, E. Michalodimitrakis, V. Ferák, S. Füredi, R. Komel, L. Beckman and R. Villems. 2004. The Western and Eastern Roots of the Saami: The Story of Genetic "Outliers" Told by Mitochondrial DNA and Y Chromosomes. *American Journal of Human Genetics* 74:661–682.

Tanner, A. 1979. *Bringing Home Animals. Religious Ideology and Mode of Production of the Mistassini Cree Hunters.* Institute of Social and Economic Research. Memorial University of Newfoundland, St. John's.

Tanner, V. 1929. *Antropogeografiska studier i Petsamoomradet. Skoltlapparna.* Fennia 49, Helsinki.

Tegengren, H. 1952. *En Utdöd Lappkultur i Kemi Lappmark.* Acta Academiae Aboensis Humaniora XIX. Åbo Academy, Åbo.

———. 1965. Hunters and Amazons: Seasonal Migrations in Older Hunting and Fishing Communities. In *Hunting and Fishing*, edited by H. Hvarfner, pp. 427–492. Norrbottens museum Luleå.

Thomas, J. 1996. *Time, Culture and Identity: An Interpretive Archaeology*. Routledge, London.

Thurenius, P. 1724 (1910). *Kort Berättelse on the Widskeppelser, som uthi Åhsilla Lappmark ännu äro i bruk.* . Utgiven av I. Fellman Handlingar 1, Umeå.

Tomasson, T. 1988. (1917) . *Några sägner, seder och bruk upptecknade efter lapparna i Åsele och Lycksele lappmark samt Herjedalen sommaren 1917* Skrifter utgivna genom Dialekt- och folkminnesarkivet i Uppsala Serie C:5.

Topham, P. B. 1977. Colonization, Growth, Succession and Competition. In *Lichen Ecology*, edited by M. R. D. Seward, pp. 32–68. Academic Press, London.

Toynbee, A. J. 1934. *A Study of History* 2. Cambridge University Press, Cambridge.

Turi, J. 1911. *En bog om Lappernes liv. Muttalus Samid Birra.* Nordiska Bokhandeln, Stockholm.

Ukkonen, P. 2002. The Early History of Seals in the Northern Baltic. *Annales Zoologici Fennici* 39:187–207.

Urbańczyk, P. 1992. *Medieval Arctic Norway*. Institute of Archaeology and Material Culture, Polish Academy of Sciences, Warsawa.

Utagawa, H. 1999. The Archaeology of Iyomante. In *Ainu: Spirit of Northern People*, edited by W. W. Fitzhugh and C. O. Dubreuil, pp. 256–260. Arctic Studies Center, National Museum of Natural History, Smithsonian Institution, Washington, D.C.

Valtonen, T. 2006. Saami Food Caches in the Báišduottar-Paistunturi Area, North Finland. In *People, Material Culture and Environment in the North. Proceedings of the 22nd Nordic Archaeological Conference, 2004*, edited by V. P. Herva, pp. 64–74. University of Oulu, Humanistinen tiedekunta, Oulun yliopisto, Oulu.

Varenius, C. 1964. Stor-Rebben. 1500 år av säsongbosättning i Piteå skärgård. *Norrbotten 1964–65*, 47–54.

———. 1978. Inventering i marginalområde: spår av primitiv kustbosättning. *Fornvännen* 73:121–133.

Vibe, C. 1970. The Arctic Ecosystem Influenced by Fluctuations in Sun-Spot and Drift-Ice Movements. In *International Union for Conservation of Nature and Natural Resources*, edited by W. A. Fuller and P. G. Kevan, pp. 115–120. New Series 16, Morger.

Vikberg, E. 1931. *Arvidsjaur.* Folkminnesuppteckningar från Arvidsjaurs parish, Lappland. Språk- och folkminnesinstitutet, Uppsala.

Viklund, K. 2000. *Utplockning och 14C-datering av kol från förmodade fornlämningar på Bureå 1:2, Bureå socken, Skellefteå kommun, Västerbotten.* Miljöarkeologiska Laboratoriet Rapport. Institutionen för arkeologi och samiska studier, Umeå universitet, Umeä.

———. 2005. Kråkbär och gravid sik- Västerbottens mångkulturella förflutna i miljöarkeologisks belysning. In *En lång historia . . . festskrift till Evert Baudou på 80-årsdagen*, edited by R. Engelmark, T. B. Larsson and L. Rathje. Archaeology and Environment 19, Kungliga Skytteanska Samfundets Handlingar 57, Umeå.

Vorren, Ø. 1968. Some Trends of the Transition from Herding to Nomadic Economy in Finnmark: Circumpolar Problems. In *Habitat, Economy and Social Relations in the Arctic*, edited by G. Berg, pp. 185–194. Wenner-Gren Center International Symposium Series 21. Pergamon Press, New York.

———. 1985. Circular Sacrificial Sites and Their Function. In *Saami Pre-Christian Religion: Studies on the Oldest Traces of Religion among the Saamis*, edited by L. Bäckman and Å. Hultkrantz, pp. 69–81. Almqvist & Wiksell International, Stockholm.

———. 1987. Sacrificial Sites, Types and Function: Saami Religion. In *Symposium on Saami Religion* Held at Åbo, Finland, 16–18 August 1984, edited by T. Ahlbäck. Skripti Instituti Donneriana Aboensis XII, Almqvist & Wiksell, Stockholm.

Vorren, Ø. and H. K. Eriksen. 1993. *Samiske offerplatser i Varanger.* Tromsø museums skrifter 24, Tromsø.

Wahlberg, M. 2003. *Svenskt ortnamnslexikon.* Språk- och folkminnesinstitutet, Uppsala.

Wallander, H. 1992. Report on the Osteological Material from the Comb Ware Site Lillberget, RAÄ 451, Överkalix, Norrbotten. In *Sedentariness during the Stone Age of Northern Sweden in the Light of the Alträsket Site, c. 5000 B.C., and the Comb Ware Site Lillberget, c. 3900 BC*, edited by O. Halén. Acta Archaeologica Lundensia 20. Lund University, Lund.

Wallerstein, I. 1974. *The Modern World-System I: Capitalist Agriculture and the Origins of the European World-Economy in the Sixteenth Century.* Academic Press, New York.

Wallerström, T. 1995. *Norrbotten, Sverige och Medeltiden. Problem kring makt och bosättning i en europeisk periferi.* Lund Studies in Medieval Archaeology 15:1–2. Almqvist & Wiksell, Stockholm.

———. 2000. The Saami between East and West in the Middle Ages: An Archaeological Contribution to the History of Reindeer Breeding. *Acta Borealia* 1:3–39.

———. 2006. *Vilka var först? En nordskandinaviisk konflikt som historiskt-arkeologiskt dilemma.* Riksantikvarieämbetet, Stockholm.

Wallin, J.-E. 1994. Den fasta jordbruksnäringens utveckling i Ångermanälvens nedre dalgång under järnålder och medeltid-en paleoekologisk undersökning. In *Järnålder i Mittnorden*, edited by K. Gullberg, pp. 127–154. Scriptum, Vasa.

———. 1995. History of Sedentary Farming in Ångermanland, Northern Sweden, during the Iron Age and Medieval Period Based on Pollen Analytical Investigations. In *Vegetational History and Archaeobotany*, pp. 301–312. Springer-Verlag, Berlin.

Welinder, S. 1977. *Ekonomiska processer i förhistorisk expansion.* Acta Archaeologica Lundensia 7, Lund.

Wennstedt, B. 1989. Kultplatser i Övre Norrlands kustland. *Oknytt* 10(3–4):23–34.
———. 2002. Reindeer Herding and History in the Mountains of Southern Sapmi. *Current Swedish Archaeology* 10:115–136.
Wennstedt Edvinger, B. and U. S. Winka. 2001. *Sydsamiska kulturmiljöer.* Skrifter utgivna av Gaaltije 1, Östersund.
Wennstedt Edvinger, B. and B. Ulfhielm. 2004. *Samer i Hälsingland: Inventering, studiecirklar, utställning.* Länsmuseet Gävleborg, Gävle.
Wennstedt Edvinger, B. and N. D. Broadbent. 2006. Saami Circular Sacrificial Sites in Northern Coastal Sweden. *Acta Borealia* 23(1):24–55.
Wennstedt, O. 1988. *Jungfruhamn och Dödmansskär. En studie över ortnamn i Lövångers sockens kustområde.* Research Reports 10. Center for Arctic Cultural Research, Umeå University, Umeå.
Werbart, B. 2002. *De osynliga identiteterna.* Studia Archaeologica Universitatis Umensis. Umeå University, Umeå.
Westberg, H. 1964. Lämningar efter gammal fångstkultur i Hornslandsområdet. *Fornvännen* 59:24–41.
Westerberg, J. O. 1988. *Säljaktens redskap. En studie av bevarade redskap från Norrbotten och Västerbotten.* Research Report 7. Center for Arctic Cultural Research, Umeå University, Umeå.
Westerdahl, C. 1989. *En kulturgräns nolaskogs.* Örnsköldsviks museums småskriftserie 20, Örnsköldsvik.
———. 1995a. Schiff-und Bootbau Samischer Bootsbau, Teil 1. *Deutsches Schiffahrtsarchiv* 18:233–260.
———. 1995b. Stone Maze Symbols and Navigation: A Hypothesis on the Origin of Coastal Mazes in the North. *International Journal of Nautical Archaeology* 24(4):267–277.
———. 2004. En gränsöverskridande folk. Sydsamer i Ångermanland och Åsele Lappmark. In *Tidsspår – Västernorrland – Sameland. Om samisk närvaro i Ångermanland och Medelpad,* edited by M. Bergvall and P. Persson, pp. 110–139. Länsmuseet Västernorrland, Härnosand.
Westerlund, E. 1965. Lapsk bosättning vid kusten? *Västerbotten* (1965):203–211.
Westin, G. 1962. *Övre Norrlands forntid.* Övre Norrlands historia 1. Norrbottens och Västerbottens landsting, Umeå.
White, R. 1991. *The Middle Ground: Indians, Empires, and Republics of the Great Lakes Region, 1650–1815.* Cambridge University Press, Cambridge.
Whittaker, I. 1980. Tacitus' "Fenni" and Ptolemy's "Phinnoi". *The Classical Journal* 75(3):215–224.
Wiklund, K. B. 1947. *Lapparna.* Albert Bonniers Förlag, Stockholm.
Williamson, C. 2004. Contact Archaeology and the Writing of Aboriginal History. In *The Archaeology of Contact in Settler Societies,* edited by T. Murray, pp. 176–199. Cambridge University Press, Cambridge.
Wolf, E. R. 1997. *Europe and the People without History.* University of California Press, Berkeley.
Yates, T. 1989. Habitus and Social Space: Some Suggestions about Meaning in the Saami (Lapp) Tent ca. 1700–1900. In *The Meaning of Things: Material Culture and Symbolic Expression,* edited by I. Hodder. Unwin Hyman, London.
Zachrisson, I. 1976. *Lapps and Scandinavians: Archaeological Finds from Northern Sweden.* Early Norrland 10. Kungliga Vitterhets Historie Antikvitets Akademien, Stockholm.
———. 1984. *De samiska metalldepåerna år 1000–1350 i ljuset av fyndet från Mörtträsket, Lappland. (The Saami Metal Deposits A.D. 1000–1350 in the light of the find from Mörtträsket, Lapland.)* Archaeology and Environment 3. Umeå universitet, Umeå.
———. 1987a. Arkeologi och etnicitet. Samisk kultur i mellersta Sverige ca 1–1500 e. Kr. *Bebyggelsehistorisk tidskrift* 14:24–41.
———. 1987b. Sjiele, Sacrifices, Oden Treasures and Saami Graves. In *Saami Religion,* edited by T. Ahlbäck, pp. 61–68. Skripti Instituti Donneriana Aboensis XII, Almqvist & Wisksell, Stockholm.
———. 1988. Arkeologi och etnicitet. Samisk kultur i mellersta Sverige ca 1–1500 e.Kr. Samer och germaner i det förhistoriska Norrland, edited by P. H. Ramqvist. *Bebyggelsehistorisk tidskrift* 14(1987):24–41.

———. 1991. The Saami Shaman Drums: Some Reflexions from an Archaeological Perspective. In *The Saami Shaman Drum,* edited by T. Ahlbäck and J. Bergman, pp. 80–95. Based on Papers Read at the Symposium on the Saami Shaman Drum Held at Åbo, Finland, 19–20 August 1988.

———. 1992. Saami Prehistory in the South Saami Area. In *Readings in Saami History, Culture and Language,* edited by R. Kvist, pp. 9–23. Miscellaneous Publications 14. Center for Arctic Cultural Research, Umeå University, Umeå.

———. 1995. Ethnicity – Conflicts on Land Use: Sámi and Norse in Central Scandinavia in the Iron Age and Middle Ages. In *'Utmark': The Outfield as Industry and Ideology in the Iron Age and the Middle Ages,* edited by S. Innselset and I. Öye, pp. 193–201. University of Bergen, UBAS International 1, University of Bergen Archaeological Series, Bergen.

———. 1997a. *Möten i gränsland. Samer och germaner i Mellan skandinavien.* Statens historiska museum monographs 4, Stockholm, Stockholm.

———. 1997b. Oral Traditions, Archaeology and Linguistics: The Early History of the Saami in Scandinavia. In *Archaeology and Language I. Theoretical and Methodological Orientations,* edited by R. Blench and M. Spriggs, pp. 371–376. One World Archaeology 27. Routledge, London and New York.

———. 2004. Archaeology and Ethics: The South Sámi Example. In *Swedish Archaeologists on Ethics,* edited by H. Karlsson, pp. 117–131. Bricoleur Press, Lindome.

———. 2006. Magiska pilar och mystiska tecken – något om samer och järn. *Med hammare och fackla (Sancte Örjens Gille)* 39:25–35.

Zachrisson, I. and E. Iregren. 1974. *Lappish Bear Graves in Northern Sweden.* Early Norrland 5. Kungliga Vitterhets Historie och Antikvitets Akademien, Stockholm.

Ågren, P.-U. 1969. Från birkarlar till träpatroner. In *Västerbotten. Ett bildverk,* pp. 45–200. Alhems Förlag, Malmö.

Åhrén, I. 2004. Frostviken – Lapparnas högkvartär. In *Tidspår – Västernorrland – Sameland. Om samisk närvaro i Ångermanland och Medelpad,* edited by M. Bergvall and P. Persson, pp. 62–88. Härnosand Museum, Härnosand.

Ångström, A. 1968. *Sveriges Klimat.* Generalstabens Litografiska Anstallts Förlag, Stockholm.

Åström, K. and O. Norberg. 1984. Förhistoriska och medeltida skidor. *Västerbotten,* 82–88.

# Index

# About the Author

Noel D. Broadbent earned his Ph.D. in 1997 at Uppsala University in Sweden. From 1983–1989, he was Director of the Center for Arctic Cultural Research at Umeå University; from 1990–1996 he was Director of the Arctic Social Sciences Program at the National Science Foundation in Washington, D.C., and from 1996–2003 held the Chair of Archaeology and Saami Studies in Umeå. Since 2004 he has been on the staff of the Arctic Studies Center in the Department of Anthropology at the Smithsonian's National Museum of Natural History. Among his awards are two NSF Director's Awards, The Antarctica Service Medal, the Svea Orden and the Hildebrand Prize of the Swedish Archaeological Society.